Promoting Cardiovascular Health in the Developing World

A Critical Challenge to Achieve Global Health

Committee on Preventing the Global Epidemic of Cardiovascular Disease:
Meeting the Challenges in Developing Countries

Board on Global Health

Valentín Fuster and Bridget B. Kelly, *Editors*

INSTITUTE OF MEDICINE
OF THE NATIONAL ACADEMIES

THE NATIONAL ACADEMIES PRESS
Washington, D.C.
www.nap.edu

THE NATIONAL ACADEMIES PRESS   500 Fifth Street, N.W.   Washington, DC 20001

NOTICE: The project that is the subject of this report was approved by the Governing Board of the National Research Council, whose members are drawn from the councils of the National Academy of Sciences, the National Academy of Engineering, and the Institute of Medicine. The members of the committee responsible for the report were chosen for their special competences and with regard for appropriate balance.

This study was supported by Contract No. N01-OD-4-2139, Task Order No. 206, between the National Academy of Sciences and the National Institutes of Health. Any opinions, findings, conclusions, or recommendations expressed in this publication are those of the author(s) and do not necessarily reflect the view of the organizations or agencies that provided support for this project.

International Standard Book Number-13: 978-0-309-14774-3
International Standard Book Number-10: 0-309-14774-3

Additional copies of this report are available from the National Academies Press, 500 Fifth Street, N.W., Lockbox 285, Washington, DC 20055; (800) 624-6242 or (202) 334-3313 (in the Washington metropolitan area); Internet, http://www.nap.edu.

For more information about the Institute of Medicine, visit the IOM home page at: www.iom.edu.

Copyright 2010 by the National Academy of Sciences. All rights reserved.

Printed in the United States of America

The serpent has been a symbol of long life, healing, and knowledge among almost all cultures and religions since the beginning of recorded history. The serpent adopted as a logotype by the Institute of Medicine is a relief carving from ancient Greece, now held by the Staatliche Museen in Berlin.

Suggested citation: IOM (Institute of Medicine). 2010. *Promoting Cardiovascular Health in the Developing World: A Critical Challenge to Achieve Global Health*. Washington, DC: The National Academies Press.

*"Knowing is not enough; we must apply.
Willing is not enough; we must do."*
—Goethe

INSTITUTE OF MEDICINE
OF THE NATIONAL ACADEMIES

Advising the Nation. Improving Health.

THE NATIONAL ACADEMIES
Advisers to the Nation on Science, Engineering, and Medicine

The **National Academy of Sciences** is a private, nonprofit, self-perpetuating society of distinguished scholars engaged in scientific and engineering research, dedicated to the furtherance of science and technology and to their use for the general welfare. Upon the authority of the charter granted to it by the Congress in 1863, the Academy has a mandate that requires it to advise the federal government on scientific and technical matters. Dr. Ralph J. Cicerone is president of the National Academy of Sciences.

The **National Academy of Engineering** was established in 1964, under the charter of the National Academy of Sciences, as a parallel organization of outstanding engineers. It is autonomous in its administration and in the selection of its members, sharing with the National Academy of Sciences the responsibility for advising the federal government. The National Academy of Engineering also sponsors engineering programs aimed at meeting national needs, encourages education and research, and recognizes the superior achievements of engineers. Dr. Charles M. Vest is president of the National Academy of Engineering.

The **Institute of Medicine** was established in 1970 by the National Academy of Sciences to secure the services of eminent members of appropriate professions in the examination of policy matters pertaining to the health of the public. The Institute acts under the responsibility given to the National Academy of Sciences by its congressional charter to be an adviser to the federal government and, upon its own initiative, to identify issues of medical care, research, and education. Dr. Harvey V. Fineberg is president of the Institute of Medicine.

The **National Research Council** was organized by the National Academy of Sciences in 1916 to associate the broad community of science and technology with the Academy's purposes of furthering knowledge and advising the federal government. Functioning in accordance with general policies determined by the Academy, the Council has become the principal operating agency of both the National Academy of Sciences and the National Academy of Engineering in providing services to the government, the public, and the scientific and engineering communities. The Council is administered jointly by both Academies and the Institute of Medicine. Dr. Ralph J. Cicerone and Dr. Charles M. Vest are chair and vice chair, respectively, of the National Research Council.

www.national-academies.org

COMMITTEE ON PREVENTING THE GLOBAL EPIDEMIC OF CARDIOVASCULAR DISEASE: MEETING THE CHALLENGES IN DEVELOPING COUNTRIES

VALENTÍN FUSTER (*Chair*), Mount Sinai Heart
ARUN CHOCKALINGAM (through January 2010), Faculty of Health Sciences, Simon Fraser University
CIRO A. DE QUADROS, Albert B. Sabin Vaccine Institute
JOHN W. FARQUHAR, Stanford Prevention Research Center, Stanford University School of Medicine
ROBERT C. HORNIK, The Annenberg School for Communication, University of Pennsylvania
FRANK B. HU, Departments of Nutrition and Epidemiology, Harvard School of Public Health
PETER R. LAMPTEY, Family Health International
JEAN CLAUDE MBANYA, Faculty of Medicine and Biomedical Sciences, University of Yaoundé I
ANNE MILLS, Department of Public Health and Policy, London School of Hygiene and Tropical Medicine
JAGAT NARULA, Division of Cardiology, University of California, Irvine School of Medicine
RACHEL A. NUGENT, Center for Global Development
JOHN W. PEABODY, Institute for Global Health, University of California, San Francisco
K. SRINATH REDDY, Public Health Foundation of India
SYLVIE STACHENKO, The School of Public Health, University of Alberta
DEREK YACH, PepsiCo

Study Staff

BRIDGET B. KELLY, Study Director/Program Officer
COLLIN WEINBERGER, Research Associate (from April 2009)
RACHEL JACKSON, Research Associate (through February 2009)
LOUISE JORDAN, Research Assistant
KRISTEN DANFORTH, Senior Program Assistant
JULIE WILTSHIRE, Financial Associate
PATRICK KELLEY, Director, Board on Global Health

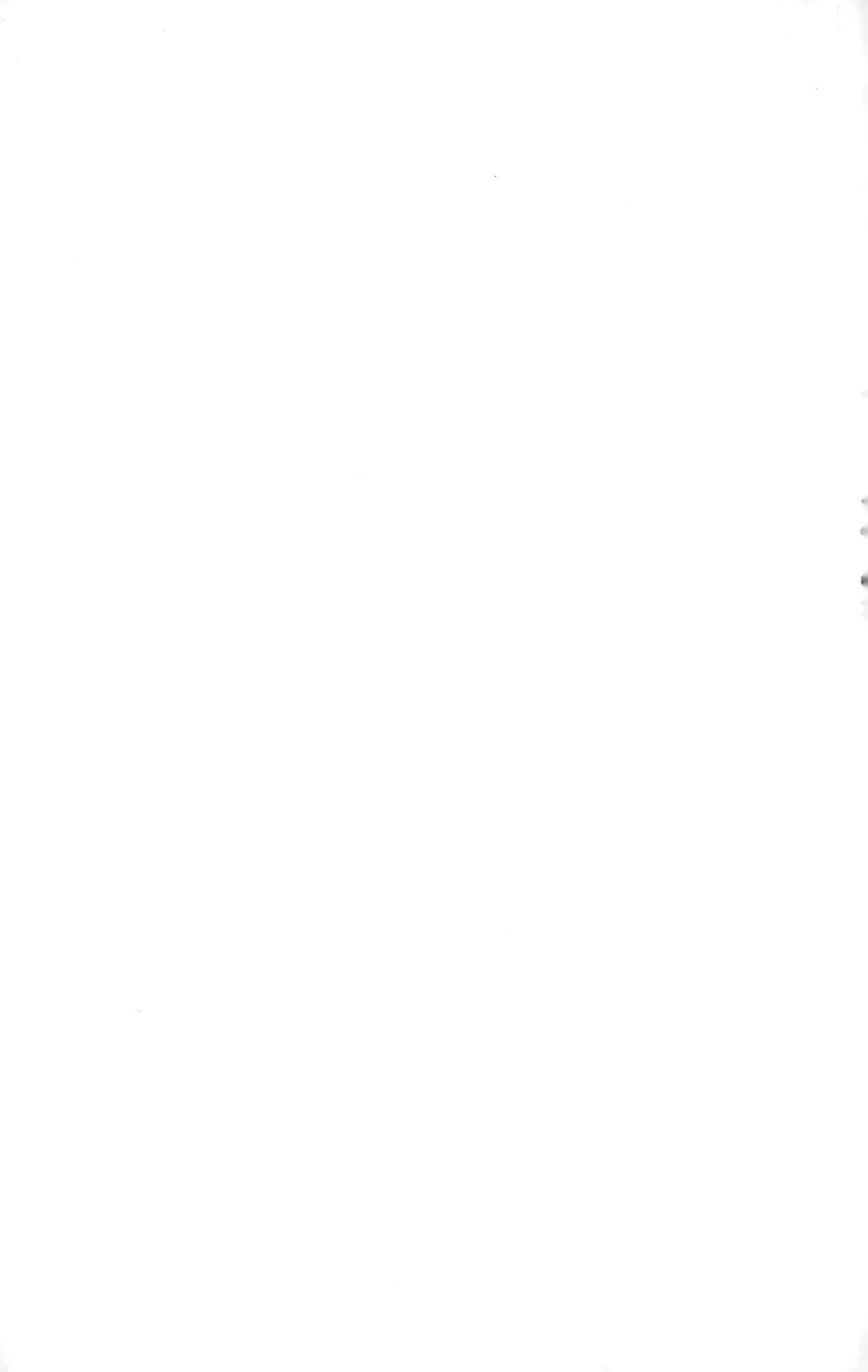

Reviewers

This report has been reviewed in draft form by individuals chosen for their diverse perspectives and technical expertise, in accordance with procedures approved by the National Research Council's Report Review Committee. The purpose of this independent review is to provide candid and critical comments that will assist the institution in making its published report as sound as possible and to ensure that the report meets institutional standards for objectivity, evidence, and responsiveness to the study charge. The review comments and draft manuscript remain confidential to protect the integrity of the deliberative process. We wish to thank the following individuals for their review of this report:

Robert Beaglehole, School of Population Health, University of Auckland, New Zealand
Tom Coates, David Geffen School of Medicine, University of California, Los Angeles
Susan J. Crockett, Bell Institute of Health and Nutrition
Martha N. Hill, Johns Hopkins University School of Nursing
James Hospedales, Pan American Health Organization/World Health Organization
Dean Jamison, Institute for Health Metrics and Evaluation, University of Washington
Katherine Marconi, Department of Management and Finance, University of Maryland University College
Bongani Mayosi, University of Capetown, Department of Medicine
Anthony Mbewu, South African Medical Research Council

Pekka Puska, National Institute for Health and Welfare, Finland
Ricardo Uauy, London School of Hygiene and Tropical Medicine
Suwit Wibulpolprasert, Ministry of Public Health, Thailand

Although the reviewers listed above have provided many constructive comments and suggestions, they were not asked to endorse the conclusions or recommendations nor did they see the final draft of the report before its release. The review of this report was overseen by **David R. Challoner,** Vice President for Health Affairs, Emeritus, University of Florida and **Harlan M. Krumholz,** Yale University School of Medicine. Appointed by the National Research Council and Institute of Medicine, they were responsible for making certain that an independent examination of this report was carried out in accordance with institutional procedures and that all review comments were carefully considered. Responsibility for the final content of this report rests entirely with the authoring committee and the institution.

Preface

About 10 years ago, in an address as the newly appointed President of the American Heart Association (AHA), I alluded to three serious challenges facing the field of cardiovascular disease: (1) How to support and energize research, which is so crucial to preventing the still-evolving epidemic of cardiovascular disease (CVD)? (2) Is it realistic to expect that this global epidemic can be lessened or avoided solely by professional and public education, or is there a need for more aggressive implementation strategies at a global level? (3) Would a more integrated and cooperative global approach, involving many if not all of the national and international organizations represented at the AHA Scientific Sessions, maximize the effectiveness of individual organizations and their volunteers?

Some of my colleagues diplomatically questioned the arguments of my speech, arguing that the AHA should focus its attention on the United States as the primary objective. At that time, my answer did not differ from the answer I would provide today, although now in much stronger terms after having been exposed even more thoroughly to the realities of the epidemic in low- and middle-income countries as President of the World Heart Federation. Over two-thirds of deaths attributable to CVD worldwide occur in low and middle income countries. Therefore, if the goal of the cardiovascular community is truly to achieve cardiovascular health, I see a clear responsibility to think and act globally, beyond the borders of high income countries.

Aging of populations, globalization, and rapid urbanization are changing disease patterns around the world. The epidemiological transition to a high chronic disease burden is occurring at a particularly rapid rate in developing countries. Thus, solutions for low and middle income countries need to be initiated within a short time frame, which represents an important public health challenge, given that these regions have fewer resources and greater health inequities than high income countries. If this challenge is not met, it will be impossible to achieve better health worldwide. Therefore, just as it is incumbent upon the cardiovascular community in high income countries to think and act globally, it is also incumbent upon the global health community to act upon the needs of cardiovascular disease.

This recognition of the need for action from leaders in both cardiovascular disease and global health served as motivation to accept the Institute of Medicine's invitation to chair this ad hoc committee, which was charged to study the evolving global epidemic of CVD and to offer conclusions and recommendations pertinent to its control. Since the inception of this study, the committee recognized that it faced a broad task and a complex problem. At our first meeting it became clear that my colleagues shared one of my primary concerns: after substantive efforts of nearly two decades in which convened committees and documents have portrayed the evolving health and economic burden of CVD, in what way could our committee contribute toward a solution? Thus, the committee took on as a driving force the task of evaluating the factors contributing to the profound mismatch or "action gap" between the compelling evidence that had been articulated in previous efforts and the lack of concrete steps to implement actions. Our goal became to identify the necessary next steps to move forward and to define a framework in which to implement these steps.

We approached the task systematically, meeting four times in person, including two public sessions in which a number of additional experts in various fields were gathered to help inform our deliberations. These meetings were supplemented by countless ongoing deliberations through phone calls and email exchanges. Since the very beginning of our "run," our outstanding study director from the IOM staff, Bridget Kelly, focused our efforts toward a limited number of feasible recommendations which, of course, progressively evolved as we reached our final conclusions over time.

This report reflects the path the committee followed. We reviewed the compelling epidemiological and economic evidence, which we found provides a clear mandate for action. We recognized the need for measurement and evaluation to truly understand the local nature of the epidemic and how best to intervene in ways that are locally relevant. We reconciled our "dream" of an ideal vision to promote cardiovascular health with our understanding of the pragmatic considerations of implementing interventions in low and middle income countries and the limited documentation and evaluation of successful strategies in these settings. Importantly, the committee chose to highlight the emerging importance of targeting mothers, children, youth, and young adults for prevention interventions in order to achieve long-term success in promoting cardiovascular health and reducing the burden of CVD.

Ultimately, the committee recognized that success in overcoming the burden of CVD will require the combined efforts of many players sustained over many years. Success is possible if the major stakeholders in CVD, related chronic diseases, and other areas of global health can be organized at global, national, and local levels to implement the necessary actions to control the global epidemic of CVD. It is the hope of all involved in this project that this report will prove to be a catalyst for action in the next stage of progress in the fight against global cardiovascular disease.

I would like to thank the members of the committee for their devotion of time and energy to this project. It was a privilege and a pleasure to work with my fellow committee members, to learn from them in their respective areas of expertise, and to engage with them in hearty discourse about the issues at hand. Many other experts also gave generously of their time and expertise to contribute to our information-gathering, and their contributions are deeply appreciated. The many other individuals who played a role in this process are listed in the acknowledgments on the following page, and I would like to add a special note of gratitude to the Institute of Medicine and especially to Bridget Kelly, Collin Weinberger, Louise Jordan, and Kristen Danforth, members of the project staff, for their laudable efforts shepherding and supporting the committee through every aspect of this process.

Valentín Fuster, *Chair*
Committee on Preventing the
Global Epidemic of Cardiovascular Disease:
Meeting the Challenges in Developing Countries

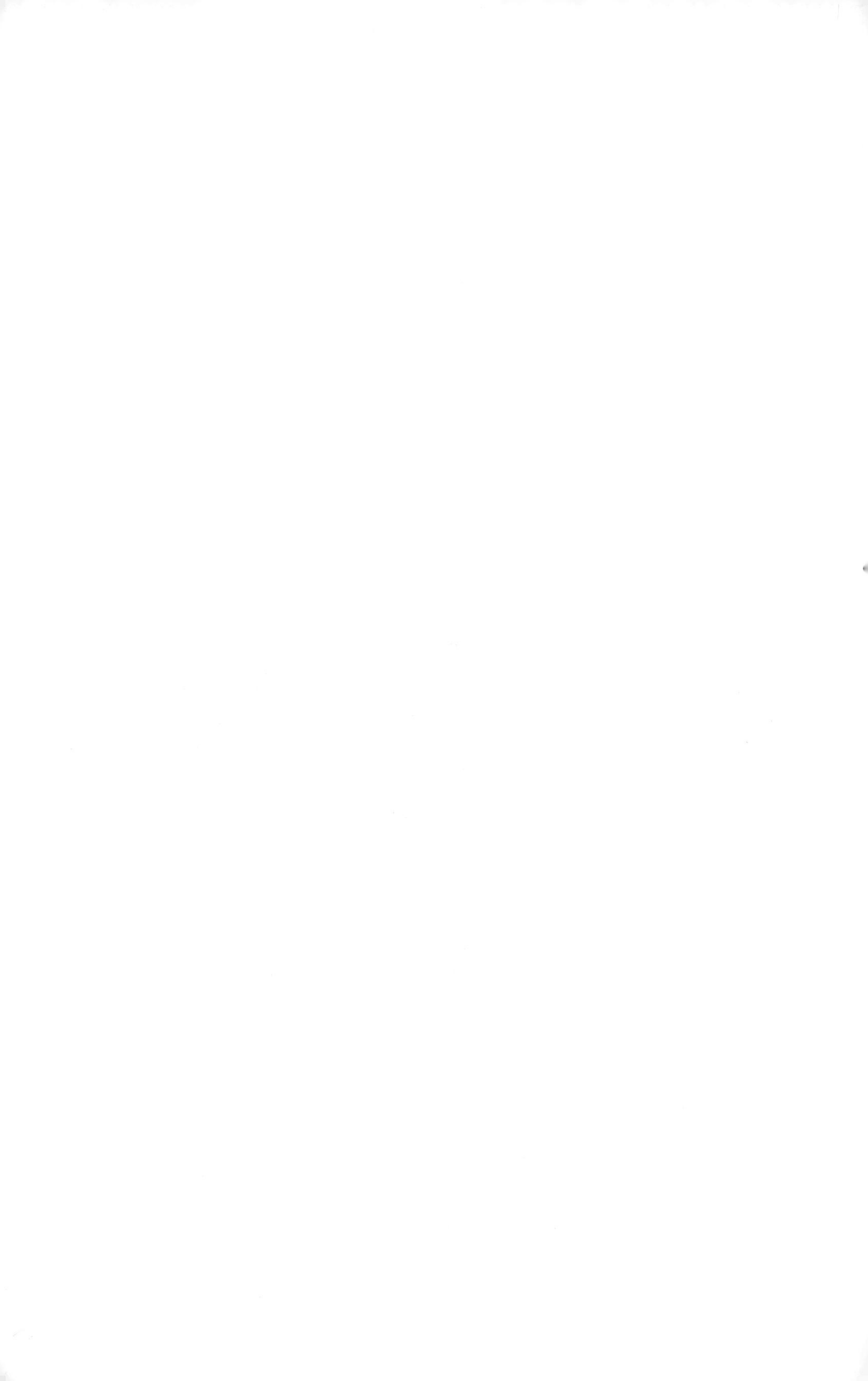

Acknowledgments

The Committee is deeply appreciative of the many valuable contributions from those who assisted with this project. First, the Committee would like to thank the National Heart, Lung, and Blood Institute for funding this study, and Zhi-Jie Zheng and Elizabeth Nabel for their guidance and support. The committee benefited enormously from the generously given time and expertise of the speakers and panelists at public information-gathering sessions. These individuals are listed in full in Appendix C. Several authors wrote papers for the committee, which were immensely helpful to the committee's deliberations: Thomas Gaziano and Grace Kim; Alejandro Jadad; Stephen Jan and Alison Hayes; Marie-Claude Jean and Louise St-Pierre; Mehmood Khan and George Mensah; Jeff Luck and Riti Shimkhada; and Marc Suhrcke, Till Boluarte, and Louis Niessen.

The committee would also like to thank Dorothy Chyung and Rajesh Vedanthan, who contributed research and writing support to committee members during this process. In addition, Morgan Heller helped in the early stages of the project as an intern at the Institute of Medicine. Belis Aladag and Laura Samuel each spent time with the committee and project staff as part of their training and education programs; both went above and beyond all expectations, and their valuable research, writing, and analytic contributions to the project were very much appreciated.

A number of individuals were crucial to the administrative and logistical success of this project. For their patience and help coordinating schedules and facilitating communication, the committee would like to thank Jennifer W. Tsai, Alanur Inal-Veith, Chellam Chellappan, Brian Shaw, Julia Addae-Mintah, Immaculate Kofie, Sarah Toming, Lucy Gonzales, Jasmine

Samuel, Lisa Nordin, Marie Viau, Ann LaBombardi, and Josie Kummer. In addition, Anthony Mavrogiannis and the staff at Kentlands Travel deserve mention for their much-appreciated persistence and problem-solving in working with the often complex travel needs and requirements of this project.

Finally, the committee conveys its gratitude and appreciation for the hard work and professionalism of the many staff of the Institute of Medicine and the National Academies who had a hand in every stage of this project. In particular, the committee would like to express its thanks for the excellent work of the study director, Bridget Kelly, and all the members of the project team who provided research, writing, analytic, and administrative support: Kristen Danforth, Louise Jordan, Collin Weinberger, Rachel Jackson, and Julie Wiltshire. The committee is also grateful for the support of Patrick Kelley, director of the Board on Global Health, who provided guidance and wisdom at critical stages of the project.

Contents

Summary		1
1	Introduction	19
2	Epidemiology of Cardiovascular Disease	49
3	Development and Cardiovascular Disease	125
4	Measurement and Evaluation	149
5	Reducing the Burden of Cardiovascular Disease: Intervention Approaches	185
6	Cardiovascular Health Promotion Early in Life	275
7	Making Choices to Reduce the Burden of Cardiovascular Disease	317
8	Framework for Action	373

APPENDIXES

A	Statement of Task	437
B	Committee and Staff Biographies	439
C	Public Session Agendas	451
D	Acronyms and Abbreviations	459
E	World Bank Income Classifications	463

Summary

Cardiovascular disease (CVD)[1] is often thought to be a problem of wealthy, industrialized nations. In fact, as the leading cause of death worldwide, CVD now has a major impact not only on developed[2] nations but also on low and middle income countries,[3] where it accounts for nearly 30 percent of all deaths. The increased prevalence of risk factors for CVD and related chronic diseases[4] in developing countries, including tobacco use, unhealthy dietary changes, reduced physical activity, increasing blood lipids, and hypertension, reflects significant global changes in behavior and lifestyle. These changes now threaten once-low-risk regions, a shift that is accelerated by industrialization, urbanization, and globalization. The potentially devastating effects of these trends are magnified by a deleterious economic impact on nations and households, where poverty can be both a contributing cause and a consequence of chronic diseases. The accelerating

---

[1] The term "cardiovascular disease" is used throughout the report to refer to cardiac disease, vascular diseases of the brain and kidney, and peripheral vascular disease. The report's main focus is on the major contributors to global CVD mortality, coronary heart disease and stroke, and on the major modifiable risk factors for cardiovascular diseases.

[2] The terms "developed" and "high income countries" are used interchangeably throughout the report to refer to countries classified by the World Bank as high income economies (see Appendix E for 2009 classifications).

[3] The terms "developing" and "low and middle income countries" are used interchangeably throughout the report to refer to countries classified by the World Bank as low, lower middle, and upper middle income economies (see Appendix E for 2009 classifications).

[4] The term "chronic diseases" is used throughout the report to refer to CVD and the following related chronic diseases that share many common risk factors: diabetes, cancer, and chronic respiratory disease.

rates of unrecognized and inadequately addressed CVD and related chronic diseases in both men and women in low and middle income countries are cause for immediate action.

In the past several decades increasing attention has been given to the emergence of chronic diseases as a threat to low and middle income countries. Substantive efforts to more accurately document and draw attention to the economic and health burden have led to a growing recognition that CVD and related chronic diseases need to be on the health agenda for all nations. At the international level, there have been several landmark documents produced to translate this recognition into calls for action and to develop strategies and policy frameworks.

Despite this progress, there remains a profound mismatch between the compelling evidence documenting the health and economic burden of CVD and the lack of concrete steps to increase investment and implement CVD prevention and disease management efforts in developing countries. To help catalyze the action needed, the U.S. National Heart, Lung, and Blood Institute (NHLBI) sponsored this study of the evolving global epidemic of CVD. The Institute of Medicine convened the Committee on Preventing the Global Epidemic of Cardiovascular Disease: Meeting the Challenges in Developing Countries to assess the current tools for CVD control and the knowledge and strategies pertinent to their implementation. The committee was charged with evaluating the available evidence to offer conclusions and recommendations to reduce the global burden of CVD, with an emphasis on developing guidance for partnership and collaborations among a range of public- and private-sector entities involved with global health and development.

In response to its charge, the committee undertook an examination of the current state of efforts to reduce the global epidemic of CVD based on a review of the available literature and of information gathered from various stakeholders in CVD and global health. In this analysis, the committee evaluated why there has not been more action to address chronic diseases and assessed the available evidence on intervention approaches to prevent and manage CVD, emphasizing knowledge and strategies pertinent to their implementation in low and middle income countries. Through careful consideration of the evidence and a thorough deliberation process, the committee drew conclusions about the necessary next steps to move forward.

Prior reports have identified general priorities and recommended a wide range of possible actions for a multitude of stakeholders; indeed, the findings and conclusions of this report reinforce many of those messages and priorities. In this report's recommendations, however, the committee has emphasized advancing the field beyond messages about broad conceptual solutions and has identified a limited set of specific actions targeted to specific stakeholders. These actions are intended to encourage a sufficient shift in the global health and development agenda to facilitate critical next steps that will build toward the eventual goal of widespread dissemination and implementation of evidence-based programs, policies, and other tools to address CVD and related chronic diseases in developing countries.

ACTIONS TO REDUCE THE GLOBAL BURDEN OF CVD

The actions needed for an individual to prevent and treat CVD are deceptively straightforward: eat a healthy diet, remain physically active throughout life, don't use tobacco, and seek health care regularly. The reality is much more complex. Behavior change is difficult, individual choices are influenced by broader social and environmental factors, and many people do not have the resources or access to seek appropriate health care.

Solutions can also seem simple at the level of governments and other organizations. Declarations have called on governments to invest more in CVD, to develop laws to protect health, and to ensure access to services to meet the cardiovascular health needs of people. International conference recommendations have demanded that food companies restrict marketing of certain products to children; eliminate transfats and reduce saturated fat, unhealthy oils, sugar, and salt in their products; and make healthy foods more affordable and available. In reality, however, governments and donors need to balance many competing priorities in the allocation of resources, and the level of capacity and infrastructure to support action varies among countries. Context is also critical; programs and policies that have worked in one environment may not work in another. The health systems infrastructure in many countries is insufficient to support chronic disease prevention, treatment, and management. Companies are obligated and motivated to meet the needs of their shareholders even when willing to collaborate to work toward public health goals. These realities have often not been fully considered in the effort to draw attention to the compelling burden of CVD and to call for action.

Along with the need to recognize these realities in the effort to implement policies and programs, the committee identified several key barriers to progress in controlling the global epidemic of CVD. There is concern that attention to CVD would detract from other health needs; there is uncertainty about the effectiveness and feasibility of policies, programs, and services in the contexts in which they need to be implemented; efforts among stakeholders are fragmented and there is a need for focused leadership and collaboration centered on clearly defined goals and outcomes; there is a lack of financial, individual, and institutional resources; and there is insufficient capacity to meet CVD needs in low and middle income countries, including health workforce and infrastructure capacity as well as implementation and enforcement capacity for policies and regulatory approaches.

The committee also identified several essential functions that are needed to overcome these barriers. These include advocacy and leadership at global and national levels, developing policy, program implementation, capacity building, research focusing on evaluating approaches in developing countries that are context specific and culturally relevant, ongoing monitoring and evaluation, and funding. Success will require resources—financial, technical, and human—and the combined efforts of many players sustained over many years. The following summarizes the committee's conclusions and recommendations about these barriers and how to overcome them by strengthening these essential functions.

Aligning Chronic Disease Needs with Health and Development Priorities

Global health and development stakeholders and national governments in the developing world face important challenges that remain far from adequately managed, such as basic economic development priorities, poverty alleviation, hunger reduction, and a range of health issues in areas such as infectious disease and maternal and child health. In addition, the state of the global economy affects the resources of both donor countries and governments in low and middle income countries. As a result, decision makers face very difficult choices about resource allocation. Rather than competing against existing priorities, leaders in the effort to reduce the burden of CVD and related chronic diseases at both global and local levels need to better communicate the importance of integrating attention to these diseases within other health and development needs. Better alignment among these priorities, as described in this report, has the potential to synergistically improve economic and health status. Furthermore, this can help ensure that current and future health and development efforts do not inadvertently worsen the growing epidemic of chronic diseases.

In order to lay the groundwork to achieve this synergy, governments in low and middle income countries, global health funders, and development agencies need to give CVD and related chronic diseases more equal footing as a development and health priority. Currently, however, most agencies providing development assistance do not include chronic diseases as an area of emphasis. Given the compelling health and economic burden, these agencies will not truly meet their goals of improving health and well-being worldwide without committing to address chronic diseases in alignment with their evolving global health priorities. Leadership in eliminating this gap at these agencies is a critical first step to encourage a greater emphasis on chronic diseases among all stakeholders.

Recommendation 1: Recognize Chronic Diseases as a Development Assistance Priority

Multilateral[5] and bilateral[6] development agencies that do not already do so should explicitly include CVD and related chronic diseases as an area of focus for technical assistance, capacity building, program implementation, impact assessment of development projects, funding, and other areas of activity.

Evidence-Based and Locally Relevant Solutions

Stakeholders of all kinds, from national governments to development agencies and other donors, who have committed to taking action to address the global burden of chronic diseases will need to carefully assess the needs of the population they are targeting, the state of current efforts, the available capacity and infrastructure, and the political will to support the available opportunities for action. This assessment will inform priorities and should lead to specific and realistic goals for intervention strategies that are adapted to local baseline capacity and burden of disease and designed to improve that baseline over time. These goals will determine choices about the implementation of both evidence-based policies and programs and also capacity building efforts. Ongoing evaluation of implemented strategies will allow policy makers and other stakeholders to determine if implemented actions are having the intended effect and meeting the defined goals, and to reassess needs, capacity, and priorities over time.

Given limited resources to allocate to CVD, developing country governments and other stakeholders will want to focus efforts on goals that promise to be economically feasible, have the highest likelihood of intervention success, and have the largest impact on morbidity. Successes in reducing the burden of CVD in many high income countries provide considerable knowledge about how to manage disease and reduce the major behavioral and biological risk factors for CVD, which are well-described and largely consistent worldwide. However, much of this knowledge is not easily translated into solutions for the developing world. Low and middle and income countries have resource constraints, cultural contexts, social structures, and social and behavioral norms that are distinct from high income countries

---

[5] The term "multilateral development agencies" is used throughout the recommendations to refer to international, multilateral entities that provide health and development assistance, such as the World Health Organization and World Bank and regional development banks.

[6] The term "bilateral development agencies" is used throughout the recommendations to refer to national agencies that provide foreign development assistance, such as the U.S. Agency for International Development (USAID) in the United States and analogous agencies in other G20 countries.

and distinct among different developing countries. The goal of simply implementing solutions drawn directly from best practices in high income countries is a siren song; this approach will not be compelling to policy makers in low and middle income countries or to the agencies that provide external assistance to these countries.

While the needs, capacity, and priorities will vary across countries, the available intervention and economic evidence suggests that substantial progress in reducing CVD can be made in the near term through strategies to reduce tobacco use; to reduce salt consumption; and to improve delivery of clinical prevention in high-risk patients. These goals have credible evidence for lowered CVD morbidity, demonstrated likelihood of cost-effectiveness, and examples of successful implementation of programs with the potential to be adapted for low and middle income countries.

To achieve successful adaptation and implementation of these priority approaches and to move toward a sufficient knowledge base to implement other promising strategies in the longer term, real work lies ahead to build on the knowledge derived from existing best practices in CVD and on practical knowledge that can be gleaned from successful implementation experience in other areas of global health. Together, these can be the basis to establish what works for CVD within local realities in relevant settings and then to disseminate those findings among countries with similar epidemics and similar infrastructure, resources, and cultural environments. To these ends, the committee makes recommendations in the following areas.

Better Local Data

A first step for governments and program implementers is to determine the extent and nature of cardiovascular risk in their local population and to assess their needs and capacity to address CVD and related chronic diseases. Improved population data are crucial to compel action, to inform local priorities, and to measure the impact of implemented policies and programs.

Recommendation 2: Improve Local Data

National and subnational governments[7] should create and maintain health surveillance systems to monitor and more effectively control chronic diseases. Ideally, these systems should report on cause-specific mortality and the primary determinants of CVD. To strengthen existing initiatives, multilateral development agencies and World Health Orga-

---

[7] The term "national and subnational governments" is used throughout the recommendations to refer to national governments and/or governments below the level of the national government, such as provinces, territories, districts, municipalities, cities, and states within federal systems.

nization (WHO) (through, for example, the Health Metrics Network and regional chronic disease network, NCDnet) as well as bilateral public health agencies[8] (such as the Centers for Disease Control and Prevention [CDC] in the United States) and bilateral development agencies (such as USAID) should support chronic disease surveillance as part of financial and technical assistance for developing and implementing health information systems. Governments should allocate funds and build capacity for long-term sustainability of disease surveillance that includes chronic diseases.

Policy Approaches Based on Local Priorities

One of the primary goals in meeting the challenges of CVD is to create environments that support and empower individual behavior choices that help prevent the acquisition and augmentation of risk. In countries that have adequate regulatory and enforcement capacity, policy makers have a range of policy solutions they can implement to target local priorities and goals. Because the determinants of CVD extend beyond the realm of the health sector, coordinated approaches are needed so that policies in nonhealth sectors of government, such as agriculture, urban planning, transportation, and education, can be developed synergistically with health policies to reduce, or at least not adversely affect, risk for CVD. In addition to coordinating among different sectors of government, policies in each of these domains can be developed with input from civil society and the private sector. This coordinated, intersectoral approach can help determine the balance of regulatory measures, incentives, and voluntary measures that is likely to be most effective and realistic in the local political and governmental context, especially when the feasibility of policy changes is challenged by economic aims that may be in conflict with goals for improving health outcomes.

A policy approach supported by a strong evidence base in high income countries is implementation of the Framework Convention for Tobacco Control, which emphasizes measures such as taxation; protection from exposure to tobacco smoke; health warnings and public awareness campaigns; tobacco cessation services; and controls on tobacco advertising, illicit trade, and sales to minors. In addition, a collection of successful strategies to reduce salt in the food supply and in consumption in high income settings could potentially be adapted to low and middle income settings and are already being initiated in some developing countries. Analogous efforts

---

[8] The term "bilateral public health agencies" is used throughout the recommendations to refer to national public health agencies such as the Centers for Disease Control and Prevention (CDC) in the United States and analogous agencies in other G20 countries.

could be explored to reduce consumption of other unhealthy dietary components, including saturated fats and transfats, unhealthy oils, and sugars. Agriculture policies could also be considered, where feasible, to avoid overproduction of meat and unhealthy oils and to encourage greater production of healthy foods such as fruits and vegetables. Finally, for those countries on the verge of rapid urbanization, policies for future urban planning could promote physical activity and improve access to healthy food sources. Many of these policies would be in synergy with aims to minimize potential negative environmental and safety effects of rapid urban development.

Health communications and education efforts at the population level are another strategy to affect CVD-related behaviors. Public communication interventions that are coordinated with the policy changes selected by government authorities can enhance the effectiveness of both approaches. In addition to promoting behavior change, communication programs and engagement with the media can be used to build public support for policy changes.

The feasibility and effectiveness of policy approaches and health communications efforts to reduce CVD in low and middle income settings must be ascertained. It is therefore crucial that government authorities, with external technical and financial assistance when needed, implement both the initiatives and the necessary mechanisms for monitoring, evaluation, and transparent reporting of their effects. This will inform ongoing action within countries and help build a global knowledge base of feasible and effective approaches.

> **Recommendation 3: Implement Policies to Promote Cardiovascular Health**
>
> **To expand current or introduce new population-wide efforts to promote cardiovascular health and to reduce risk for CVD and related chronic diseases, national and subnational governments should adapt and implement evidence-based, effective policies based on local priorities. These policies may include laws, regulations, changes to fiscal policy, and incentives to encourage private-sector alignment. To maximize impact, efforts to introduce policies should be accompanied by sustained health communication campaigns focused on the same targets of intervention as the selected policies.**

Improved Health Care Delivery

Clinical interventions can provide treatment for CVD as well as control of biological risk factors such as elevated blood pressure, blood lipids, and blood glucose for both individuals already diagnosed with CVD and those at high risk, ideally in the context of a supportive environment created by policy and health communication initiatives to address behavioral risk by promoting healthy individual choices and appropriate self-care. However, implementation of these effective approaches requires an adequate system of organizations, institutions, and resources to meet health needs. Many countries lack this health systems infrastructure. In this aspect, strategies to reduce the burden of chronic diseases can be coordinated with, rather than compete against, efforts in other areas of global health. Therefore, the CVD community should seek opportunities to create stronger interactions with existing major global initiatives that are increasing support for broad health systems strengthening as part of their current mission, such as the International Health Partnership; the U.S. HIV/AIDS programs implemented under the President's Emergency Plan for AIDS Relief; the Global Fund for AIDS, Tuberculosis and Malaria; and the Global Alliance for Vaccines and Immunization. Such an integrated approach dovetails with current efforts to transition from costly, disease-specific approaches toward more efficient approaches that promote better primary health care to meet a range of health needs. It also fits into a shift in the global health paradigm from acute, short-term interventions to longer-term investments in overall health.

In particular, a critical component to make it feasible to reduce the burden of CVD is an adequate and appropriately trained local workforce to initiate and sustain intervention efforts. Therefore, as part of current and future strategies to strengthen the overall health and public health workforce in low and middle income countries, international and national CVD stakeholders need to work to build capacity in the areas of cardiovascular health promotion, CVD prevention, CVD clinical services, and CVD-related research. In particular, capacity building could include enhancing curricular development to include chronic diseases in training programs in clinical, public health, research, economic, epidemiology, behavioral, health promotion, and health communications disciplines.

In addition to building local workforce capacity, strengthening health systems to better meet the needs of both chronic disease and other health needs in low and middle income countries will require low-cost approaches to deliver high-quality care by improving equitable access to affordable health services and essential medicines, diagnostics, and technologies for prevention and treatment; monitoring clinical practice and improving the quality of care; introducing risk-pooling mechanisms for financing health services; and using information technologies.

In addition, the chronic disease community needs to actively engage in current and future health systems strengthening efforts in low and middle income countries not only to improve prevention and care for CVD and related chronic diseases but also to contribute chronic care expertise to help develop solutions for infectious diseases that require chronic management, such as HIV/AIDS and tuberculosis.

Recommendation 4: Include Chronic Diseases in Health Systems Strengthening

Current and future efforts to strengthen health systems and health care delivery funded and implemented by multilateral agencies, bilateral public health and development agencies, leading international nongovernmental organizations (NGOs),[9] and national and subnational health authorities should include attention to evidence-based prevention, diagnosis, and management of CVD. This should include developing and evaluating approaches to build local workforce capacity and to implement services for CVD that are integrated with primary health care services, management of chronic infectious diseases, and maternal and child health.

Coordination of National and Subnational Approaches

The breadth of the many determinants that affect CVD means that these efforts must extend beyond the public health and health care sectors to include authorities throughout the whole of government in a coordinated intersectoral approach. For example, strategies to reduce tobacco use or salt consumption will require actions by a range of governmental agencies (health, agriculture, finance, broadcasting, education) as well as private-sector producers and retailers. The political will to support and the expertise to implement such a broad effort cannot depend on the Ministry of Health alone. To coordinate these efforts, ensure the allocation of necessary resources, and have the best chance for real impact requires a mechanism at a level that is insulated from the relative influence of different ministries within the government. Coordination and communication within a whole-of-government approach also needs to include legislatures in order to pass laws needed to implement policies and, in some cases, to initiate changes in the activities of executive agencies. In addition, these efforts must be coordinated with stakeholders in the private sector and civil society as well as donors and agencies providing external development assistance. A useful model for this approach comes from successful efforts to achieve national coordination of efforts in the fight against HIV/AIDS.

---

[9] The term "leading international nongovernmental organizations" is used throughout the recommendations to refer to NGOs with a mission to address CVD and/or related chronic diseases, such as the World Heart Federation and the World Hypertension League, as well as those with a mission to advance global health more broadly, such as the International Union for Health Promotion and Education and the Global Forum for Health Research.

Recommendation 5: Improve National Coordination for Chronic Diseases

National governments should establish a commission that reports to a high-level cabinet authority with the specific aim of coordinating the implementation of efforts to address the needs of chronic care and chronic disease in all policies. This authority should serve as a mechanism for communicating and coordinating among relevant executive agencies (e.g., health, agriculture, education, and transportation) as well as legislative bodies, civil society, the private sector, and foreign development assistance agencies. These commissions should be modeled on current national HIV/AIDS commissions and could be integrated with these commissions where they already exist.

Generating Evidence for Locally Relevant CVD Programs

Local realities affect the planning, implementation, effectiveness, and sustainability of approaches to prevent and manage CVD. High-quality evaluations of programs are needed in settings that are analogous to those in which they are intended to be implemented in order to generate knowledge about what is not only effective but also feasible. The approaches that need to be evaluated are broad and include population surveillance methods; population-based health promotion and CVD prevention approaches; health education; financing of health care, interventions and incentives to improve the quality of care, models for efficient delivery, and integration of health care services; and integrated community-based approaches.

The health sector and public health community in high income countries also stand to learn from what works in resource-constrained contexts in low and middle income countries. Developed countries are urgently in need of effective and affordable solutions for CVD, which remains a major health burden, especially for those populations most susceptible to health disparities.

Recommendation 6: Research to Assess What Works in Different Settings

The National Heart, Lung, and Blood Institute (NHLBI) and its partners in the newly created Global Alliance for Chronic Disease, along with other research funders[10] and bilateral public health agencies, should prioritize research to determine what intervention approaches will be most

---

[10] The term "research funders" is used throughout the recommendations to refer to multilateral and bilateral health agencies as well as foundations and other nongovernmental organizations that fund global health research.

effective and feasible to implement in low and middle income countries, including adaptations based on demonstrated success in high income countries. Using appropriate rigorous evaluation methodologies, this research should be conducted in partnership with local governments, academic and public health researchers, nongovernmental organizations, and communities. This will serve to promote appropriate intervention approaches for local cultural contexts and resource constraints and to strengthen local research capacity.

A. Implementation research should be a priority in research funding for global chronic disease.
B. Research support for intervention and implementation research should include explicit funding for economic evaluation.
C. Research should include assessments of and approaches to improve clinical, public health, and research training programs in both developed and developing countries to ultimately improve the status of global chronic disease training.
D. Research should involve multiple disciplines, such as agriculture, environment, urban planning, and behavioral and social sciences, through integrated funding sources with research funders in these disciplines. A goal of this multidisciplinary research should be to advance intersectoral evaluation methodologies.
E. In the interests of developing better models for prevention and care in the United States, U.S. agencies that support research and program implementation should coordinate to evaluate the potential for interventions funded through their global health activities to be adapted and applied in the United States.

Dissemination and Practice-Based Evidence

Efforts to address CVD are being implemented in many developing countries. These efforts offer the potential to contribute to the available knowledge base of feasible and effective solutions for CVD in low and middle income countries. However, there is insufficient evaluation and reporting of these programs and policies, and inadequate systematic mechanisms for disseminating what has worked in one context to other similar contexts. Regional coordination can provide a much-needed mechanism for countries to build their knowledge base through innovation and evaluation, to share knowledge and technical capacity among countries with similar epidemics, resources, and cultural conditions, and to help build international support for national-based solutions.

Recommendation 7: Disseminate Knowledge and Innovation Among Similar Countries

Regional organizations, such as professional organizations, WHO observatories and chronic disease networks, regional and subregional development banks, and regional political and economic organizations should continue and expand regional[11] mechanisms for reporting on trends in CVD and disseminating successful intervention approaches. These efforts should be supported by leading international NGOs, development and public health agencies, and research funders (including the Global Alliance for Chronic Disease). The goal should be to maximize communication and coordination among countries with similar epidemics, resources, and cultural conditions in order to encourage and standardize evaluation, help determine locally appropriate best practices, encourage innovation, and promote dissemination of knowledge. These mechanisms may include, for example, regional meetings for researchers, program managers, and policy makers; regionally focused publications; and registries of practice-based evidence.

Prevention Early in Life

Accumulation of cardiovascular risk begins early in life, and evidence on rising rates of childhood obesity and youth smoking in low and middle income countries as well as emerging evidence on the effects of early nutrition on later cardiovascular health support the value of starting health promotion efforts during pregnancy and early childhood and continuing prevention efforts throughout the life course. Thus, prevention early in life warrants special attention within the implementation of many of the recommendations in this report, especially those focusing on research efforts and integration with existing health systems strengthening efforts. This will allow progress toward a true life-course approach to promoting cardiovascular health. In particular, maternal and child health programs offer an opportunity to provide care that not only takes into account shorter-term childhood outcomes but also includes greater attention to future lifelong health, including cardiovascular health. In addition to efforts to reduce risk for child obesity and prevent initiation of tobacco use, emerging evidence on the effects of early nutrition on later cardiovascular health means that the CVD and maternal and child health communities need to work together more closely to ensure that food and nutrition programs for undernourished children do not inadvertently contribute to long-term chronic disease

---

[11] The term "regional" is not meant to limit mechanisms for coordination and dissemination to geographical groupings. These mechanisms could, where appropriate, also include groupings by, for example, risk profile, political system, or economic development status.

risk. Reproductive health and family planning programs are also an avenue both to address prenatal risks for CVD and to promote cardiovascular health among women. Other approaches with some success in high income countries and emerging potential for low and middle income countries include education initiatives targeted to children and school-based programs, which need to be an area of emphasis in future research efforts. Adolescents and young adults could also be targeted to take advantage of their potential to serve as powerful advocates for change.

Organizing Global Solutions

Although the importance of local solutions cannot be overstated, active engagement of international partners is also critical to the success of global CVD control efforts. The process of translating goals into action is a complex, difficult, and long-term effort that succeeds when groups work together. Successful partnerships should include a clear articulation of roles, agreement on targets, and transparent monitoring. Such partnerships have proven highly effective at mobilizing commitments toward the prevention and treatment of infectious diseases. Current global efforts toward CVD prevention and control, however, lack widespread, coordinated action.

A broad vision for collaboration and partnership is now required to elevate CVD within the global health agenda and to effectively organize the many committed stakeholders to implement and be accountable for action. This vision is centered on the need to accommodate the realities of tight global health budgets and multiple competing priorities and to strike a balance between integrated and disease-specific approaches. Many chronic diseases, such as diabetes, cancer, and chronic respiratory illnesses, share common behavioral risk factors with CVD, including tobacco use, dietary factors, and physical inactivity. Organizations focused on these chronic diseases can jointly support approaches for reduction of shared risk factors, while at the same time retaining disease-specific programs, especially in the areas of research and technical expertise for clinical prevention and treatment.

Most chronic diseases—and indeed many communicable diseases—also share the same social determinants. In addition, as described earlier, the determinants of CVD and related chronic diseases extend beyond the realm of the health sector. Thus, an integrated approach focused on health promotion is warranted, with partnerships across sectors such as health, agriculture, development, civil society, and the private sector. The common goals of shared risk-factor reduction and modifying social determinants for health promotion thus create a frame in which CVD and non-CVD organizations can concentrate their efforts and maximize the impact of their resources.

Role of the Private Sector

Many intervention approaches designed to change the interrelated determinants that affect chronic diseases are more likely to succeed if public education and government policies and regulations are complemented by the voluntary collaboration of the private sector. These collaborations can serve to achieve health aims if agreements and negotiations are conducted transparently on public health terms under clear ethical guidelines, and if they establish defined goals and timelines that are assessed using independent monitoring mechanisms. Under these circumstances, motivated private-sector leaders at the multinational, national, and local levels in the food industry; in the pharmaceutical, biotechnology, and medical device industry; and in the business community have the potential to be powerful partners in the public health challenge to reduce the burden of CVD. The food industry (including manufacturers, retailers, and food service companies) can be engaged to expand and intensify collaboration with international public-sector efforts to reduce dietary intake of salt, saturated fats, transfats, unhealthy oils, and sugars in both adults and children, and to fully implement marketing restrictions on unhealthy products. Pharmaceutical, biotechnology, medical device, and information technology companies can be enlisted to develop, provide, and distribute safe, effective, and affordable diagnostics, therapeutics, and other technologies to improve prevention, detection, and treatment of CVD in low and middle income countries. Global and local businesses can also provide support for implementation of worksite prevention programs.

Recommendation 8: Collaborate to Improve Diets

WHO, the World Heart Federation, the International Food and Beverage Association, and the World Economic Forum, in conjunction with select leading international NGOs and select governments from developed and developing countries, should coordinate an international effort to develop collaborative strategies to reduce dietary intake of salt, sugar, saturated fats, and transfats in both adults and children. This process should include stakeholders from the public health community and multinational food corporations as well as the food services industry and retailers. This effort should include strategies that take into account local food production and sales.

Recommendation 9: Collaborate to Improve Access to CVD Diagnostics, Medicines, and Technologies

National and subnational governments should lead, negotiate, and implement a plan to reduce the costs of and ensure equitable access to

affordable diagnostics, essential medicines, and other preventive and treatment technologies for CVD. This process should involve stakeholders from multilateral and bilateral development agencies; CVD-related professional societies; public and private payers; pharmaceutical, biotechnology, medical device, and information technology companies; and experts on health care systems and financing. Deliberate attention should be given to public–private partnerships and to ensuring appropriate, rational use of these technologies.

Increased Resources

Increasing the allocation of resources for chronic diseases will be fundamental to an advancement of the global scope and scale necessary to control the CVD epidemic. Most organizations investing in global health currently focus the vast majority of funds toward acute health needs and chronic infectious diseases. However, given the alarming trends in disease burden, funders need to take chronic noncommunicable diseases into account to truly improve health globally. This investment could occur as an expansion of their primary global health mission and also as part of existing programs where objectives overlap and minimal new investment would be needed, such as early prevention maternal and child health programs; chronic care models for infectious and noninfectious disease; health systems strengthening; and health and economic development. In order to marshal the resources needed to implement actions that are aligned with the priorities outlined in this report, CVD and other chronic disease stakeholders need to build a case for investment by more effectively communicating with existing and potential new funders.

Recommendation 10: Advocate for Chronic Diseases as a Funding Priority

Leading international and national NGOs and professional societies related to CVD and other chronic diseases should work together to advocate to private foundations, charities, governmental agencies, and private donors to prioritize funding and other resources for specific initiatives to control the global epidemic of CVD and related chronic diseases. To advocate successfully, these organizations should consider (1) raising awareness about the population health and economic impact and the potential for improved outcomes with health promotion and chronic disease prevention and treatment initiatives, (2) advocating for health promotion and chronic disease prevention policies at national and subnational levels of government, (3) engaging the media about policy priorities related to chronic disease control, and (4) highlighting the importance of translating research into effective individual- and population-level interventions.

To support these efforts to better mobilize and align resources to meet the pressing burden of CVD and related chronic diseases, the level of investment required for this critical priority in global health needs to be defined more clearly. There is a need for high-quality analyses of the gap between current resources and intervention efforts and future needs and intervention opportunities. This will help inform the best balance of intervention approaches for future investments and resource allocation, including health promotion, prevention, treatment, and disease management. Conducting such analysis at the country level in low and middle income countries will be an important planning tool for national and subnational governments as well as for funders and development agencies.

Recommendation 11: Define Resource Needs

The Global Alliance for Chronic Disease should commission and coordinate case studies of the CVD financing needs for five to seven countries representing different geographical regions, stages of the CVD epidemic, and stages of development. These studies should require a comprehensive assessment of the future financial and other resource needs within the health, public health, and agricultural systems to prevent and reduce the burden of CVD and related chronic diseases. Several scenarios for different prevention and treatment efforts, training and capacity building efforts, technology choices, and demographic trends should be evaluated. These assessments should explicitly establish the gap between current investments and future investment needs, focusing on how to maximize population health gains. These initial case studies should establish an analytical framework with the goal of expanding beyond the initial pilot countries.

Global Reporting and Dialog

Progress on CVD requires that many players better coordinate their efforts, define clear goals, communicate shared messages through multiple channels from the community to the global level, and take decisive action together on the areas identified in this report. Although regional, national, and subnational actions will be the foundation for successful implementation of efforts to reduce the burden of CVD, global coordination is also critical. To accomplish this, a consistent reporting mechanism at the global level is needed to track progress, to stimulate ongoing dialog about strategies and priorities, and to continue to galvanize stakeholders at all levels.

This global mechanism can be built upon ongoing efforts by WHO to report on the global status of noncommunicable diseases, including developing guidance for surveillance systems and standardizing core indicators.

Recommendation 12: Report on Global Progress

WHO should produce and present to the World Health Assembly a biannual World Heart Health Report within the existing framework of reporting mechanisms for its Action Plan for the Global Strategy for the Prevention and Control of Noncommunicable Diseases. The goal of this report should be to provide objective data to track progress in the global effort against CVD and to stimulate policy dialog. These efforts should be designed not only for global monitoring but also to build capacity and support planning and evaluation at the national level in low and middle income countries. Financial support should come from the Global Alliance for Chronic Disease, with operational support from the CDC. The reporting process should involve national governments from high, middle, and low income countries; leading international NGOs; industry alliances; and development agencies. An initial goal of this global reporting mechanism should be to develop or select standardized indicators and methods for measurement, leveraging existing instruments where available. These would be recommended to countries, health systems, and prevention programs to maximize the global comparability of the data they collect.

CONCLUSION

Ultimately, the committee concluded that better control of CVD and related chronic diseases worldwide, and particularly in developing countries, is eminently possible. However, to achieve that goal will require sustained efforts, strong leadership, collaboration among stakeholders based on clearly defined goals and outcomes, and an investment of financial, technical, and human resources. Rather than competing against other global health and development priorities, the CVD community needs to engage policy makers and global health colleagues to integrate attention to CVD within existing global health missions and efforts because, given the high and growing burden, it will be impossible to achieve global health without better efforts to promote cardiovascular health.

1

Introduction

As the leading cause of death worldwide, cardiovascular disease (CVD) has a major impact on both developed and developing nations. Although the spotlight is more often on the global burden of mortality associated with malaria, tuberculosis, and HIV/AIDS, CVD causes more than three times the annual deaths of these three diseases combined. Indeed, nearly 30 percent of all deaths in low and middle income countries are attributable to CVD, and more than 80 percent of CVD-related deaths worldwide now occur in low and middle income countries (WHO, 2008b). This health burden is accompanied by a deleterious economic impact. However, despite the significant and growing health and economic burden in low and middle income countries, CVD and related chronic diseases are not included by most stakeholders in their investments and commitments to improving the health of the world's people.

CVD and related chronic diseases were once considered to be diseases of industrialized nations. However, in recent years an increasingly robust body of epidemiological evidence has highlighted the proliferation of CVD risk factors worldwide, including obesity, hypertension, and diabetes. The worsening of cardiovascular health around the world—and most notably in developing countries—reflects significant global changes in behavior and lifestyle. The "westernization" of dietary habits, decreased levels of physical activity, increased childhood obesity, and increased tobacco consumption—accelerated by industrialization, urbanization, and globalization—now threaten once-low-risk regions. In addition, the decline in infectious diseases and improved childhood nutrition have contributed to the aging of populations in many low and middle income countries, resulting in an increasing number of individuals who survive to the age at which risk factors they accrued throughout childhood and early adulthood manifest as chronic diseases. This has resulted in an epidemic that is "old" in its similarity to the rise in CVD that occurred in the developed world in previous decades, yet brings with it new characteristics that are a result of contemporary global circumstances.

STUDY CHARGE, APPROACH, AND SCOPE

Over the past several decades, a considerable amount has been learned about the determinants of CVD as well as how to reduce CVD incidence and mortality. Building on this knowledge and the emerging evidence of the growing burden of CVD in developing countries, there has been a steady escalation of international reports, declarations, and resolutions calling attention to the growing threat of the global CVD epidemic. These are summarized in Figure 1.1 and Box 1.1 later in this chapter, where they are discussed in more detail to set the historical context for this report.

These declarations, reports, and resolutions have resulted in a growing recognition that CVD, and chronic noncommunicable diseases more broadly, are a worldwide problem whose burden is increasingly felt by low and middle income countries. In the past several years, this recognition has begun to translate into guidance for action. However, despite examples from the developed world that demonstrate promise and hope for the reduction of disease burden on a national level, the burden of CVD has continued to grow and concrete steps toward scaling up CVD treatment and prevention efforts in developing countries have been slow to materialize. Recognizing a need to help catalyze progress from guidance and strategies to actions, the National Heart, Lung, and Blood Institute (NHLBI) sponsored this study by the Institute of Medicine (IOM), and an ad hoc committee was convened to study the evolving global epidemic of CVD and offer conclusions and recommendations pertinent to its control.

Study Charge

The full Statement of Task for the Committee on Preventing the Global Epidemic of Cardiovascular Disease: Meeting the Challenges in Developing Countries can be found in Appendix A. In summary, the committee was charged with synthesizing and expanding relevant evidence and knowledge based on research findings, with an emphasis on developing concepts of global partnership and collaborations, and on recommending actions targeted at global governmental organizations, nongovernmental organizations (NGOs), policy and decision makers, funding agencies, academic and research institutions, and the general public.

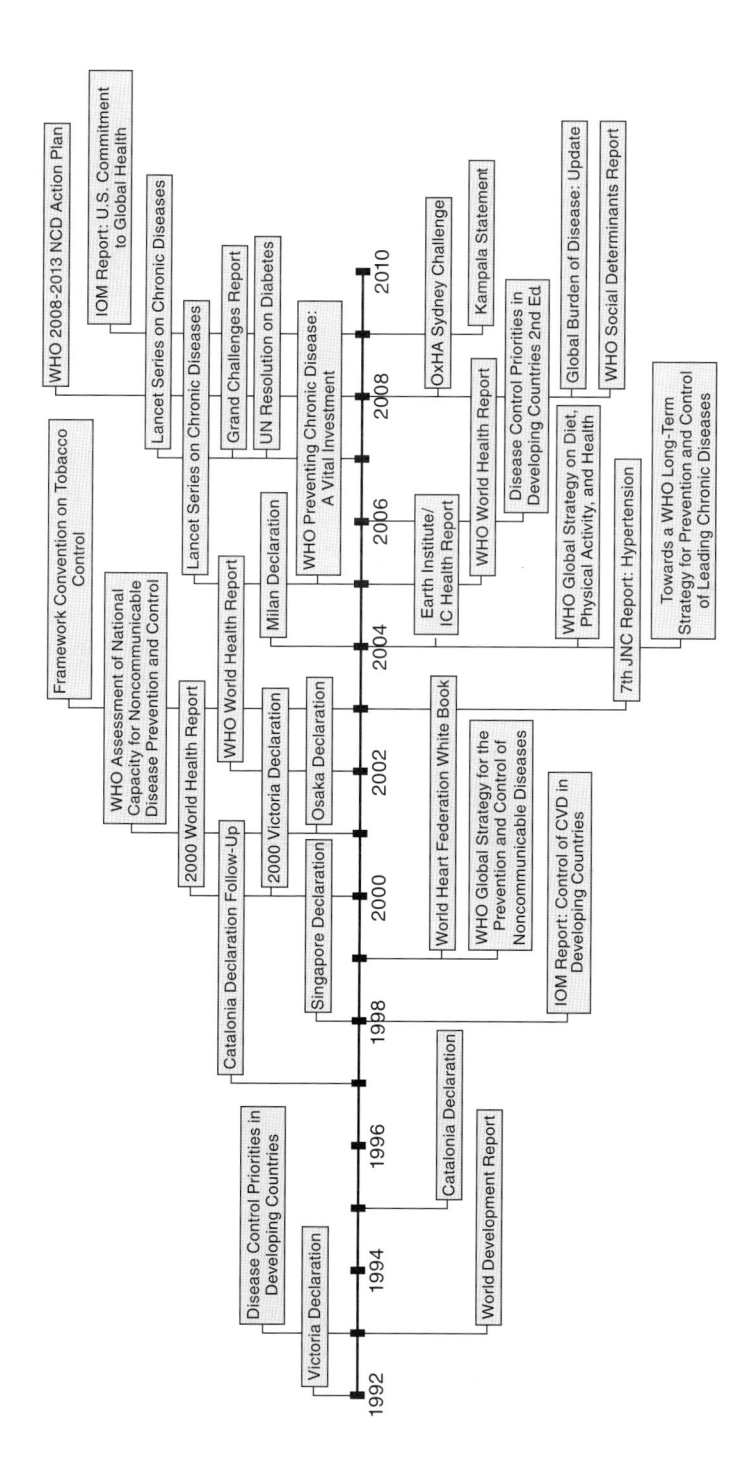

FIGURE 1.1 Timeline of major documents related to global CVD.

In response to its charge, the committee undertook an analysis of the current state of efforts to reduce the global epidemic of CVD based on a review of the available literature and of information gathered from various stakeholders in CVD and global health. In this analysis, the committee evaluated why there has not been more action to address CVD; assessed the available evidence on intervention approaches to prevent and manage CVD, including knowledge and strategies pertinent to their implementation in low and middle income countries; and drew conclusions about the necessary next steps to move forward.

Prior reports have identified general priorities and recommended a wide range of possible actions for a multitude of stakeholders; indeed, the findings and conclusions of this report reinforce many of those messages and priorities. In this report's recommendations, however, the committee has emphasized advancing the field beyond messages about broad conceptual solutions and has identified a limited set of specific actions targeted to specific stakeholders. These actions are intended to encourage a sufficient shift in the global health and development agenda to facilitate critical next steps that will build toward the eventual goal of widespread dissemination and implementation of evidence-based programs, policies, and other tools to address CVD and related chronic diseases in developing countries.

Study Approach

The committee met four times to deliberate in person, and conducted additional deliberations by teleconference and electronic communications. Public information-gathering sessions were held in conjunction with the second and third meetings; the complete agendas for these sessions can be found in Appendix C. The committee also commissioned several papers that informed the study; these are referenced within the report.

The committee reviewed literature and information from a range of disciplines and sources. A comprehensive systematic review of all primary literature relevant to the study's broad charge was not within the scope of the study. Instead, this report represents a summative description of the key evidence, with illustrative research examples discussed in more detail. In order to limit the length of this document and to avoid replication of existing work, the committee sought existing relevant, high-quality systematic and narrative reviews. In content areas where these were available, the report includes summaries of key findings, but otherwise refers the reader to the available resources for more detailed information.

For intervention approaches to reduce the burden of disease, the committee reviewed the literature to identify relevant examples of interventions, programs, or policies that target CVD and related CVD-risk factors, as well as to identify areas in which relatively little applicable intervention research has been conducted. The committee's approach to the analysis of intervention evidence is described in full in Chapter 5. In summary, the committee emphasized effectiveness, contextual generalizability, feasibility, and relevance for real-world implementation. Therefore, the focus was on identifying intervention approaches for CVD with evidence in developing countries. Where this evidence was limited, examples were sought that offer generalizable lessons from interventions with evidence from both CVD-specific approaches in developed countries and developing country evidence for non-CVD health outcomes.

Using this approach, the report strives to move the field beyond a discussion of general intervention approaches and policy priorities in the broad terms of prior reports, such as "reduce salt consumption," "improve diets," "reduce tobacco use," "increase physical activity," and "screen and treat biological risk factors and disease." The report achieves this by offering a pragmatic review of the available evidence in the context of potential for implementation of interventions and strategies, while recognizing the complexities of heterogeneity and variability in capacity among different low and middle income countries. Indeed, the committee's goal was to go beyond the relatively few well-known intervention examples that appear in many preceding reports to instead gather information of sufficient depth, breadth, and specificity on actual intervention implementation in order to realistically inform resource prioritization in real-world, country-specific decision making.

Applying this approach revealed significant gaps in the evidence base and led to greater specificity and clarity in defining the needs to transition from knowledge to action, which has resulted in a research agenda focusing on implementation research and additional economic analysis. However, the committee does not intend that the findings highlighting ongoing research priorities be taken as a suggestion of inaction. A principle throughout the report is one of being action oriented based on available findings.

Study Scope and Audiences

This committee was tasked by the sponsor to focus on cardiovascular disease, which is the largest contributor to the global burden of chronic disease (WHO, 2008b). This focus was clearly mandated by the Statement of Task, but with the understanding that the report should consider CVD in the context of other related chronic diseases that share common risk factors and intervention approaches, especially diabetes, cancer, and chronic respiratory disease (Nabel, 2009). The term cardiovascular disease can encompass a wide range of diseases, such as coronary heart disease, congestive heart failure, vascular diseases of the brain and kidney, peripheral vascular disease, congenital heart defects, and infectious cardiac disease. As evidenced in Chapter 2, the committee focused its attention primarily on the major contributors to global CVD mortality, coronary heart disease and stroke, and on the major modifiable risk factors for cardiovascular diseases, especially tobacco use, unhealthy diet, physical inactivity, obesity, hypertension, dyslipidemia, and elevated blood glucose as well as broader determinants associated with risk for CVD. In addition, although not the major emphasis of the report, in some regions there continues to be a high burden of infectious cardiac disease, particularly rheumatic heart disease and Chagas disease (Muna, 1993; WHO, 2003b; WHO Study Group and WHO, 2004). Therefore, these are also reviewed briefly in Chapter 2 of the report, along with pericarditis and cardiomyopathies caused by tuberculosis (TB) and HIV.

In order to identify steps to prevent and mitigate the growing burden of cardiovascular disease, the committee was charged by the sponsor to study CVD "prevention and management." In the course of its deliberations among experts from a range of disciplines that have a role in addressing cardiovascular disease, such as public health, health communications, and cardiology, the committee found that different fields often use different terms and definitions to categorize similar intervention approaches and that many intervention approaches do not fall into clearly delineated categories. The committee felt that it was not in its mandate nor was it feasible within the study scope and timeline to come to consensus definitions of terms and their subcategories. Therefore, to prevent confusion and to avoid detracting from key messages with discussions of nomenclature, the committee refers broadly to health promotion, prevention, treatment, and disease management, but whenever possible the committee refers to specific intervention approaches descriptively rather than categorically and makes no attempt to assign them to further subcategories.

Furthermore, the committee views health promotion, prevention, treatment, and disease management as part of a continuous spectrum. The committee interpreted its charge to be inclusive of this spectrum of approaches rather than as a mandate to recommend choices among them, and the committee found that the entire range warrants attention in order to truly address CVD and related chronic diseases. Indeed, the totality of the available intervention and economic evidence supports a balanced approach in which promotion and prevention is emphasized, but which also recognizes the need for effective, appropriate, quality delivery of medical interventions for risk reduction and treatment. The appropriate balance of investment in different intervention approaches across this spectrum is a challenge for evidenced-base policy decisions that is discussed in Chapter 7.

The sponsor's charge to the committee clearly anticipated that the very nature of the problem necessitates concerted action by a wide range of stakeholders. As articulated in the committee's Framework for Action (Chapter 8), the committee also recognizes the need to be broad in the approach to the problem, and thus the report has messages and recommendations aimed at multilateral and bilateral development and health agencies, national and subnational governments in low and middle income countries, nongovernmental organizations, professional societies, research and training institutions, and the private sector (see Figure 8.2 in Chapter 8).

However, unlike many of the preceding documents in the field of global chronic diseases, this report was initiated by a specific stakeholder with the will and resources to act upon its recommendations. Therefore, the committee viewed this study as first and foremost an opportunity to provide independent, external guidance to NHLBI to inform and support its emerging investments in global CVD and to help set goals and priorities that will ensure the success of current and future endeavors to incorporate global health into its activities, including its strategic partnerships with other relevant stakeholders within the United States and internationally. The committee also viewed the report as an opportunity to identify ways in which the U.S. global health agenda, along with the international global health agenda, can evolve to be more inclusive of chronic diseases, providing elaboration on a mandate that was issued in the 2009 IOM report *The U.S. Commitment to Global Health* (IOM, 2009).

As a result, the committee focused many of its recommendations on the fundamental goal of identifying actions that could be taken or supported by the study sponsor, NHLBI, and its potential partners within the U.S. government. As the ultimate recommendation language indicates, many of these actions would also be appropriate for other stakeholders, and many are recommended in the context of collaborative strategies. This relative emphasis on the U.S. government as a key target for the report's messages does not reflect a judgment on the part of the committee that the needed worldwide actions should be centered in the United States, but simply reflects an emphasis on the logical primary and receptive audience for a report sponsored by a U.S. government agency and conducted by the U.S. Institute of Medicine. This capacity to convey credible messages to the U.S. government gives this report the potential to have an unprecedented influence compared to prior reports on this topic. This is especially the case given its timely publication during a process of reflection and evolution of U.S. global health priorities, evidenced by the current administration's emerging Global Health Initiative (U.S. Department of State, 2010).

HISTORICAL CONTEXT

A Growing Focus on Global Health

The past decade has seen increased recognition that the international community must take action to improve the health of all people worldwide. In 1997, the IOM released its report *America's Vital Interest in Global*

Health, which emphasized that the United States has a vital and direct stake in the health of people around the globe and that it should increase investments in foreign aid to improve health (IOM, 1997). Since then, the U.S. government has significantly increased its development spending on health. U.S. Agency for International Development (USAID) and U.S. State Department global health program funding grew by 350 percent between 2001 and 2008, and by 2006 health aid made up 23 percent of total U.S. allocable aid (IOM, 2009; OECD, 2008). This pattern of increased funding for global health by the United States can be expected to continue for the next 6 years as President Obama requested that Congress allocate $63 billion to global health between 2009 and 2014 for his new Global Health Initiative (U.S. Department of State, 2010). At the international level, the establishment of the Global Fund to Fight AIDS, Tuberculosis and Malaria; the Global Alliance for Vaccines and Immunizations; and the Millennium Development Goals were examples of important steps in bringing global health issues to the forefront. Finally, the establishment of major private funders such as the Bill & Melinda Gates Foundation and the William J. Clinton Foundation infused significant new capital into the fight against the causes of disease and suffering.

While these new investments and commitments to improving the health of the world's people were unprecedented and have undoubtedly saved millions of lives, the majority of these efforts have largely ignored CVD and other chronic noncommunicable diseases. This extends to the Millennium Development Goals, in which chronic diseases are not explicitly mentioned and are instead relegated to Millennium Development Goal 6, grouped into the catchall category of "other diseases."

International Realization of CVD Burden

Although not emphasized in most major global health efforts, the increasing burden of CVD in developing countries was first recognized on the international stage at least as long ago as the first international declaration on CVD in 1956, when India proposed a resolution on CVD and hypertension at the Ninth World Health Assembly (WHO, 1956). The growing burden of chronic diseases was further highlighted by the World Bank's 1984 report *China: Health Sector*, which noted the increasing burden of CVD among China's health challenges (World Bank, 1984). However, evidence of the growing chronic disease burden more broadly in low and middle income countries did not begin to gain significant notice until the early 1990s. At this time, advances in epidemiological methods and metrics as well as more accurate data allowed for novel analyses of worldwide disease burden (Jamison et al., 1993). These analyses shed light on the truly global impact of CVD and other chronic diseases and helped

INTRODUCTION 27

instigate a number of international reports, declarations, and resolutions calling attention to the growing threat of the global CVD epidemic. These efforts from the past two decades are described briefly here and summarized in Figure 1.1 and Box 1.1.

Documentation of the Disease Burden

One of the first such publications to highlight the global burden of CVD and chronic diseases was the 1993 World Development Report by the World Bank. This report focused on the critical role that investments in health play in international development, also emphasizing the rising burden of chronic diseases in low and middle income countries. The report also introduced the Global Burden of Disease study, which definitively established that chronic diseases are responsible for more deaths worldwide than any other cause (Murray and Lopez, 1996; WHO, 2003b).

As the realization of the true global burden of CVD began to grow among the international public health community, several major reports examined national capacities to implement CVD prevention and treatment programs. These reports, most notably the 1999 World Heart Federation White Book on the Impending Global Pandemic of Cardiovascular Diseases (Achutti et al., 1999) and the 2001 World Health Organization (WHO) Assessment of National Capacity for Noncommunicable Disease Prevention and Control (Alwan et al., 2001), found that the majority of countries did not have chronic disease control policies, programs, funding, or the will to take action. As a result, there was little prevention or control under way.

A series of reports from multilateral organizations further examined the growing burden of CVD and other chronic diseases in developing countries. These included the 2000, 2002, and 2005 World Health Reports and the Global Burden of Disease Reports from 1996, 2006, and 2008 (Lopez and Disease Control Priorities Project, 2006; Murray and Lopez, 1996; WHO, 2000, 2002, 2008b, 2008c). In addition, the 2004 Earth Institute/IC Health Report, which examined the social and macroeconomic impact of the growing CVD epidemic, concluded that the burden of cardiovascular mortality and disability was likely to drastically affect working-age adults in developing countries, leading to substantial reductions in productivity and ensuing economic losses (Leeder et al., 2004).

Taken together, these reports established that CVD is the number one cause of death worldwide, that about 80 percent of these deaths occur in low and middle income countries, that the disease burden will only increase in the coming decades, that it will likely have detrimental economic impacts on low and middle income countries, and that control efforts are not sufficient to address the disease burden. These data and projections forced the realization that the global health agenda must expand beyond infectious diseases and maternal and child health to include CVD and other chronic diseases. These reports also recognized that global CVD is a complex problem, influenced by interdependent factors that involve many sectors and stakeholders extending far beyond the realm of health and public health systems.

Calls for Action

As the new disease burden data were making the true worldwide toll of CVD increasingly clear, calls for action were issued from a number of sources. In 1998 the IOM released a report titled *Control of Cardiovascular Diseases in Developing Countries: Research, Development, and Institutional Strengthening*. It offered recommendations to better document the magnitude of cardiovascular disease burden, use case-control studies to develop prevention strategies, address risk factors such as hypertension and tobacco use, evaluate low-cost drug regimens, improve the affordability of care for CVD, build research and development capacity, and develop institutional mechanisms to facilitate CVD prevention and control (IOM, 1998).

In a series of declarations from the International Heart Health Conferences, the cardiovascular community called on multinational organizations, governments, civil society, and communities to take immediate action on CVD prevention and control. The first of these was the Victoria Declaration in 1992, which was subsequently followed by the Catalonia Declaration (released in 1995 with a follow-up in report in 1997), the Singapore Declaration in 1998, the second Victoria Declaration in 2000, the Osaka Declaration in 2001, and most recently the Milan Declaration in 2004 (Advisory Board of the Fifth International Heart Health Conference, 2004; Advisory Board of the First International Conference on Women, Heart Diseases, and Stroke, 2000; Advisory Board of the Fourth International Heart Health Conference, 2001; Advisory Board of the International Heart Health Conference, 1992; Advisory Board of the Second International Heart Health Conference, 1995; Grabowsky et al., 1997; Pearson et al., 1998).

In addition to the declarations of the International Heart Health Conferences, a number of other reports and resolutions highlighted the growing worldwide epidemic of CVD and related chronic diseases and issued additional calls to action for its prevention and control. These included the United Nations (UN) Resolution on Diabetes announced in 2007, the 2008 Sydney Resolution and Sydney Challenge from the Oxford Health Alliance Summit, and the 2009 Kampala Statement (Chronic Disease Summit, 2009; The Sydney Resolution, 2008; United Nations General Assembly, 2006). In

2009, the IOM report *The U.S. Commitment to Global Health* also recognized the need to apply resources to chronic diseases in the developing world as part of the global health agenda (IOM, 2009).

Taken together, these publications shone a brighter spotlight on the burden of CVD, placed increasing pressure on national governments and the international community, and offered recommendations to tackle the issue of CVD. However, despite these calls for action, implementation of CVD prevention and control programs in developing countries has been slow to materialize.

New Strategies, Policies, and Partnerships

To try to initiate implementation of these calls for action, the international community has begun to take steps to develop strategies and plans for action. While serving as director general of WHO, Gro Harlem Brundtland elevated the treatment and control of chronic diseases to the same level of urgency as infectious diseases. In 1999, Brundtland presented the WHO Executive Board with a draft Global Strategy for the Prevention and Control of Noncommunicable Diseases, which emphasized improving chronic disease surveillance, addressing common risk factors, and improving primary care services worldwide (Brundtland, 1999). This Global Strategy was later discussed at the Fifty-Third World Health Assembly, where the Assembly called on the Director General to continue prioritizing chronic diseases and urged Member States to redouble their noncommunicable disease surveillance, prevention, and control efforts (WHA, 2000).

In 2003, after 5 years of unprecedented negotiation, the Member States of WHO unanimously adopted the Framework Convention on Tobacco Control, the first and only legally binding treaty ever adopted by WHO. This treaty called for the implementation of tobacco reduction strategies and new regulatory policies, and a formal reporting mechanism on progress is being implemented (WHO, 2003a). This was followed by the 2004 WHO Global Strategy on Diet, Physical Activity, and Health as well as the 2007 Grand Challenges in Global Health report in *Nature* (Daar et al., 2007; WHO, 2004), which outlined research and policy priorities for chronic diseases. The 2008 release of the WHO 2008-2013 Action Plan for the Global Strategy for the Prevention and Control of Noncommunicable Diseases (WHO, 2008a) established a policy framework for action, with specific recommendations for WHO, Member States, and civil society. However, this action plan does not specify who will act on specific recommendations, what resources they need, and to whom governments would be accountable for inaction.

THE CHALLENGES OF TAKING ACTION

As part of its charge, the committee assessed why there has not been more concrete action to address global CVD despite the considerable progress in delineating strategies and policies. One of the challenges is the lack of awareness and understanding of the growing burden of CVD in the developing world. Indeed, the formerly pervasive perspective, expressed by the World Bank in 1999, was that CVD is a problem that afflicts only the affluent, that addressing CVD does not need to be on the health agenda for nonindustrialized nations, and that resources dedicated to CVD would potentially serve to increase the gap between the rich and poor (Gwatkin and Guillot, 1999). However, because of the intense efforts described above to more accurately document and draw attention to the economic and health burden of CVD, this misperception has been recognized and is beginning to be reversed. Indeed, the past declarations and recent global strategies provide a welcome sign that the international community is more aware of the importance of CVD and chronic diseases. This was demonstrated by the very different perspective articulated more recently by the World Bank (2007), which recognized the very real effects of chronic diseases on the poor and in developing countries and acknowledged chronic noncommunicable diseases as a development priority. As a result of the significant progress in raising awareness among major global health stakeholders, this report has the advantage of being released in a climate of greater receptivity to its messages than previous documents. Nevertheless, there remains a gap between the burden of disease and the level of awareness, and this report offers an additional tool to further equip those working in this field to continue their laudable efforts to increase attention to the problem.

In addition, even with an increasing recognition by the global health community of the health and economic burden of CVD in the developing world, there remain significant barriers to effective action. These barriers include the perception of CVD as a competitor to other health needs, causing it to remain a low priority and resulting in a lack of financial, individual, and institutional resources; insufficient capacity to meet CVD needs, including health workforce and infrastructure capacity as well as implementation and enforcement capacity for policies and regulatory approaches; insufficient knowledge of the effectiveness and feasibility of programs and policies in contexts similar to those in which they need to be implemented; a high degree of fragmentation of efforts by various players; and a lack of clear leadership and collaboration focused on defined goals and outcomes.

Although the prevailing attitudes about the importance of CVD are changing, both global health funders and national governments of low and middle income countries have yet to elevate action to address CVD as a priority. This is in part because of very important and legitimate high-priority development needs, as outlined in the Millennium Development Goals. Global health and development stakeholders and national governments in the developing world face very real and critical challenges that remain far from adequately addressed in the areas of poverty and hunger reduction, basic development priorities, and a range of health issues in areas such as infectious disease and maternal and child health.

This report is timely in its publication during a period of serious discussions among most stakeholders revisiting the priorities of the global health agenda. However, the realities of competing priorities persist. Therefore, the committee felt that the current climate of both transition and greater receptivity to chronic disease needs can best be converted into action by identifying opportunities to invest in the components of solutions for global CVD that are best aligned with the existing primary missions and developing strategic approaches of global health stakeholders. With this in mind, the report advances the issue of the global epidemic of cardiovascular disease by focusing less on an independent call for action to address CVD, but rather on identifying entry points for CVD to be a part of the current and future global health agenda as it continues to evolve.

Thus, rather than competing against existing priorities, leaders in the CVD community need to better communicate the importance of integrating attention to CVD within these priorities to policy and decision makers. Better alignment among these priorities has the potential to synergistically improve economic and health status. Furthermore, this can help ensure that current and future health and development efforts do not inadvertently worsen the growing epidemic of chronic diseases. Without a new approach that includes chronic diseases, the health dividend gained from progress in other areas of global health could be squandered as one set of problems is tackled while a new set is allowed to grow.

Recognizing the importance of including CVD in the development and global health agendas of international stakeholders and national governments in low and middle income countries is a crucial factor in increasing the allocation of resources that can be applied to chronic noncommunicable diseases. However, more resources alone will not solve the problem of the growing epidemic of CVD. There is a need for progress and increased capacity at the policy, institutional, and research levels so that CVD prevention and control can be implemented in developing countries.

There is also a gap in knowledge about how to transfer the considerable body of knowledge on etiology and modifiable risk factors into feasible large-scale efforts within the context-specific needs of developing countries. The epidemiological evidence is strong, but evidence for specific interventions implemented in low and middle income countries showing the benefits of improving CVD outcomes, or even in changing risk factors, is largely unavailable. This gap within the field of global CVD presents an additional barrier to action and is a critical area to tackle in order to have the capacity to act as the previously described barriers of political will and lack of resources are overcome.

Therefore, to fill this knowledge gap and thus to effectively prevent and control CVD in the developing world, there is a need for an increased focus on policy research, health systems research, and implementation research to provide the necessary knowledge to solve the challenges associated with intervention programs, workforce capacity, and other needs. This research will further help ensure that health and public health systems can deliver interventions at clinical, community, and population levels. It is imperative that the results of research be transformed into effective disease control programs, and that best practices from communities that have had a head start on tackling the CVD epidemic be more effectively evaluated and adapted for implementation. Lessons learned in controlling infectious diseases also need to be applied for the purpose of bringing down rates of CVD. The current emphasis in the global health community on developing health systems capacity also provides a window of opportunity to improve capacity for delivery of preventive and therapeutic care for chronic diseases. In addition, policies in nonhealth sectors of government and the private sector need to be developed synergistically to reduce, or at least not adversely affect, risk for CVD.

Finally, the stakeholders and global partnerships that are emerging to tackle CVD need to be more effectively marshaled and coordinated to support the implementation of actions to address the problem. Many players share the responsibility to address CVD. They include international, regional, national, and local players. While different stakeholders will have different relative strengths and different appropriate contributions to a worldwide effort to address the rising disease burden, each player that commits to taking action has in common the need to plan strategically as current efforts are continued and expanded or new ones are adopted. The process of translating goals into action is a complex, difficult, and long-term effort that succeeds when groups work together as part of their strategic planning and implementation of efforts. It would not be practical, efficient, or effective for a single mechanism of coordination to govern all actions to reduce the global burden of disease. However, sustainable progress on CVD and related chronic diseases can be enhanced if there is greater communication among stakeholders to avoid unnecessary duplication of efforts and if players with complementary functions and goals define shared messages and coordinate better to take decisive action together. Many emerging mechanisms for coordination at global, regional, and national levels can be strengthened to serve this purpose, while new alliances and partnerships can also be sought. Such partnerships have proven highly effective at mobilizing commitments toward the prevention and treatment of infectious diseases such as AIDS, tuberculosis, malaria, measles, and polio, especially when built on the principles of establishing trust, agreeing on priorities and outcomes, and implementing transparent reporting and monitoring.

A FRAMEWORK FOR ACTION

The ultimate goal in meeting the challenges of CVD in the developing world is to first create environments that promote health and help prevent the acquisition and augmentation of risk. Second is to build systems and implement programs to effectively detect and reduce risk and to manage CVD. The committee has identified several "essential functions" that are required to meet these goals. These include advocacy and leadership at global and national levels, developing policy, program implementation, capacity building, research focusing on evaluating approaches in developing countries that are context specific and culturally relevant, ongoing monitoring and evaluation, and funding. Successfully carrying out these functions will require resources—financial, technical, and human—and the combined efforts of many players over long periods of time.

Thus, in response to its charge to offer conclusions and recommendations pertinent to the control of the evolving epidemic of CVD in developing countries, in this report the committee articulates a framework for action to reduce the economic and health burden of CVD and related chronic diseases. As outlined in Figure 1.2, the chapters that follow present the committee's analysis in support of this framework.

Chapters 2 and 3 describe the determinants of global CVD and its increasing impact, along with related chronic diseases, on the health, welfare, and economies of low and middle income countries, thus providing a clear mandate for action. Chapter 4 describes measurement and evaluation as a fundamental element for the framework and as a means to develop, implement, and sustain effective approaches to reduce the burden of disease. Chapter 5 discusses intervention approaches to reduce the burden of disease, and Chapter 6 more specifically relates the importance of targeting mothers, children, youth, and young adults for prevention interventions in order to achieve long-term success in promoting cardiovascular health and reducing the burden of CVD. Chapter 7 describes the economic analyses that help inform policy decisions about prioritization of investments. Finally, Chapter 8 brings together all the preceding components to describe the essential functions that are needed to address global CVD and how the major stakeholders in CVD, in related chronic diseases, and in global health and development can be organized at global, national, and local levels to create a framework for implementing the necessary actions to control the global epidemic of CVD.

Drivers
- ② Epidemiology
- ③ Development

Approaches
- ⑤ Intervention Approaches
  - ⑥ Health Promotion Early in Life

⑦ Prioritization

Response
- ⑧ Framework for Action

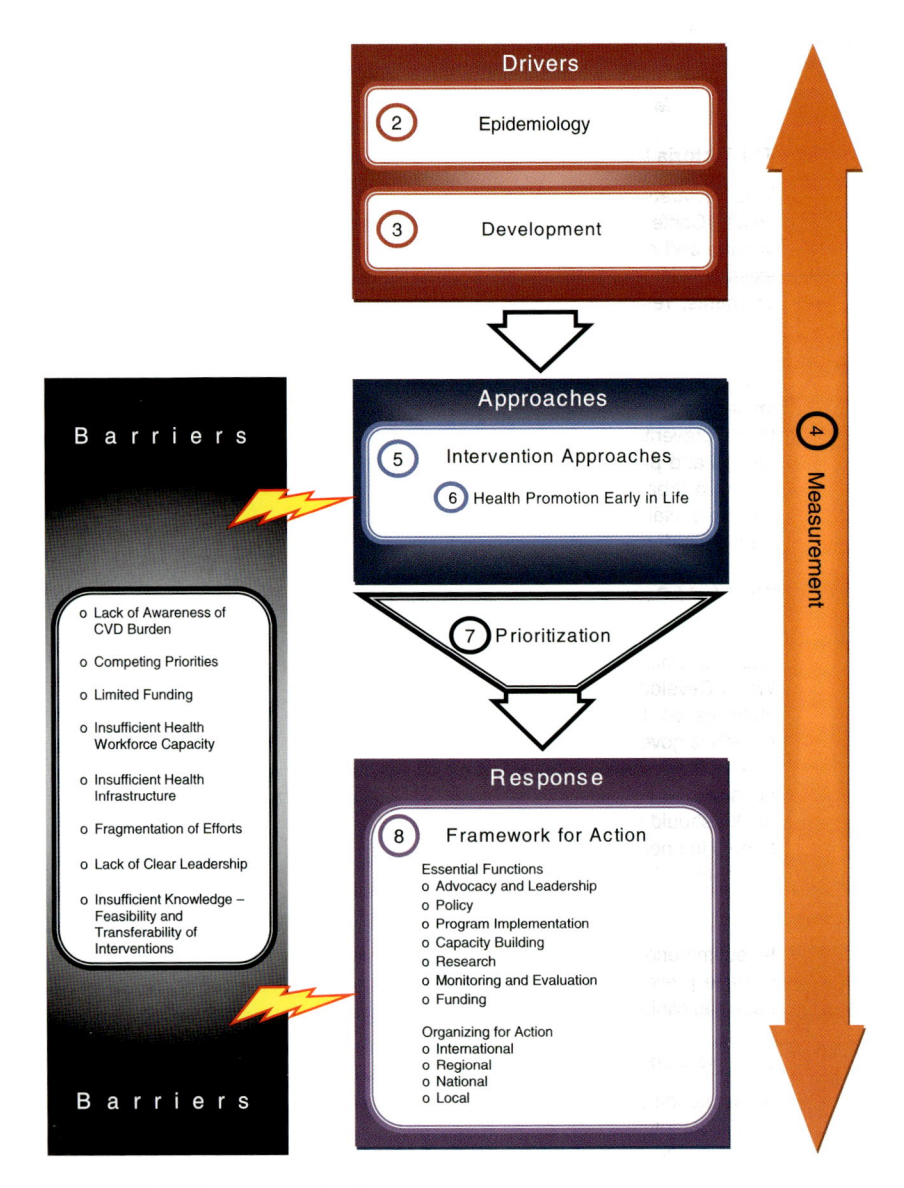

Essential Functions
- Advocacy and Leadership
- Policy
- Program Implementation
- Capacity Building
- Research
- Monitoring and Evaluation
- Funding

Organizing for Action
- International
- Regional
- National
- Local

Barriers
- Lack of Awareness of CVD Burden
- Competing Priorities
- Limited Funding
- Insufficient Health Workforce Capacity
- Insufficient Health Infrastructure
- Fragmentation of Efforts
- Lack of Clear Leadership
- Insufficient Knowledge – Feasibility and Transferability of Interventions

④ Measurement

FIGURE 1.2 Report organization.

BOX 1.1
Major Prior Global CVD Documents

1992 The Victoria Declaration on Heart Health

This declaration, which was issued following the First International Heart Health Conference, was intended to give a sense of urgency to the prevention and control of CVD. It focused on exploring methods of applying existing knowledge about CVD prevention on a global scale, urging governments, research institutions, scientists, the media, and civil society to join forces in eliminating the CVD epidemic by adopting new policies, making regulatory changes, and implementing new population-level health promotion and CVD prevention programs. It further specified that the policy implementation should consist of the adoption of a public health approach to the prevention and control of CVD that was inclusive of all population groups and promoted "four cornerstones" of heart health (healthy dietary habits, a tobacco-free lifestyle, regular physical activity and a supportive psycho-social environment) (Advisory Board of the International Heart Health Conference, 1992).

1993 The World Bank *World Development Report: Investing in Health*

This report examined the interplay among human health, health policy, and economic development. Like its predecessors, this report included the World Development Indicators, which offer selected social and economic statistics on 127 countries. This report advocated a three-pronged approach to government policies for improving health in developing countries. First, governments need to foster an economic environment that enables households to improve their own health. Second, government spending on health should be redirected to more cost-effective programs that do more to help the poor. Third, governments need to promote greater diversity and competition in the financing and delivery of health services. The report also highlighted the need to promote tobacco control and acknowledged the rising burden of chronic diseases in low and middle income countries. It recommended that basic public health interventions including chronic disease prevention could be a part of low and middle income countries' essential clinical package (World Bank, 1993).

1993 *Disease Control Priorities in Developing Countries* (DCP)

A companion document to the 1993 *World Development Report*, this book used a variety of measures to evaluate the effectiveness of interventions, including an important new metric for measuring disease outcomes: the disability-adjusted life year (DALY). The use of DALYs in both this document and the subsequent *Global Burden of Disease* report dramatically altered the way researchers measured disease burden because it quantified the toll of disabilities associated with diseases. This helped researchers fully realize the tremendous burden of chronic diseases, which cause years of disability and impair an individual's ability to lead a healthy life. The report also provided quantitative evidence on demographic transition and the resulting growth in CVD in developing countries. It also generated initial estimates of

continued

**BOX 1.1
Continued**

the cost-effectiveness of primary prevention, of secondary prevention (using low-cost drugs) and of treatment of angina, diabetes and acute myocardial infarction (Jamison et al., 1993; Murray and Lopez, 1996).

1995 The Catalonia Declaration: Investing in Heart Health (40 case studies)

Issued after the Second International Heart Health Conference, this declaration sought to support efforts of the Victoria Declaration by examining the economic realities of implementing CVD prevention on a global scale. It provided concrete examples of policies and programs for CVD prevention that succeeded in saving both lives and money in an effort to prove that investing in heart health now will save money in the long term. It also presented 12 recommendations for promoting heart health, described resources for and barriers to implementing CVD prevention programs, and highlighted 41 successful projects that have been implemented in a range of countries (Advisory Board of the Second International Heart Health Conference, 1995).

1997 Worldwide Efforts to Improve Heart Health: A Follow-up to the Catalonia Declaration—Selected Program Descriptions

This companion document further explored case studies presented in the Catalonia Declaration and discussed additional programs designed to promote heart health. It gathered diverse information related to CVD prevention and described 83 projects in 6 continents and more than 30 countries (Grabowsky et al., 1997).

1998 The Singapore Declaration: Forging the Will for Heart Health in the Next Millennium

This declaration, built on the Victoria and Catalonia declarations, focused on the need to build capacity to create heart health. It provided guidance on how to develop an infrastructure for heart health at the international, national, and local levels, focusing on identifying leadership, policy, economic, scientific, technical, and physical considerations and creating individual, organizational, and political will for implementation (Pearson et al., 1998).

1998 The IOM Report: *Control of Cardiovascular Diseases in Developing Countries*

This report established priorities for research and development (R&D) investment to control CVD in developing countries and offered recommendations for R&D investment in several broad areas for the control of CVD. These areas included determining the magnitude of CVD burden in low and middle income countries; developing targeted and effective prevention strategies using case-control studies; reducing tobacco use; detecting and treating hypertension; starting pilot studies to evaluate essential vascular packages of effective and low-cost drugs; developing algorithms for affordable clinical CVD care; building R&D capacity; and developing institutional mechanisms that facilitate CVD prevention and control (IOM, 1998).

1999 World Heart Federation *White Book*

This book was designed to define the problems posed by the present and projected burden of CVD, to document the resources available to combat CVD, and to develop appropriate strategies for international action. It provided a framework of action for the World Heart Federation to galvanize the efforts of relevant stakeholders at the global level. The book urged a global approach to CVD, emphasizing coordination among global, regional, and local programs. It also emphasized that prevention programs must be designed to address risk factors across the entire lifespan, starting in childhood (Achutti et al., 1999).

1999 *Global Strategy for the Prevention and Control of Noncommunicable Diseases: Report by the Director-General*

This report by WHO Director-General Gro Harlem Brundtland called attention to the growing burden of noncommunicable diseases in low and middle income countries and cited the increasingly strong epidemiological evidence linking these diseases to common risk factors. It briefly reviewed lessons learned in chronic disease prevention and control and, based on these lessons, called for improved surveillance of emerging noncommunicable disease epidemics and their determinants, a redoubling of efforts to reduce the exposure to major determinants of CVD, and continued emphasis on primary care capacity strengthening (Brundtland, 1999). The report became the basis for future WHO strategies for chronic disease control such as the Global Strategy on Diet, Physical Activity, and Health and the 2008 Action Plan for the Global Strategy for the Prevention and Control of Noncommunicable Diseases (WHO, 2004, 2008a).

2000 The 2000 Victoria Declaration

This declaration highlighted the high burden of CVD among women worldwide, calling upon governments, research institutions, NGOs, multinational organizations, and civil society to invest resources and develop targeted CVD prevention and treatment programs for women. While describing "the policies, community action programs and services required to support heart disease and stroke prevention and management, [the declaration emphasized] using the values of health as a human right, equity, solidarity, participation and accountability." The declaration also emphasized the importance of the psychosocial and socioeconomic determinants of women's heart disease and stroke (Advisory Board of the First International Conference on Women, Heart Diseases, and Stroke, 2000, p. 3).

2000 *2000 World Health Report*

The *2000 World Health Report* focused on strengthening health systems. It emphasized that health systems (and their supporting governments) have four vital functions: service provision, resource generation, financing and, most important, stewardship. The report stressed that it is the responsibility of national governments to ensure that health systems are providing both fair and good health care to the entire population—standards that require governments to devise essential care packages that ensure high-quality care for all. The report is significant for CVD because it is evidence of the shifting priorities of the international health

continued

**BOX 1.1
Continued**

community from vertical, disease-specific initiatives to a more horizontal, health systems strengthening emphasis. Furthermore, the report estimated that noncommunicable diseases together contributed to almost 60 percent of global mortality (33.5 million deaths) and 43 percent of the global burden of disease in 1999 (WHO, 2000).

2001 The Osaka Declaration: Health, Economics and Political Action: Stemming the Global Tide of Cardiovascular Disease

This declaration furthered the process started by previous heart health declarations by reviewing the factors outside of the health sector, specifically social, economic, and political factors, that have contributed to the lack of progress in CVD prevention and promotion globally. It also argued for the crucial advocacy role for health professionals and their organizations to influence health system governance and address systemic barriers to achieving health. The declaration also examined global forces beyond the health system that affect the awareness, understanding, and commitment to take global action on CVD prevention (Advisory Board of the Fourth International Heart Health Conference, 2001).

2001 WHO *Assessment of National Capacity for Noncommunicable Disease Prevention and Control*

This report described the national capacity for noncommunicable disease prevention and control in WHO Member States based on a survey conducted in 2001. The survey found that fewer than half the WHO Member States had chronic disease policies and that only about two-thirds of the countries had tobacco or food and nutrition legislation. Furthermore, fewer than two-thirds of the countries had a chronic disease unit in their ministries of health, and fewer than 40 percent had a specific chronic disease budget line. The report highlights the traditional lack of attention that chronic diseases receive in many countries around the world despite their increasing prevalence and responsibility for morbidity and mortality. The report identifies a number of areas in which WHO could provide technical support and emphasized the need for countries and the international community to strengthen their capacity to prevent and treat chronic diseases (Alwan et al., 2001).

2002 *2002 World Health Report*

The *2002 World Health Report* focused on reducing risks and promoting healthy lives. The report highlighted the world's 10 leading risk factors that account for more than one-third of deaths worldwide. It went on to suggest effective and efficient strategies governments and the international community can employ to reduce the prevalence of these risk factors, thus saving millions of lives. Five of the risk factors highlighted in the report—hypertension, tobacco consumption, alcohol consumption, high cholesterol, and obesity—are key cardiovascular risk factors. The report emphasizes the increasing global burden of CVD, especially its rise in low and middle income countries, citing the dual epidemics of infectious and noncommunicable diseases that many developing countries are now facing. The report's focus on risk-factor reduction and its prominent use of key

CVD risk factors provides further validation of the gravity of the worldwide CVD epidemic and signals the growing recognition from the global health community of the importance of addressing CVD in developing countries (WHO, 2002).

2003 Framework Convention on Tobacco Control

This treaty, adopted by the World Health Assembly on May 21, 2003, was the first negotiated under the auspices of the World Health Organization and has since become one of the most rapidly adopted international treaties in history, having been ratified by nearly 170 countries. The treaty was developed in response to the global tobacco epidemic and represents a shift in the way the world addresses regulation of addictive substances by stressing the importance of reducing demand for tobacco. The treaty encourages countries to strengthen their tobacco control policies by enacting price, tax, regulatory, and social measures to reduce demand. The treaty represents a major milestone in the global fight to reduce chronic disease risk factors and has prompted previously unseen international collaboration around tobacco control (WHO, 2003a, 2010).

2003 *Seventh Report of the Joint National Committee on Prevention, Detection, Evaluation, and Treatment of High Blood Pressure*

The JNC7 report summarized the available scientific evidence on hypertension and offers guidance to primary care clinicians. The report specified hypertensive risk thresholds for adults and offered guidelines for appropriate treatment with antihypertensive medication. The report cited the significant success in awareness and reduction of hypertension in the United States, with awareness increasing from 51 to 70 percent by 1999-2000. It also reported that since 1972, age-adjusted death rates from stroke and coronary heart disease (CHD) had declined by approximately 60 and 50 percent, respectively. This provides evidence that CVD mortality can be significantly reduced with comprehensive treatment and prevention programs (Joint National Committee on Prevention, Detection, Evaluation, and Treatment of High Blood Pressure, 2003).

2004 *Towards a WHO Long-Term Strategy for Prevention and Control of Leading Chronic Diseases*

This report recommended seven strategic initiatives for action by WHO. It described the health and economic impacts of chronic diseases and the long-term drivers underlying their spread, and it analyzed the deeply entrenched policy responses to the epidemic of chronic diseases. The resulting strategy builds on the existing efforts of the WHO noncommunicable disease cluster and takes a long-term, strategic global view (Yach and Hawkes, 2004).

2004 *WHO Global Strategy on Diet, Physical Activity and Health*

The goal of this report was to guide the development of environments that enable sustainable actions at individual, community, national, and global levels that, when taken together, will lead to reduced rates of disease and death that are related to unhealthy diet and physical inactivity. These actions would have potential for public health gains worldwide and would support the UN Millen-

continued

BOX 1.1
Continued

nium Development Goals. The Global Strategy sought to help reduce chronic disease risk factors stemming from poor diet and lack of physical activity through essential health action; increase overall awareness of the influences of diet and physical activity on health; encourage the development, strengthening, and implementation of policies and action plans to improve diets and increase physical activity; and monitor scientific data and support research on diet and physical activity (WHO, 2004).

2004 The Milan Declaration: Positioning Technology to Serve Global Heart Health

This declaration followed up on the previous International Heart Health Declarations by calling for the international community to mobilize new and existing technologies to improve heart health. The declaration examined a range of technologies—including health promotion and disease prevention, information and communication technology, food technology, medical technology, and biotechnology—and their potential to reduce the burden of CVD. A key consideration identified for all governments was balancing highly technical and expensive technologies that benefit a small number of individuals and population-level strategies that enhance the health status of the entire population. The declaration stressed that a comprehensive range of treatment and prevention strategies is essential to control the global CVD epidemic and that treatment technology options need to be effective but also sustainable and affordable (Advisory Board of the Fifth International Heart Health Conference, 2004).

2004 *Earth Institute/IC Health Report*

This report examined the social and economic impact of CVD, now and for the next 40 years, in one low income and four middle income countries. It also reviewed existing data on the costs and benefits of strategies for the prevention of CVD. The report offered six conclusions emphasizing the need to put CVD in low and middle income countries on the international health and development agendas, more accurately document the prevalence and costs of CVD worldwide, develop partnerships at the macroeconomic level with national governments in key developing countries, establish health worker training programs about CVD, undertake trial treatment and prevention interventions, and establish a long-term research base for CVD interventions (Leeder et al., 2004).

2005 *WHO Preventing Chronic Disease: A Vital Investment*

This report made the case for urgent action to halt and reverse the course of the growing chronic disease epidemic worldwide. It sought to dispel the misperception that chronic diseases are diseases of the affluent and do not affect those in low and middle income countries. It estimated 80 percent of chronic disease-related deaths in 2005 to be in low and middle income countries and in younger people than in high income countries. The report stressed that the growing threat of chronic diseases can be overcome using existing knowledge and highly cost-effective interventions and provided suggestions for how countries can implement interventions to reduce and prevent chronic diseases (WHO, 2005a).

2005 ***2005 World Health Report***

This World Health Report highlighted maternal and child health issues. One of the major foci of the report was achieving universal access to health services, which the report stressed could be achieved through health systems strengthening. The report emphasized that this strengthening needed to occur at the infrastructure, workforce, and health systems funding levels. The report also tied maternal and child health efforts to chronic diseases by recognizing that the antecedents of many of these diseases occur in early life, and, as such, improving health early in life is an important component of preventing the early onset of chronic diseases (WHO, 2005b).

2005 ***Lancet* Series on Chronic Diseases**

The first of two *Lancet* series on chronic diseases, this set of articles called attention to the major gap in the global health discourse regarding chronic diseases. The series noted that chronic diseases were not listed in the Millennium Development Goals and warned that if they continue to be ignored by the global health community, the progress gained from reducing the burden of infectious diseases would be eclipsed by a rising burden of chronic diseases in developing countries (Epping-Jordan et al., 2005; Fuster and Voûte, 2005; Horton, 2005; Reddy et al., 2005; Strong et al., 2005; Wang et al., 2005).

2006 ***Disease Control Priorities in Developing Countries* 2nd Edition (DCP2)**

This follow-up to the original *Disease Control Priorities in Developing Countries* brought together 350 specialists from diverse fields and proposed context-sensitive policy recommendations to significantly reduce the burden of disease in developing countries. The book included a chapter that specifically discussed CVD and further called into focus the sizable burden of the disease in developing countries. It estimated the economic burden of CVD in low and middle income countries and updated and expanded the cost-effectiveness estimates for prevention and treatment interventions from the 1993 report (Jamison et al., 2006; World Bank, 2006).

2007 ***Lancet* Series on Chronic Diseases**

The second *Lancet* series on chronic diseases noted the increasing recognition of the importance of chronic diseases within the global health community. It also provided a deeper, more nuanced examination of the burden of chronic diseases and predicted the reductions in burden at the population and individual level that could be achieved through prevention and treatment interventions (Abegunde et al., 2007; Asaria et al., 2007; Beaglehole et al., 2007; Gaziano et al., 2007; Horton, 2007; Lim et al., 2007).

2007 UN Resolution on Diabetes

In January 2007, the United Nations established November 14 World Diabetes Day, as an official United Nations Day. The resolution recognized diabetes as a widespread and serious chronic disease that threatens international development and the achievement of the Millennium Development Goals. It also recognized that diabetes prevention and control should be included in health-system

continued

BOX 1.1
Continued

strengthening efforts. The resolution is important because it was an additional sign that the international health community was increasingly recognizing the threat posed by noncommunicable diseases and the necessity to invest in their prevention and control (United Nations General Assembly, 2006).

2007 Grand Challenges in Chronic Non-communicable Diseases

This article identified the top 20 policy and research priorities for chronic noncommunicable diseases. These grand challenges are intended to guide policy and research in an evidence-based manner and make the case for worldwide debate, support, and funding. The authors asserted that with concerted action following the blueprint outlined in the article, 36 million premature deaths from chronic noncommunicable diseases can be averted by 2015 (Daar et al., 2007).

2008 *Closing the Gap in a Generation: Health Equity Through Action on the Social Determinants of Health. Final Report of the WHO Commission on Social Determinants of Health*

This report of the Commission on Social Determinants of Health examined how health-damaging experiences are unequally distributed within and across societies as a result of unfair economic arrangements, poor social policies, and discriminatory politics. The report calls on the international community to close the health gap in a generation, setting out key areas—daily living conditions, social and cultural inequalities, and the need for governments committed to equity—in which action is needed. It provided analysis of these social determinants of health and concrete examples of types of action that have proven effective in improving health and health equity in countries at all levels of socioeconomic development (CSDH, 2008).

2008 Oxford Health Alliance Sydney Resolution and Sydney Challenge (The Sydney Resolution)

The Sydney Resolution and Challenge were the outcomes of the 2008 Oxford Health Alliance Summit and served as a call to action for the international community to make healthier choices to turn back the rising tide of preventable chronic diseases. The resolution explained that 50 percent of the world's deaths are caused by four preventable chronic diseases: CVD, diabetes, chronic lung disease, and cancer. The resolution stressed that these four diseases place immense costs on society, threaten economic stability, and push individuals further into poverty. The resolution challenged the international community to take urgent action and prioritize health-promoting decisions in urban planning, food manufacturing and policy, business decisions, and public policy (The Sydney Resolution, 2008).

2008 *Global Burden of Disease* 2004 Update

This update to the *Global Burden of Disease* report, based on 2004 data, revised previous estimates of the burden of ischemic heart disease (IHD) and diabetes based on more accurate data, resulting in a significantly increased estimate of the global burden of these chronic diseases. These revisions increased the estimated disability-adjusted life years for IHD by 7 percent. The report also used new data to recalibrate the long-term case fatality rates for cerebrovascular disease, decreasing the prevalence of stroke survivors and, as a result, decreasing the estimate of global years lost to disability due to cerebrovascular disease by 30 percent. The report stressed that of every 10 deaths globally 6 are caused by noncommunicable diseases and that CVD was the leading cause of death worldwide. CVD was responsible for 32 percent of global deaths in women and 27 percent of the deaths in men in 2004. The report also affirmed that IHD and cerebrovascular disease were the number one and two causes of death in high and middle income countries, and that IHD was the number two cause of death in low income countries. Furthermore, the update projected that CVD burden would continue to increase in low and middle income countries (WHO, 2008b).

2008 WHO 2008-2013 Action Plan for the Global Strategy for the Prevention and Control of Noncommunicable Diseases

This action plan, directed at the international development community as well as government and civil society, makes the case for urgent action to enact chronic disease prevention and control programs. The document provides a policy framework for action, outlining a series of objectives and action items for key stakeholder groups at varying levels of the global health system. It further urges WHO Member States to develop national policy frameworks, establish prevention and control programs, and share their experiences and build capacity internationally to address chronic diseases. Recognizing that 80 percent of the chronic disease burden is in developing countries and that the disease burden is projected to increase over the next 10 years, the plan places particular focus on low and middle income countries. The action plan was endorsed by all 193 Member States during the World Health Assembly in May 2008 (WHO, 2008a).

2009 The IOM Report: *The U.S. Commitment to Global Health*

This report examined the U.S. commitment to global health and articulated a vision for future U.S. investments and activities in this area. Coinciding with the U.S. presidential transition, the report outlined how the U.S. global health enterprise, which includes both government agencies and nongovernmental organizations, can improve global health under the leadership of a new administration. The report identified five key areas for action by the U.S. global health enterprise: scaling up existing interventions; generating and sharing knowledge to address health problems endemic to the global poor; investing in people, institutions, and capacity building with global partners; increasing the U.S. financial commitments to global health; and setting an example of engaging in partnerships. The report also included an emphasis on the rising tide of noncommunicable diseases in low and middle income countries, specifically recommending that the United States increase attention to chronic diseases and adopt a leadership role in reducing deaths from chronic diseases and tobacco-related illnesses (IOM, 2009).

continued

> **BOX 1.1**
> **Continued**
>
> **2009 Kampala Statement**
>
> This statement was a product of a summit, Preparing Communities: Chronic Diseases in the Developing Regions of Africa and Asia hosted by the Aga Khan Development Network, in Kampala, Uganda. In the Statement the Assembly of Kampala agreed: "1) to implement the WHO Action Plan . . . and create the basis for a multisectoral chronic disease alliance in Asia-Africa, and to accelerate progress by sharing resources, expertise, and experiences to promote an integrated and evidence-based approach to reducing the health and economic burdens of chronic diseases; 2) that governments and multisectoral partners at all levels will provide the leadership vital to further refine and advance the directions developed during this summit; and 3) to build upon and expand the momentum generated at this summit and monitor and report back on progress in 2011 in New Delhi, India" (Chronic Diseases Summit, 2009).

REFERENCES

Abegunde, D. O., C. D. Mathers, T. Adam, M. Ortegon, and K. Strong. 2007. The burden and costs of chronic diseases in low-income and middle-income countries. *Lancet* 370(9603):1929-1938.

Achutti, A., I. Balaguer-Vintro, A. B. d. Luna, J. Chalmers, A. Chockalingam, E. Farinaro, R. Lauzon, I. Martin, J. G. Papp, A. Postiglione, and K. S. Reddy. 1999. *The world heart federation's white book: Impending global pandemic of cardiovascular diseases: Challenges and opportunities for the prevention and control of cardiovascular diseases in developing countries and economies in transition.* Edited by A. Chockalingam and I. Balaguer-Vintro. Spain: Prous Science.

Advisory Board of the Fifth International Heart Health Conference. 2004. *The Milan Declaration: Positioning technology to serve global heart health.* http://www.internationalhearthealth.org/Publications/milan_declaration.pdf (accessed February 5, 2009).

Advisory Board of the First International Conference on Women, Heart Diseases, and Stroke. 2000. *The 2000 Victoria Declaration—women, heart disease and stroke: Science and policy in action.* http://www.internationalhearthealth.org/Publications/victoria_eng_2000.pdf (accessed February 5, 2009).

Advisory Board of the Fourth International Heart Health Conference. 2001. *The Osaka Declaration: Health, economics and political action: Stemming the global tide of cardiovascular disease.* http://www.internationalhearthealth.org/Publications/Osaka2001.pdf (accessed February 5, 2009).

Advisory Board of the International Heart Health Conference. 1992. *The Victoria Declaration on Heart Health.* http://www.internationalhearthealth.org/Publications/victoria_eng_1992.pdf (accessed February 5, 2009).

Advisory Board of the Second International Heart Health Conference. 1995. *The Catalonia Declaration: Investing in heart health.* http://www.internationalhearthealth.org/Publications/catalonia1995.pdf (accessed February 5, 2009).

Alwan, A. D., David Maclean, and Ahmed Mandil. 2001. *Assessment of national capacity for noncommunicable disease prevention and control: The report of a global survey.* Geneva: World Health Organization.

Asaria, P., D. Chisholm, C. Mathers, M. Ezzati, and R. Beaglehole. 2007. Chronic disease prevention: Health effects and financial costs of strategies to reduce salt intake and control tobacco use. *Lancet* 370(9604):2044-2053.

Beaglehole, R., S. Ebrahim, S. Reddy, J. Voute, and S. Leeder. 2007. Prevention of chronic diseases: A call to action. *Lancet* 370(9605):2152-2157.

Brundtland, G. H. 1999. *Global strategy for the prevention and control of noncommunicable diseases: Report by the director-general.* Geneva: World Health Organization.

Chronic Diseases Summit. 2009. Kampala statement: Preparing communities: Chronic diseases in Africa and Asia. Kampala, Uganda.

CSDH (WHO Commission on Social Determinants of Health). 2008. *Closing the gap in a generation: Health equity through action on the social determinants of health.* Final report of the Commission on Social Determinants of Health. Geneva: World Health Organization.

Daar, A. S., P. A. Singer, D. L. Persad, S. K. Pramming, D. R. Matthews, R. Beaglehole, A. Bernstein, L. K. Borysiewicz, S. Colagiuri, N. Ganguly, R. I. Glass, D. T. Finegood, J. Koplan, E. G. Nabel, G. Sarna, N. Sarrafzadegan, R. Smith, D. Yach, and J. Bell. 2007. Grand challenges in chronic non-communicable diseases. *Nature* 450(7169):494-496.

Epping-Jordan, J. E., G. Galea, C. Tukuitonga, and R. Beaglehole. 2005. Preventing chronic diseases: Taking stepwise action. *Lancet* 366(9497):1667-1671.

Fuster, V., and J. Voûte. 2005. MDGs: Chronic diseases are not on the agenda. *Lancet* 366(9496):1512-1514.

Gaziano, T. A., G. Galea, and K. S. Reddy. 2007. Scaling up interventions for chronic disease prevention: The evidence. *Lancet* 370(9603):1939-1946.

Grabowsky, T. A., J. W. Farquhar, K. R. Sunnarborg, V. S. Bales, and Stanford University School of Medicine. 1997. *Worldwide efforts to improve heart health: A follow-up to the Catalonia Declaration—selected program descriptions.* http://www.international hearthealth.org/Publications/catalonia.pdf (accessed February 5, 2009).

Gwatkin, D. R., and M. Guillot. 1999. *The burden of disease among the global poor: Current situation, future trends, and implications for strategy.* Washington, DC: World Bank.

Horton, R. 2005. The neglected epidemic of chronic disease. *Lancet* 366(9496):1514.

Horton, R. 2007. Chronic diseases: The case for urgent global action. *Lancet* 370(9603): 1881-1882.

IOM (Institute of Medicine). 1997. *America's vital interest in global health: Protecting our people, enhancing our economy, and advancing our international interests.* Washington, DC: National Academy Press.

IOM. 1998. *Control of cardiovascular diseases in developing countries.* Washington, DC: National Academy Press.

IOM. 2009. *The U.S. commitment to global health: Recommendations for the new administration.* Washington, DC: The National Academies Press.

Jamison, D. T., H. W. Mosley, A. R. Measham, and J. L. Bobadilla, eds. 1993. *Disease control priorities in developing countries.* 1st ed. New York: Oxford University Press.

Jamison, D. T., J. G. Breman, A. R. Measham, G. Alleyne, M. Claeson, D. B. Evans, P. Jha, A. Mills, and P. Musgrove, eds. 2006. *Disease control priorities in developing countries.* 2nd ed. New York: Oxford University Press.

Joint National Committee on Prevention, Detection, Evaluation, and Treatment of High Blood Pressure. 2003. *The seventh report of the joint national committee on prevention, detection, evaluation, and treatment of high blood pressure.* Bethesda, MD: National Heart, Lung, and Blood Institute, NIH, HHS.

Leeder, S., S. Raymond, and H. Greenberg. 2004. *A race against time: The challenge of cardiovascular disease in developing economies.* Edited by The Earth Institute. New York: Trustees of Columbia University.

Lim, S. S., T. A. Gaziano, E. Gakidou, K. S. Reddy, F. Farzadfar, R. Lozano, and A. Rodgers. 2007. Prevention of cardiovascular disease in high-risk individuals in low-income and middle-income countries: Health effects and costs. *Lancet* 370(9604):2054-2062.

Lopez, A. D., and Disease Control Priorities Project. 2006. Global burden of disease and risk factors. Oxford University Press; Washington, DC: World Bank.

Muna, W. F. T. 1993. Cardiovascular disorders in Africa. *World Health Statistics Quarterly* 46(2):125-133.

Murray, C. J. L., and A. D. Lopez, ed. 1996. *The global burden of disease*. Cambridge, MA: Harvard University Press.

Murray, C. J. L., A. D. Lopez, World Health Organization, World Bank, and Harvard School of Public Health. 1996. *The global burden of disease: A comprehensive assessment of mortality and disability from diseases, injuries, and risk factors in 1990 and projected to 2020, Summary.* Geneva: World Health Organization.

Nabel, E. G. 2009. Sponsor perspective on institute of medicine committee on preventing the global epidemic of cardiovascular disease. Presentation at the Public Information Gathering Session for the Institute of Medicine Committee on Preventing the Global Epidemic of Cardiovascular Disease, Washington, DC.

OECD (Organisation for Economic Co-operation and Development). 2008. *Measuring aid to health*. Paris, France: OECD.

Pearson, T. A., V. S. Bales, L. Blair, S. C. Emmanuel, J. W. Farquhar, L. P. Low, L. J. MacGregor, D. R. MacLean, B. O'Connor, H. Pardell, and A. Petrasovits. 1998. The Singapore Declaration: Forging the will for heart health in the next millennium. *CVD Prevention* 1(3):182-199.

Reddy, K. S., B. Shah, C. Varghese, and A. Ramadoss. 2005. Responding to the threat of chronic diseases in India. *Lancet* 366(9498):1744-1749.

Strong, K., C. Mathers, S. Leeder, and R. Beaglehole. 2005. Preventing chronic diseases: How many lives can we save? *Lancet* 366(9496):1578-1582.

The Sydney Resolution. 2008. Paper read at Oxford Health Alliance 2008 Summit, Syndey Australia.

United Nations General Assembly. 2006. *Resolution adopted by the General Assembly: World Diabetes Day.* Sixty-first session.

U.S. Department of State. 2010. *Implementation of the global health initiative: Consultation document.* Washington, DC: U.S. Department of State.

Wang, L., L. Kong, F. Wu, Y. Bai, and R. Burton. 2005. Preventing chronic diseases in China. *Lancet* 366(9499):1821-1824.

WHA (World Health Assembly). 2000. *Prevention and control of noncommunicable diseases.* Geneva: World Health Organization.

WHO (World Health Organization). 1956. Cardiovascular diseases and hypertension. In *Program of the ninth World Health Assembly*. Geneva: World Health Organization.

WHO. 2000. *The world health report 2000—health systems: Improving performance*. Geneva: World Health Organization.

WHO. 2002. *The world health report 2002—reducing risks, promoting healthy life*. Geneva: World Health Organization.

WHO. 2003a. *WHO framework convention on tobacco control*. Geneva: World Health Organization.

WHO. 2003b. *The world health report: 2003: Shaping the future*. Geneva: World Health Organization.

WHO. 2004. *Global strategy on diet, physical activity and health*. Geneva: World Health Organization.

WHO. 2005a. *Preventing chronic diseases: A vital investment.* http://www.who.int/chp/chronic_disease_report/full_report.pdf (accessed April 23, 2009).

WHO. 2005b. *The world health report 2005—make every mother and child count*. Geneva: World Health Organization.
WHO. 2008a. *2008-2013 action plan for the global strategy for the prevention and control of noncommunicable diseases*. Geneva: World Health Organization.
WHO. 2008b. *The global burden of disease: 2004 update*. Geneva: World Health Organization.
WHO. 2008c. *The world health report 2008—primary health care: now more than ever*. Geneva: World Health Organization.
WHO. 2010. WHO framework convention on tobacco control. http://www.who.int/fctc/en/ (accessed May 26, 2010).
WHO Study Group on Rheumatic Fever and Rheumatic Heart Disease, and WHO. 2004. *Rheumatic fever and rheumatic heart disease: Report of a WHO expert consultation, Geneva, 20 October-1 November 2001, World Health Organization technical report series*. Geneva: World Health Organization.
World Bank. 1984. *China: The health sector*. Washington, DC: World Bank.
World Bank. 1993. *World development report 1993: Investing in health*. New York: Oxford University Press.
World Bank. 2006. Disease control priorities project. http://www.dcp2.org/main/Home.html (accessed May 26, 2010).
World Bank. 2007. *World development report 2007*. Washington, DC: World Bank.
Yach, D., and C. Hawkes. 2004 (unpublished). *Towards a WHO long-term strategy for prevention and control of leading chronic diseases*. Geneva: World Health Organization.

2

Epidemiology of Cardiovascular Disease

In recent years, the dominance of chronic diseases as major contributors to total global mortality has emerged and has been previously described in detail elsewhere (Adeyi et al., 2007; WHO, 2008b). By 2005, the total number of cardiovascular disease (CVD) deaths (mainly coronary heart disease, stroke, and rheumatic heart disease) had increased globally to 17.5 million from 14.4 million in 1990. Of these, 7.6 million were attributed to coronary heart disease and 5.7 million to stroke. More than 80 percent of the deaths occurred in low and middle income countries (WHO, 2009e). The World Health Organization (WHO) estimates there will be about 20 million CVD deaths in 2015, accounting for 30 percent of all deaths worldwide (WHO, 2005). The projected trends in CVD mortality and the expected shifts from infectious to chronic diseases over the next few decades are shown in Figure 2.1. By 2030, researchers project that noncommunicable diseases will account for more than three-quarters of deaths worldwide; CVD alone will be responsible for more deaths in low income countries than infectious diseases (including HIV/AIDS, tuberculosis, and malaria), maternal and perinatal conditions, and nutritional disorders combined (Beaglehole and Bonita, 2008). Thus, CVD is today the largest single contributor to global mortality and will continue to dominate mortality trends in the future (WHO, 2009e).

This chapter describes the incidence and trends over time of CVD globally, as well as in specific regions and nations throughout the world. Moreover, it lays out the major individual risk factors associated with acquisition and augmentation of risk for coronary heart disease and stroke throughout the life course. Furthermore, infectious causes of CVD and

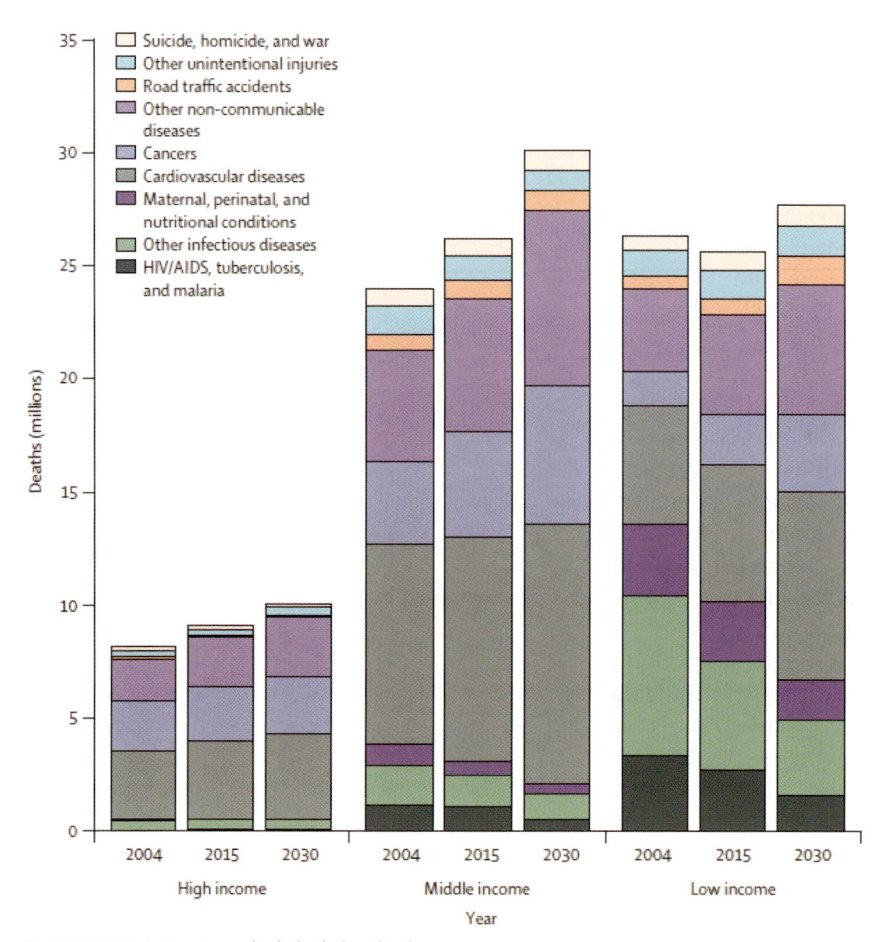

FIGURE 2.1 Projected global deaths by cause.
SOURCE: Beaglehole and Bonita, 2008.

the interface between chronic infectious diseases and CVD risk are briefly discussed later in this chapter. Broad systemic drivers that contribute to the global burden of CVD, such as urbanization and globalization, are referred to in this chapter where they relate to trends in CVD burden and to the classically defined individual risk factors. These are then discussed in more detail in Chapter 3, which focuses on the relationship between CVD and development. Together, these two chapters describe the drivers and trends in CVD worldwide, providing a compelling rationale for the need to act. The remainder of the report proceeds to discuss approaches to influence these factors in order to reduce the burden of disease.

GLOBAL TRENDS IN CVD BURDEN

Global trends in CVD are based on models that use country-specific data from a diverse range of developed and developing countries including those of the European Union (HEM Project Team, 2008; Kotseva et al., 2009a), Saudi Arabia (Al-Hamdan et al., 2005), Pakistan (Nishtar et al., 2004), South Africa (Steyn, 2006), China (Yang et al., 2008), Indonesia (Ng, 2006; Ng et al., 2006), Mexico (Fernald and Neufeld, 2007), India (Goyal and Yusuf, 2006; Reddy, 2007), and the United States (Danaei et al., 2009; Flegal et al., 2007). Over the past decade, the quality and availability of country-specific data on CVD risks, incidence, and mortality has increased in accordance with one of the major recommendations of the 1998 IOM report. What emerges are nationally derived data on risks and CVD outcomes. Therefore, in many developing countries, the lack of country-specific data on risks and CVD outcomes that was prominently highlighted in the 1998 IOM report is less of an impediment to policy development and action.

Nonetheless, before beginning a discussion of CVD trends and risk factor incidence around the world and in specific countries and regions, it is important to note several persistent limitations with the available data. Although many countries have established health surveillance systems with death registration data, the quality of the data collected varies substantially across countries. In many countries—especially in low and middle income countries—health statistics are often based on surveillance that does not cover all areas of the country, is incomplete in the areas it does cover, or is collected by undertrained staff who do not, or cannot, accurately report the pertinent data. These realities limit the reliability of some country health data (Mathers et al., 2005; Rao et al., 2005). Despite these limitations, WHO and country health statistics are often the most complete, comparable, or only data available and thus remain a key tool for evaluating the status of a CVD epidemic within and between countries. The importance of country-level epidemiological data and the ongoing need to standardize methodologies, increase data collection capacity, and improve the accuracy of national reporting are discussed further in Chapter 4.

This chapter uses the most recent data available in each area discussed below, such as deaths by cause, contributions of risk factors to deaths by cause, the composition by risk factor of deaths by a specific cause, and risk factor levels. This introduces some inconsistencies as not all data cited comes from a single source. However, there is available data that is more recent for some of these measures than for others, and this was valued above the consistency of a single data source. Wherever possible, this chapter references burden, incidence, and prevalence data from countries' national health statistics, WHO country and global statistics (which are based on national health statistics provided by Member States), or the latest *Global Burden of Disease: 2004 Update* data (also based on WHO country data) (2008a).

Global Cardiovascular Mortality

Globally, there is an uneven distribution of age-adjusted CVD mortality that is mapped in Figure 2.2. The lowest age-adjusted mortality rates are in the advanced industrialized countries and parts of Latin America, whereas the highest rates today are found in Eastern Europe and a number of low and middle income countries. For example, age-standardized mortality rates for CVD are in excess of 500 per 100,000 in Russia and Egypt; between 400 and 450 for South Africa, India and Saudi Arabia; and around 300 for Brazil and China. This is in contrast to rates of between 100 and 200 per 100,000 for Australia, Japan, France, and the United States. Overall, age-adjusted CVD death rates are today higher in major low and middle income countries than in developed countries (WHO, 2008b).

Examination of coronary heart disease (CHD) mortality trends across countries reveals considerable variability in the shape and magnitude of CHD epidemics since the 1950s. Trends are not consistent even among countries within the same geographic region. In general, three trending patterns of CHD mortality can be observed: a rise-and-fall pattern where mortality rates increased, peaked, and then fell significantly; a rising pattern, where rates have steadily increased indicating an ongoing epidemic; and a flat pattern, where CHD mortality rates have remained relatively low and stable. The rise-and-fall pattern is most notable in high income Anglo-Celtic, Nordic, and Northwestern Continental European countries as well as in the United States and Australia. In these countries, CHD mortality rates peaked in the 1960s or early 1970s and have since fallen precipitously, by an average of about 50 percent (Beaglehole, 1999; Hardoon et al., 2008; Mirzaei et al., 2009; Unal et al., 2004). The rising pattern of CHD is most notable in Eastern European and former Soviet countries, where mortality rates have continued to increase at an alarming pace and where the highest mortality rates ever recorded are currently being observed. By contrast, CHD mortality rates in Japan and several European Mediterranean countries have remained relatively low, following the flat pattern (Beaglehole, 1999; Mirzaei et al., 2009).

Mortality rates generally appear to be most closely linked to a country's stage of epidemiological transition. Epidemiological transition, a concept first proposed by Abdel Omran in the 1970s (Omran, 1971), refers to the changes in the predominant forms of disease and mortality burdening a population that occur as its economy and health system develops. In underdeveloped countries at the early stages of epidemiological transition,

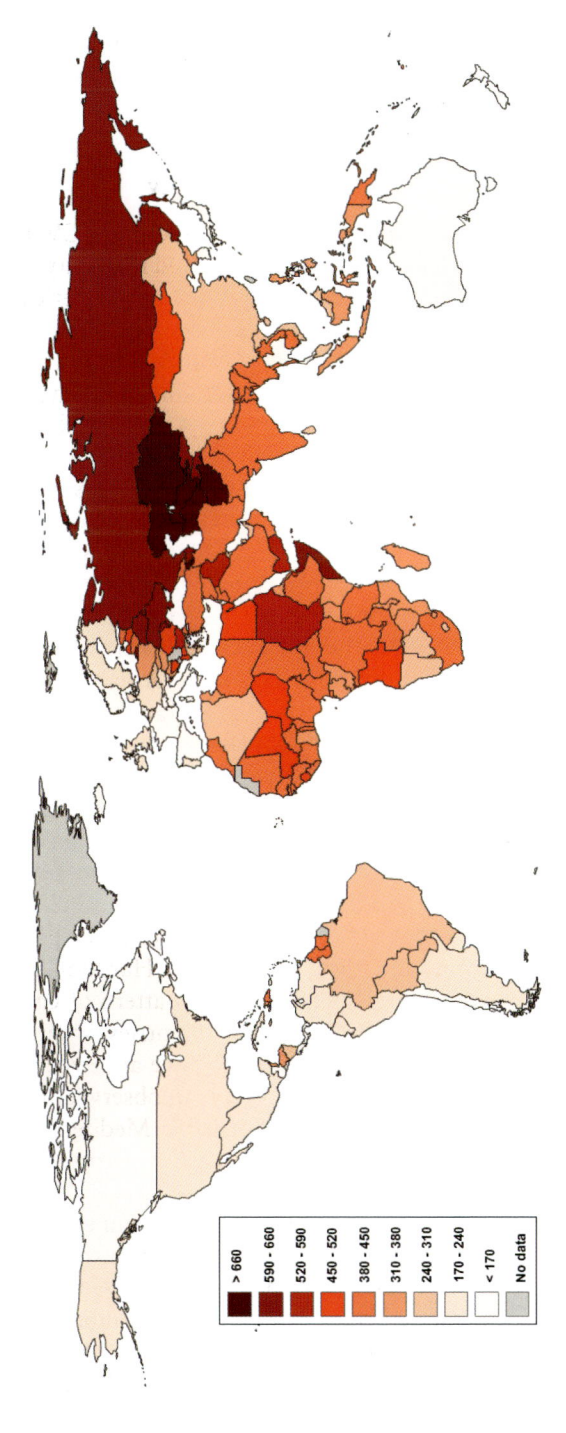

FIGURE 2.2 Age-standardized deaths due to cardiovascular disease (rate per 100,000), 2004.
NOTE: Rates are age-standardized to WHO's world standard population.
SOURCES: WHO, 2009e; map created with StatPlanet (van Cappelle, 2009).

infectious diseases predominate, but as the economy, development status, and health systems of these countries improve, the population moves to a later stage of epidemiological transition, and chronic noncommunicable diseases become the predominant causes of death and disease (Gaziano et al., 2006).

Although this general pattern connecting trends in causes of mortality and stage of development can be observed, it is difficult to make generalized observations about CHD mortality trends for most low and middle income regions. This is due to limited trending data from many low and middle income countries as well as considerable country-to-country variability within regions. The data are strongest from Latin America, where several countries—specifically Argentina, Brazil, Chile, and Cuba—have experienced declines in CHD mortality rates in the past several decades. However, with the exception of Argentina, where rates declined by more than 60 percent between 1970 and 2000, the declines have generally occurred more recently (in the 1980s and 1990s) and have been less dramatic (between 20 and 45 percent) than those in high income countries. By contrast, the epidemic in Mexico appears to be worsening, with CHD mortality rates increasing by more than 90 percent between 1970 and 2000 (Mirzaei et al., 2009; Rodriguez et al., 2006). Mortality rates in Peru have remained relatively low, following the flat pattern. In Asia, some high income countries—such as Singapore—have followed the rise-and-fall pattern, while CHD deaths in other countries (such as the Philippines and urban China) appear to be rising (Mirzaei et al., 2009). Although trending data for most of Africa is not available, Mayosi et al. (2009) report that mortality rates for CVD and diabetes are rising in South Africa. Because there can be so much variability in the nature of CVD epidemics within regions, Mirzaei et al. (2009) conclude that the most prudent strategy when grouping countries in similar epidemiological situations is to group according to CVD mortality pattern rather than by geographic region.

Conclusion 2.1: *Chronic diseases are now the dominant contributors to the global burden of disease, and CVD is the largest contributor to the chronic disease cluster. Although CVD death rates are declining in most high income countries, trends are increasing in most low and middle income countries.*

Age at Death from CVD

Not only do age-adjusted CVD death rates tend to be higher in developing countries, but a significantly higher percentage of cardiovascular deaths also occur in younger people in the developing world than in developed countries. For example, the proportion of CVD deaths reported for 35 to

64 years is 41 percent in South Africa, 35 percent in India, and 28 percent in Brazil, compared to only 12 percent in the United States and 9 percent in Portugal (Leeder et al., 2004).

The median age of heart attack and first stroke and the median age at death from ischemic heart disease (IHD) and stroke offer a means to compare countries and groups in terms of their population experiences of CVD. The WHO 2004 Global Burden of Disease study estimated these variables for countries across the development spectrum. The results for selected countries are summarized in Figure 2.3. As a general trend, men and women in countries with higher development status (measured in terms of gross domestic product [GDP] per capita) experience CVD events older and die much later than in less developed countries. For example, in Japan, Australia, France, and Sweden, the median age at death from IHD averages 85 years in women and 77 years in men. Men in these countries experience an acute myocardial infarction (AMI) more than a decade before their median age at death (WHO, 2009a). Indeed, the survival of individuals after a cardiovascular event has increased in high income countries. This trend of increased survival with CVD has caused an increased prevalence of CVD in many high income countries despite decreasing incidence over time (Davies et al., 2007).

A second set of countries experienced median events at much younger ages despite having among the highest measures of GDP growth in the world. They include many Middle Eastern countries with considerable oil wealth. A third set of countries at intermediate levels of GDP per capita achieved above-average median ages at AMI and first stroke occurrence and death. They include Malaysia, Nicaragua, China, and Jamaica. In contrast, Brazil and South Africa, in the same development group as the preceding countries but with higher degrees of social inequality (United Nations Development Program [UNDP], 2007), achieved worse cardiovascular outcomes. Thus, even with countries at similar levels of development, some achieve substantially better CVD outcomes than others. These relative success stories give some indication of how preventable and treatable CVD can be. Comparative studies across countries are needed to build a better understanding of the factors that lead to the relative successes in these countries and to help inform the development of more effective approaches to control CVD.

REASONS FOR CVD TRENDS OVER TIME

A continuing understanding of how trends in CVD change over time is important, as knowledge evolves about the underlying causes of CVD and their relative impact. The empirical base for understanding the specific reasons for changes in CVD trends over time comes from two different

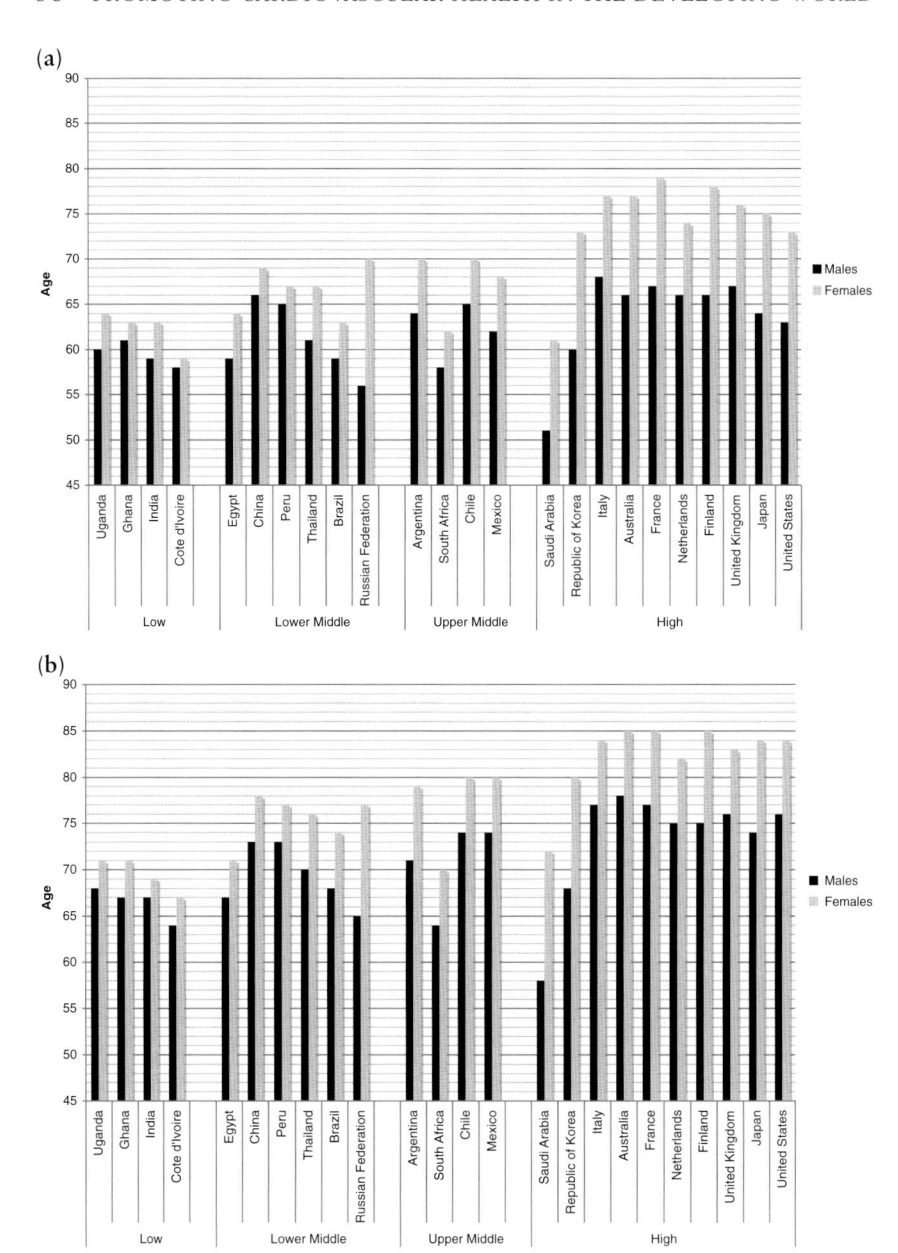

FIGURE 2.3 Median age (a) at acute myocardial infarction, (b) of ischemic heart disease deaths, (c) at first stroke, and (d) of stroke deaths, by country.
SOURCE: Data from WHO, 2009a.

EPIDEMIOLOGY OF CARDIOVASCULAR DISEASE

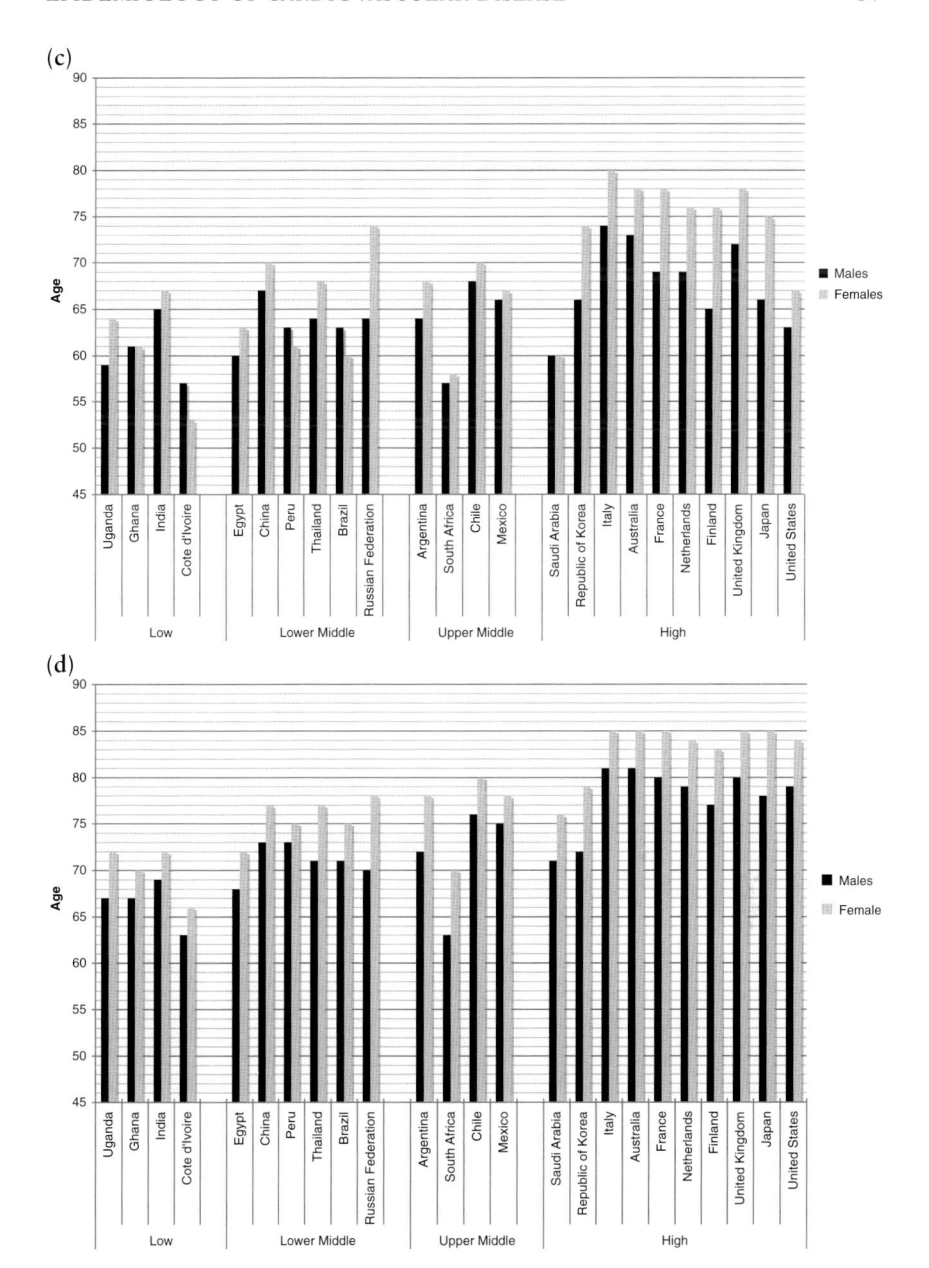

(c)

(d)

sets of observations and studies. First, there are those that investigate the causes for the increases in CVD death and incidence rates being experienced in many developing countries. Second, there are others that have analyzed the reasons for the substantive decline experienced in developed countries over the past few decades. As described below, the same set of major risk factors consistently play a large role in explaining trends in CVD incidence and death across the world. Taken together, the data indicate that poor diet, tobacco use, physical inactivity, excess alcohol use, and psychosocial factors are the major contributors to CVD increases (Anand et al., 2008; Clarke et al., 2009; Critchley et al., 2004; Lopez-Jaramillo et al., 2008; Mayosi et al., 2009; Rosengren et al., 2004; Stein et al., 2005; Yusuf et al., 2004). However, the reasons for the increase or decrease of these risks in various parts of the world are more complex. This section describes the trends in these risks, and subsequent sections of this chapter describe the nature of the relationship between these factors and risk for CVD in more detail.

Causes of the Ascent in CVD Mortality and Incidence

Data are limited on the specific causes of the increases in CVD incidence and mortality that occurred in developed countries in the early 20th century and in developing countries more recently. It is clear that by 1920 CVD was already the leading cause of death in the United States. Scientific articles from the 1930s and 1940s suggest hypertension, cholesterol, poor nutrition, obesity, smoking, physical inactivity, and psychosocial stress as the leading factors contributing to heart disease, but they do not provide strong evidence to support this assertion (Ellis, 1948; Gager, 1931; Heart disease likely fate, 1937). The original publications outlining the rationale for the Framingham Study also cite these potential risk factors, although, again, they do not provide specific supporting evidence (Dawber and Kannel, 1958; Dawber et al., 1951, 1957). Tobacco use has been the most reliably documented, and historical trends in CVD mortality and tobacco use in the United States from 1900 to 1990 closely mirror each other, with both rates increasing through the 1950s, followed by a precipitous fall beginning in the 1960s (Fox et al., 2004; Mirzaei et al., 2009; Shopland, 1995). In the United Kingdom, a 38-year follow-up of men showed that baseline differences in tobacco use, high blood pressure, and cholesterol were associated with a 10- to 15-year shorter life expectancy from age 50 (Clarke et al., 2009). The study has significance for developing countries since many of the baseline levels of risk common in the late 1960s in the United Kingdom are the norm in many developing countries today.

There are a few studies that provide more direct insight into the causes of recent increases in CVD incidence and mortality in low and middle income countries. For example, in their study on the rise of CHD mortality in Beijing from 1984 to 1990, Critchley et al. found that blood lipid increases were the largest contributor—responsible for 77 percent of increased CHD mortality (Critchley et al., 2004).

Another likely contributor is a rise in smoking. There has been a steady rise in global cigarette consumption since the 1970s, which is expected to continue over the next decade if current trends continue. In 2010, researchers estimate that 6.3 trillion cigarettes—or more than 900 cigarettes for every person on the earth—will be consumed. This increase in the total number of smokers around the world is driven predominantly by global population growth and is expected to continue unless smoking rates are drastically reduced. By 2020, if current smoking and population growth trends continue, the global annual cigarette consumption could rise to between 6.7 and 6.8 trillion cigarettes (ERC, 2007; Guindon and Boisclair, 2003; Shafey et al., 2009). This growing burden of tobacco is increasingly falling on low and middle income countries. In fact, three of the top five cigarette-consuming countries are low or middle income countries (China, the Russian Federation, and Indonesia). China alone consumes approximately 2.163 trillion cigarettes every year—37 percent of the world's annual consumption (ERC, 2007; Guindon and Boisclair, 2003; Shafey et al., 2009). By 2030, WHO projects that more than 80 percent of tobacco-related deaths will occur in developing countries (Shafey et al., 2009; WHO, 2008c). In addition to increasing consumption trends, the amount of tobacco produced globally has nearly doubled since 1960, with production increasing more than 300 percent in low and middle income countries, where by 2007, approximately 85 percent of tobacco was grown (Shafey et al., 2009). In addition, as tobacco use has declined in rich countries, transnational tobacco companies have increasingly focused on expanding markets for their products in low and middle income countries (Bump et al., 2009; Chelala, 1998; Connolly, 1992; Holzman, 1997; Mackay, 1992; Mackay and Eriksen, 2002; Martinez and Grise, 1990; Wagner and Romano, 1994).

An emerging body of evidence suggests that rapid dietary changes associated with nutritional transition, along with a decrease in levels of physical activity in many rapidly urbanizing societies, also may play a particularly important role in the rise of CVD observed in developing countries (Stein et al., 2005). The nutritional transition currently occurring in many low and middle income countries has created a new phenomenon in which it is not uncommon to see both undernutrition and obesity coexist in the same populations (Caballero, 2005; Dangour and Uauy, 2006; Reddy et al., 2003). Undernutrition has been the hallmark of the low and middle income countries of Africa, Latin America, and South Asia for decades. This situation is progressively being replaced by a distinct trend at the other end of the spectrum. While the global undernourished population is plateauing, obesity and other chronic diseases have been increasing exponentially as a result of lifestyle and behavior change, resulting in a transition from communicable to noncommunicable diseases. WHO has estimated that while the undernourished global population has declined to approximately 1.2 billion, the overweight population has increased to the same figure. Of these, an estimated 300 million are clinically obese (Misra and Khurana, 2008). As an associated problem, the global prevalence of overweight in children between the ages of 5 and 17 years is 10 percent, varying from under 2 percent in Sub-Saharan Africa to more than 30 percent in the United States (Bhardwaj et al., 2008).

Epidemiological evidence suggests that dietary changes associated with the nutritional transition, specifically the increasing consumption of energy-dense diets high in unhealthy fats, oils, sodium, and sugars, have contributed to an increase in CVD incidence in low and middle income countries (Hu, 2008). Traditionally, monitoring of dietary consumption trends in low and middle income countries has been difficult due to poor availability of quality data. The Food and Agricultural Organization (FAO) of the United Nations examines trends in the amounts of various foods that are produced, which can serve as a rough proxy for consumption. This measure usually overestimates consumption, but trends remain valid indicators of the broad changes underway. FAO data indicate that the total kilocaloric intake per capita per day (KCD) in many low and middle income countries as well as the consumption of animal products and some tropical oils (e.g., palm oil)—major sources of saturated fat—have been increasing.

To illustrate these trends, kilocaloric intake from selected food groups in China, India, Mexico, Egypt, and South Africa from 1980 to 1982 were compared to kilocaloric intake in 2001 to 2003 using data derived from FAOSTAT (Food and Agriculture Organization of the United Nations Statistical Database) (see Table 2.1). In China, total KCD increased from 2,327 kilocalories to 2,940 kilocalories, and meat consumption increased by more than 246 percent during the period.

There was also a significant increase in the intake of oils in China, with three types of oils increasing more than 100 percent: palm oil (+640 percent), soybean oil (+635 percent), and vegetable oils (+259 percent). On the positive side, the intake of fruits and vegetables also skyrocketed—by 600 and 367 percent, respectively—over the same period. On balance, these changes provided the Chinese with a mix of healthier calories; however, increased risks brought about by the increased consumption of meat and foods cooked in tropical oils are associated with adverse blood lipid changes. A similar picture was repeated in India, Mexico, and South Africa, with soaring kilocalorie intake of palm oil reported.

The exponential growth in the use of tropical oils (specifically palm oil) and partially hydrogenated soybean oil in low and middle income countries

TABLE 2.1 Percentage Change in Consumption by Kilocalories per Capita per Day in Selected Countries from 1980 to 2003

Food Type	China	Egypt	India	Mexico	South Africa
Total Kilocalories	26.3	16.2	25.7	1.5	5.7
Meat	247	48.3	40.0	18.3	6.9
Cereals	–13.9	17.6	13.8	–1.4	4.7
Sugar and Sweeteners	51.9	8.8	27.2	2.4	–18.3
Fruits	600	103	60.0	19.4	33.3
Vegetables	367	10.3	37.5	40.7	0.0
Palm Oil	640	No Data	730	2100	2400
Soybean Oil	635	35.5	48.2	50.0	189
Vegetable Oil	259	–47.8	84.6	14.7	75.4

SOURCE: FAOSTAT food consumption data.

is troubling because both these oils contain high levels of fatty acids that are atherogenic and linked to an increased risk of MI. Palm oil has a saturated fatty acid content of 45 percent, and partially hydrogenated soybean oil, although much lower in saturated fat, contains transfatty acids introduced as a byproduct of hydrogenation (see Figure 2.5 later in this chapter for a comparison of the fatty acid composition of selected cooking oils). Globally, from 1980-1981 until the present, FAO estimates that there has been a 780 percent increase in palm oil production, a 286 percent increase in soybean production, and a 400 percent increase in rapeseed production. By contrast, olive oil production has increased by only 58 percent during this period (Khan and Mensah, 2009). Although the effects of unhealthy oils on CVD risk have been established (mainly in developed countries), the population consequences for CVD of these very steep and rapid production trends have yet to be directly quantified in developing countries. Gaining a better understanding of the implications of oil production trends as well as those for several other food categories that impact CVD risk is necessary to better inform current and future actions to address CVD, including those related to agricultural policy.

Causes of the Decline in CVD Mortality and Incidence in Developed Countries

Relative Contributions of Risk-Factor Reduction and Treatment

The causes of the decline in CVD in developed countries offer potential lessons for achieving similar results in developing countries. Taken together, studies examining the causes of the decline in CHD mortality and incidence observed in developed countries since the mid-1960s suggest that risk-factor reductions and treatment each account for between 40 and 60 percent of the reduction in CVD mortality, with undetermined causes accounting for between 0 and 10 percent of additional reduction. The majority of these studies, described in more detail below, included all risk factor-reducing medications (such as statins for dyslipidemia) in the treatment category; thus, the data on risk-factor reduction are the result of lifestyle rather than medical interventions.

Several studies from Western Europe and New Zealand attributed a slightly higher percentage of the decline to the reduction of risk factors (Beaglehole, 1999; Capewell et al., 1999, 2000; Unal et al., 2004). This was particularly marked in Finland and New Zealand, where studies attributed more than 50 percent of the decline to risk-factor reductions (Laatikainen et al., 2005; Unal et al., 2004; Vartiainen et al., 1994b). Indeed, both studies from Finland found that treatments accounted for less than 25 percent of the reduction (Laatikainen et al., 2005; Vartiainen et al., 1994b), although the average declines occurred in an era of less effective treatments than are available today. Similarly, one study in the United Kingdom identified the contribution of improved treatment options in that country to be responsible for 40 percent of the reduction in mortality, with a concurrent reduction in risk factors accounting for the majority of the decline (Davies et al., 2007).

In contrast, reports from WHO's Multinational Monitoring of Trends and Determinants in Cardiovascular Disease study have suggested the role of treatment was significantly higher, accounting for the majority of the decline (Davies et al., 2007). In the United States, some studies have attributed a slightly higher percentage to treatment than to risk-factor reductions (Goraya et al., 2003; Hunink et al., 1997), although a number of other studies found that risk-factor reduction and treatment strategies contribute evenly (approximately 50 percent each) to the decline in CVD mortality rates (Ford et al., 2007; Hardoon et al., 2008).

Importantly, with each decade, the relative impact of treatment versus prevention has increased (Ford et al., 2007). This effect could be due to the increasing availability of more effective diagnostics and treatment, higher population uptake of treatment, or the relative failure to fully implement effective prevention programs at a population level.

These data reinforce the importance of a balanced approach to combating CVD that includes both treatment and prevention. Better diagnosis and treatment can extend and improve the lives of those individuals who have established disease or high risk, but successful prevention of CVD and CVD risk factors will be required to reduce the incidence of CVD. This will require successful prevention. The need for this balance leads to important cost considerations for developed and developing countries in order to limit potential inflation of medical care costs as well as to develop and implement affordable primary prevention programs. Chapters 3 and 5 discuss further the potential feasibility and relevance in developing countries of medication and other technologically based treatments versus behavioral or lifestyle risk-reduction approaches to reduce CVD burden.

Major Contributors to Risk Factor–Based Reductions in CVD

Although the numbers from each study differ, the body of evidence suggests that smoking, blood lipids, and blood pressure were the three most important risk factors in reducing CHD mortality and incidence in developed countries. In the various studies, cholesterol reductions were responsible for between 0.4 and 50 percent of the reductions and population-level blood pressure reductions were responsible for between 6 and 21 percent of the reductions (Capewell et al., 1999, 2000; Ford et al., 2007; Hunink et al., 1997; Laatikainen et al., 2005; Unal et al., 2004; Vartiainen et al., 1994b). Smoking reduction alone was responsible for between 6 and 56 percent of the reductions in the various studies.

Several studies have also provided analyses of the role that dietary changes may have played in the reduction of CHD mortality and incidence. Slattery and Randall (1988) reviewed dietary trends in the decades prior to the decline of CVD in the United States and found a series of changes in eating patterns that occurred 10 to 20 years before the decline and could have contributed to it. This is supported further by Hu et al. (2000), who found that improvements in diet accounted for a 16 percent decline in CHD incidence from 1980 to 1994 in the women in the Nurses' Health Study. In Finland, Pietenin et al. (1996) found that dietary changes instituted in the 1970s explained nearly all the reduction in cholesterol observed in the Finnish population. This is significant because the reduction in cholesterol was the most important factor in the overall reduction of CHD mortality in Finland between the 1970s and early 1990s (Laatikainen et al., 2005; Vartiainen et al., 1994b).

Indeed, few countries have documented their declines in CVD risk and CVD mortality as well as Finland. Since the 1970s both stroke and CHD mortality in Finland have declined 75 to 80 percent and the average life expectancy has increased by 5 to 6 years (Karppanen and Mervaala, 2006). These declines came about when government, health professionals, farmers, food companies, and local nongovernmental organizations invested decades of sustained work implementing efforts to support a more healthful diet (reducing saturated fat and sodium consumption, increasing fruit and vegetable consumption), reduce smoking prevalence, and promote the use of risk factor-reducing medications where indicated. As a result of these comprehensive efforts to reduce CVD risk, between 1972 and 2007, serum cholesterol declined 21 percent among men and 23 percent among women, systolic blood pressure declined by 10.1 mmHg in men and 18.6 mmHg in women, and male smoking prevalence declined from 52 to 31 percent in the North Karelia Province (Puska et al., 2009). These results have implications as a potential model for intervention, which is discussed further in Chapter 5.

> ***Conclusion 2.2:*** *The broad causes for the rise and, in some countries, the decline in CVD over time are well described. The key contributors to the rise across countries at all stages of development include tobacco use and abnormal blood lipid levels, along with unhealthy dietary changes (especially related to fats and oils, salt, and increased calories) and reduced physical activity. Key contributors to the decline in some countries include declines in tobacco use and exposure, healthful dietary shifts, population-wide prevention efforts, and treatment interventions.*

In summary, examination of global trends in CVD burden and mortality as well as analysis of the causal factors driving these trends provide a compelling argument in support of the prioritization of CVD prevention and reduction efforts worldwide—and especially in low and middle income countries. Countries and regions are either currently experiencing high CVD burden and mortality rates or they can expect to see CVD burden and mortality rates increase because of disturbing trends in the prevalence of well-established CVD risk factors in their population. Even countries that have been successful in reducing the burden of CVD over the past 40 years cannot be complacent, as certain risk factors, such as the prevalence of overweight and obesity, continue to grow despite successes in the reduction of other risk factors.

A LIFE-COURSE PERSPECTIVE ON CVD

The life-course perspective to chronic disease recognizes that CVD and other chronic diseases are the result of risks that accumulate throughout an individual's lifetime. The perspective further recognizes that these risks can and must be reduced and prevented at all stages of life (Aboderin et al., 2002). In keeping with this principle, risk for CVD begins to accumulate as early as fetal life and continues to do so through infancy, childhood, adolescence, and adult life.

The 1998 IOM report sounded the alarm about the possible role that early factors in infancy play in increasing CVD incidence later in life and the growing worldwide recognition—based on new data from prospective cohort studies—of the importance of the fetal and early childhood stages to the later onset of CVD (IOM, 1998; Victora et al., 2008; Walker and

George, 2007). Since the 1998 report, there has been a large body of evidence linking undernutrition in early life to increased chronic disease risk later in life. Gluckman and Hanson (2008) have described how important it is for infants to be of optimal weight; when they are either under or overweight, they are at risk for a higher incidence of CVD in later life. In addition, low birth weight (LBW) and rapid weight gain after infancy are now recognized to increase the risk of CVD and diabetes in adulthood (Barker et al., 2005; Prentice and Moore, 2005). These findings raise important considerations for addressing global CVD as LBW and exposure to undernutrition in utero are common in many developing countries (Caballero, 2009; Kelishadi, 2007). A consensus has not yet emerged on what constitutes optimal nutrition and growth, but greater consideration of lifetime risk in nutrition programs currently implemented in many maternal and child health programs is an opportunity to promote cardiovascular health early in life. The influences of these factors in pregnancy and early childhood on risk for CVD are discussed in greater detail in Chapter 6.

Many major risk factors for CVD are established in childhood and adolescence (Barker et al., 1993; Celermajer and Ayer, 2006; Freedman et al., 2001; Strong et al., 1999). These include tobacco use, dietary and physical activity behaviors, overweight and obesity, and adverse childhood experiences (Celermajer and Ayer, 2006; Dong et al., 2004; Freedman et al., 2001). Poor social circumstances in childhood have also been linked to CVD later in life in a number of different cohorts conducted in the United States and Europe (Davey Smith et al., 2001; Galobardes et al., 2006). The acquisition and augmentation of risk for CVD in childhood and adolescence are also discussed in more detail in Chapter 6.

By middle age, many individuals have often already accumulated significant risk, yet the potential for ongoing accumulation exists. This is demonstrated by the effectiveness of rigorous prevention and reduction of risk factors during middle age, including continued management of blood pressure, blood lipids, and diabetes; promotion of exercise and healthful eating; and quitting smoking (Goldman et al., 2009; Kalache et al., 2002). Aside from preventing the onset of disease and premature death, another key goal of risk factor reduction efforts, especially in middle age, is to prevent premature morbidity and disability (Fries, 1980; Kalache et al., 2002; Olshansky and Ault, 1986).

The accumulation of risk in later life is especially important given that, over the past 150 years, life expectancies in most parts of the world have increased dramatically (WHO, 1999). All indications suggest that this trend will continue through the 21st century, making it likely that most babies born in countries with long life expectancies since 2000 will live to see their 100th birthday (Christensen et al., 2009). This rise in the elderly population is not only occurring in developed countries. Demographers predict that by

2020, 70 percent of the world's elderly population will be living in developing countries (Kalache, 1999). As more and more people live into old age, an emphasis on delaying the onset of disability due to chronic diseases becomes increasingly important. Research has found that CVD is the second leading cause of disability among Americans aged 65 years and older, and that even subclinical CVD can significantly increase frailty, hospitalizations, and institutionalizations. However, research also indicates that ongoing risk factor-reduction efforts, particularly the promotion of increasing levels of physical activity, can significantly reduce disability and help prevent adverse cardiovascular outcomes among the elderly (Rich and Mensah, 2009, 2010; Sattelmair et al., 2009). Studies of nonagenarians, centenarians, and supercentanarians (individuals aged 110 to 119 years) reveal that it is possible to live independently and without significant assistance into the 10th and 11th decades of life; however, minimizing the accumulation of risks throughout the life course through health promotion is critical to this postponement of disability (Christensen et al., 2009).

Taken together, the evidence reinforces the need for a rigorous, life-course approach to the prevention of CVD that starts in utero and continues throughout life. The acquisition and augmentation of risk throughout the life course underscores the importance of building an array of health-promoting and disease prevention strategies that address specific age-sensitive periods of life and have long-term impacts over decades. This unifies CVD prevention with early childhood development as well as with efforts to promote healthy aging. Opportunities for interventions throughout the life course are discussed in more detail in Chapters 5 and 6.

INDIVIDUAL RISKS FOR CVD

Proximal risks for CVD include those associated with consumption patterns (mainly linked to diets, tobacco and alcohol use), activity patterns, and health service use as well as biological risk factors such as increased cholesterol, blood pressure, blood glucose, and clinical disease. The Framingham Study first centered attention on the concept of "risk factors" associated with CVD, and most recently reported substantial 30-year risk data showing the accumulation of risk over time (Pencina et al., 2009). Importantly, risk factors for the incidence of CVD and those associated with CVD severity or mortality are not synonymous. Risk factors for incidence become important starting very early in life and accumulate with behavioral, social, and economic factors over the life course to culminate in biological risks for CVD such as increased cholesterol, blood pressure, blood glucose, and clinical disease. Over the past few decades, the effectiveness of early screening and long-term treatment for biological risks or early disease has contributed to the sharp declines in CVD mortality seen in many countries (Hunink et al., 1997).

This section focuses on these proximal behavioral and biological risks for CVD, while Chapter 3 includes a more detailed discussion of broad systemic drivers of CVD.

Better Data on Individual Risk Factors

The recent WHO *Global Health Risks Report of 2009* (Lopez et al., 2006) and the earlier *World Health Report of 2002* provide comparable and robust estimates of the contribution of risks to total mortality and measures of disability (Mathers et al., 2003; WHO, 2002, 2009b). This kind of data, which was explicitly called for in the 1998 IOM report, allows policy makers to shift their focus upstream from diseases and deaths to risks. Relatively few major behavioral and biological risk factors account for CVD incidence around the world. Tobacco use, diet (including alcohol, total calorie intake, and specific nutrients) and physical inactivity serve as the three major behavioral risks. Between them, they account for a significant proportion of cancer, diabetes, and chronic respiratory disease incidence in addition to CVD (Hu et al., 2001; van Dam et al., 2008; WHO, 2002; Yach et al., 2004, 2005). Concerted action focused on these behavioral risks, along with biological risks such as high blood pressure, high blood lipids, and high blood glucose, would have a wide impact on the global incidence and burden of disease (WHO, 2009b).

Reflecting the predominant role of CVD and its related risk factors in global mortality, Table 2.2 highlights the role of these biological and behavioral factors as the leading global risks for mortality from all causes. High blood pressure, tobacco use, elevated blood glucose, physical inactivity, and overweight and obesity are the five leading factors globally. In middle income countries, alcohol replaces high blood glucose in the top five; in low income countries, a lack of safe water, unsafe sex, and undernutrition are important. These latter points are discussed further in this report in relation to both the role of early childhood nutrition in the later onset of CVD as well as the need to integrate the management of HIV/AIDS more closely with CVD in low income countries (WHO, 2009b).

The *Global Burden of Disease and Risk Factors* report provides additional analysis of the relative contribution of individual risk factors specifically to CVD burden. Using 2001 data, the report estimates the percentage decrease in IHD and stroke burden that could be expected if population exposure to a risk factor were reduced to zero by calculating the population attributable fraction for each of the key CVD risk factors. This analysis is summarized in Table 2.3 and Figure 2.4. The report found that hypertension, high cholesterol, overweight and obesity, smoking, low fruit

TABLE 2.2 Ranking of 10 Selected Risk-Factor Causes of Death by Income Group, 2004

Region	Rank	Risk Factor	Deaths (Millions)	% of Total
World	1	High Blood Pressure	7.5	12.8
	2	Tobacco Use	5.1	8.7
	3	High Blood Glucose	3.4	5.8
	4	Physical Inactivity	3.2	5.5
	5	Overweight and Obesity	2.8	4.8
	6	High Cholesterol	2.6	4.5
	7	Unsafe Sex	2.4	4.0
	8	Alcohol Use	2.3	3.8
	9	Childhood Underweight	2.2	3.8
	10	Indoor Smoke from Solid Fuels	2.0	3.3
High Income Countries[a]	1	Tobacco Use	1.5	17.9
	2	High Blood Pressure	1.4	16.8
	3	Overweight and Obesity	0.7	8.4
	4	Physical Inactivity	0.6	7.7
	5	High Blood Glucose	0.6	7.0
	6	High Cholesterol	0.5	5.8
	7	Low Fruit and Vegetable Intake	0.2	2.5
	8	Urban Outdoor Air Pollution	0.2	2.5
	9	Alcohol Use	0.1	1.6
	10	Occupational Risks	0.1	1.1
Middle Income Countries[a]	1	High Blood Pressure	4.2	17.2
	2	Tobacco Use	2.6	10.8
	3	Overweight and Obesity	1.6	6.7
	4	Physical Inactivity	1.6	6.6
	5	Alcohol Use	1.6	6.4
	6	High Blood Glucose	1.5	6.3
	7	High Cholesterol	1.3	5.2
	8	Low Fruit and Vegetable Intake	0.9	3.9
	9	Indoor Smoke from Solid Fuels	0.7	2.8
	10	Urban Outdoor Air Pollution	0.7	2.8
Low Income Countries[a]	1	Childhood Underweight	2.0	7.8
	2	High Blood Pressure	2.0	7.5
	3	Unsafe Sex	1.7	6.6
	4	Unsafe Water, Sanitation, Hygiene	1.6	6.1
	5	High Blood Glucose	1.3	4.9
	6	Indoor Smoke from Solid Fuels	1.3	4.8
	7	Tobacco Use	1.0	3.9
	8	Physical Inactivity	1.0	3.8
	9	Suboptimal Breastfeeding	1.0	3.7
	10	High Cholesterol	0.9	3.4

[a] Countries grouped by gross national income per capita—low income ($825 or less), high income ($10,066 or more).
SOURCE: Adapted from WHO, 2009b.

and vegetable intake, and physical inactivity were the leading contributors to IHD and stroke burden worldwide (Lopez et al., 2006). These findings are consistent with other large-scale studies of risk-factor contributions to overall CVD burden (see the discussion of the INTERHEART study in the following paragraphs); however, it should be noted that the report did not examine the role of elevated blood glucose in its analyses.

In addition to calling for better global data on CVD risks, the 1998 IOM report also recommended the use of case-control studies to establish the role of major risks for CVD (IOM, 1998). The INTERHEART study was an important response to this call (Iqbal et al., 2008; Yusuf et al., 2004). It enrolled approximately 15,000 cases and 15,000 controls from 52 countries in Western, Central, and Eastern Europe; the Middle East; Asia; and Africa to examine the impact of risk factors on incidence of AMI. Although there are limitations in comparing the INTERHEART study, a case-control study, to a classical prospective cohort study, its major findings are reminiscent of the conclusions of the original Framingham Study several decades ago as well as its 30-year follow-up studies (Yusuf et al., 2004). The INTERHEART study found that abnormal blood lipids are the most important contributors to CVD globally. Tobacco was the second most important risk factor, coequal to lipids in men but lower in women. Other key risk factors included abdominal obesity, psychosocial factors, hypertension, and diabetes (Yusuf et al., 2004).

While the INTERHEART study showed that the top risk factors contributing to CVD are generally consistent globally, the study also found distinct regional differences, much like the data described previously on the rising trends in CVD prevalence over time. For example, while abdominal obesity was the greatest or second-greatest contributor to CVD risk in 8 of the 10 regions studied, it was the smallest contributor in China. In addition, while psychosocial factors were among the top three risk factors by both population attributable risk and odds ratio (measures of risk-factor burden and impact, respectively) in Western Europe, the Middle East, China, and North America, they appeared to be much less influential in Central and Eastern Europe and South Asia (Iqbal et al., 2008; Yusuf et al., 2004).

Few studies have quantified the consequent impact of these risks on the risk of stroke in developing country populations. However, findings from a study in the United Kingdom are informative. A cohort of 20,040 people was followed over 11 years to determine the risk of stroke incidence. Four measures of health behaviors combined—smoking, low physical activity, low plasma vitamin C levels (used as a proxy for fruit and vegetable intake), and not drinking alcohol in moderation (abstaining from alcohol or consuming more than 14 drinks per week)—predicted more than a two-fold increase in stroke incidence (Myint et al., 2009). This is consistent with prior findings in large cohorts of men and women in the United States that

TABLE 2.3 Contribution of Selected Risk Factors (by Population Attributable Fractions [PAF]) to IHD and Stroke Burdens, 2001

	Risk Factor	World	High Income Countries	Low and Middle Income Countries
Ischemic Heart Disease	High Blood Pressure	45%	48%	44%
	High Cholesterol	48%	57%	46%
	Overweight and Obesity	18%	27%	16%
	Low Fruit and Vegetable Intake	28%	19%	30%
	Physical Inactivity	21%	21%	21%
	Smoking	17%	23%	15%
	Alcohol Use	2%	−13%	4%
	Urban Air Pollution[a]	2%	1%	2%
Stroke	High Blood Pressure	54%	56%	54%
	High Cholesterol	16%	25%	15%
	Overweight and Obesity	12%	20%	10%
	Low Fruit and Vegetable Intake	11%	9%	11%
	Physical Inactivity	7%	8%	6%
	Smoking	13%	21%	12%
	Alcohol Use	3%	−11%	5%
	Urban Air Pollution[a]	3%	1%	4%

[a] PAFs for Urban Air Pollution have large uncertainty.
SOURCE: Data from Lopez et al., 2006.

a healthful diet and lifestyle—not smoking, regular exercise, moderate alcohol consumption, and not being overweight—was associated with nearly 80 percent lower risk of ischemic stroke compared to having none of these healthy lifestyle components (Chiuve et al., 2008).

> ***Conclusion 2.3:*** *The major contributing individual risk factors for CVD are generally consistent across the globe and include abnormal blood lipids, tobacco use and exposure, abdominal obesity, psychosocial factors, hypertension, and diabetes. However, the detailed underlying risk profile differs across populations and varies over time. Interventions and prevention strategies need to focus on current local risk profiles to ensure they are adapted to the specific settings where they will be applied.*

Major Proximal Risk Factors for CVD

This section described the major risk factors for CVD in more detail. The section begins with behavioral risk factors, including tobacco use, di-

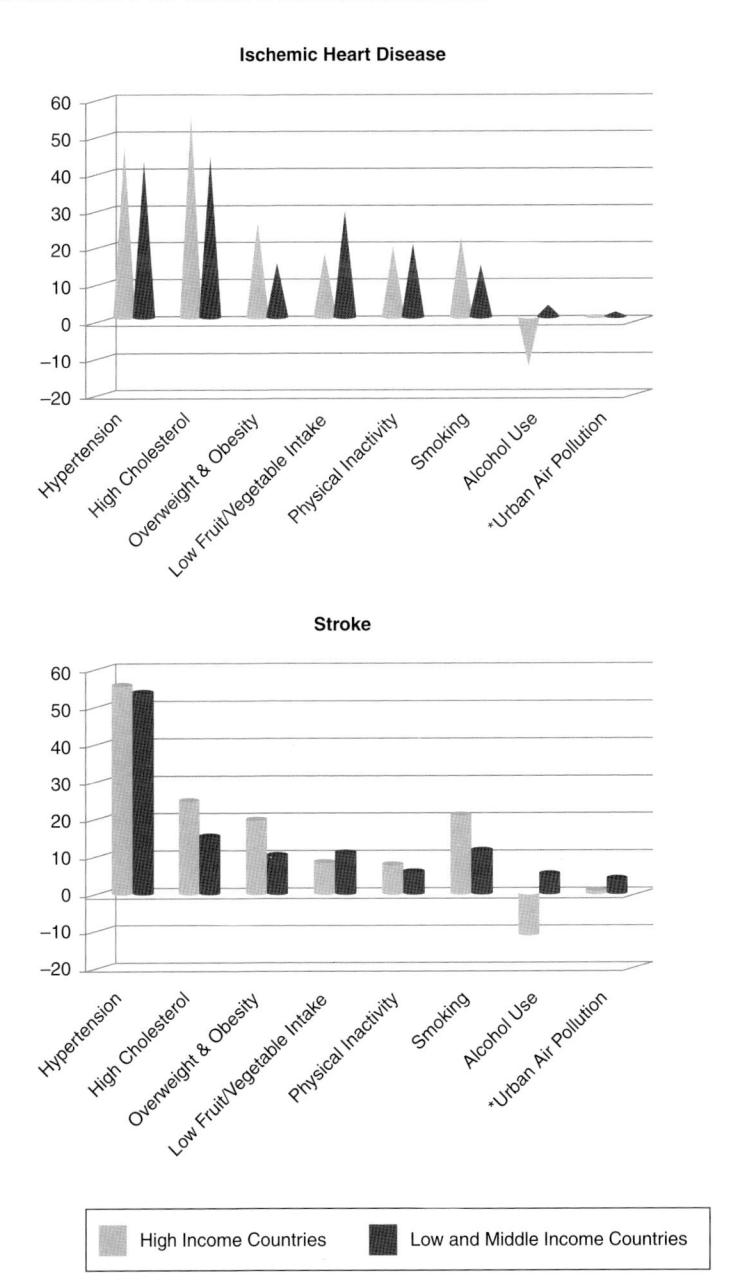

FIGURE 2.4 Contribution of selected risk factors (by PAF) to IHD and stroke burdens, 2001.
*PAFs for urban air pollution have high uncertainty.
SOURCE: Data from Lopez et al., 2006.

etary factors, alcohol, and physical activity. This is followed by the major biological risk factors that mediate the role of these behaviors in leading to CVD, including obesity, blood pressure, blood lipids, and diabetes. Finally, additional contributing factors are also discussed, including mental health, genetics, and air pollution.

Tobacco

There are currently more than 1 billion smokers worldwide. Although use of tobacco products is decreasing in high income countries, it is increasing globally, with more than 80 percent of the world's smokers now living in low and middle income countries (Jha and Chaloupka, 1999). In China alone, there are 303 million adult smokers and 530 million people passively exposed to secondhand smoke (Yang et al., 2008). Tobacco use kills 5.4 million people a year—more than the annual deaths due to tuberculosis (TB), HIV/AIDS, and malaria combined—and accounts for 1 in 10 adult deaths worldwide (Mathers and Loncar, 2006; WHO, 2009e). In the 20th century 100 million deaths were caused by tobacco, and, if current trends continue, there will be up to 1 billion deaths in the 21st century (WHO, 2008c). By 2030, researchers estimate that 80 percent of tobacco-related deaths will occur in low and middle income countries (Mathers and Loncar, 2006).

In the Global Burden of Disease study, Lopez et al. (2006) estimated that in 2000, 880,000 deaths from CHD and 412,000 deaths from stroke were attributable to tobacco. These data are based on updated estimates of the relative risk of death among smokers for CHD, stroke, and hypertensive heart disease. The relative risks are highest in young people (as found by the INTERHEART study and described earlier). However, the most common type of tobacco-related CVD deaths varies around the world. For example, in India, a higher proportion of smokers die from CHD; in China, tobacco kills more through stroke (Ezzati et al., 2005).

Smoking cessation has been shown to have significant impacts on reducing CHD. In a major review of the evidence, Critchley and Capewell (2003) determined that successful smoking cessation reduced CHD mortality risk by up to 36 percent. Smoking cessation leads to significantly lower rates of reinfarction within 1 year among patients who have had a heart attack and reduces the risk of sudden cardiac death among patients with CHD (Gritz et al., 2007). There is consensus in the literature that CVD risk drops precipitously within the first 2 to 3 years of smoking cessation. Although the specific timeline of risk reduction depends on the number of years as a smoker and the quantity of tobacco smoked daily, it is conceivable that, over time, former smokers' CVD risk can drop to levels similar to that of someone who has never smoked (Gritz et al., 2007; Mackay and Eriksen, 2002).

Two major trends are of real concern with respect to the future of tobacco-related CVD. First, in most parts of the world, the smoking rates are higher among the poorest populations (WHO, 2008c). The second worrisome trend is in smoking among girls. The disparity in smoking prevalence between boys and girls in their teenage years is much less than the ratio reported among adults from the same regions (Brands and Yach, 2002). In most parts of the developing world, women smoke at a significantly lower rate than men, a disparity that could help explain the lower rates of cardiovascular mortality among women (see the discussion of gender differences in CVD later in this chapter) (Pilote et al., 2007). However, the Global Youth Tobacco Survey found that girls smoked at the same rate as boys in more than 60 percent of the countries included in the survey (Shafey et al., 2009; Warren, 2003; Warren et al., 2008). If future generations of girls catch up to boys and smoke at the rates that men do today, CVD and associated tobacco-related death rates will rise sharply. On the other hand, if policies could instead bring both men's and women's smoking rates to below those of women today, the preventive gain would be immense.

In addition to active smoking, it has become increasingly apparent that exposure to secondhand smoke significantly increases cardiovascular risk. A recent IOM review of the effects of secondhand smoke exposure concluded that exposure to secondhand smoke significantly increases cardiovascular risk and that public smoking bans can significantly reduce the rate of heart attacks. The report concluded that secondhand smoke exposure increases cardiovascular risk by 25 to 30 percent and that there is sufficient evidence to support a causal relationship between secondhand smoke exposure and AMI. This causality was reinforced by the report's conclusion that smoking bans significantly reduce the rate of AMIs, with declines ranging from 6 to 47 percent (IOM, 2009).

Dietary Factors

The relationship between CVD and diet is one of the most studied relationships in epidemiology. Several key relationships identified decades ago remain valid, while others have evolved in the light of better-quality research. For example, current evidence does not support the use of general terms like "lipids" or "fats" without qualifying their type and considering the amount used in the diet. Although nutritional research has traditionally focused on the effect of individual food groups or nutrients on CVD, there has been a shift in recent years toward comparing how different types of dietary patterns in their entirety affect CVD risk. The following sections reflect this shift by first discussing research on oils and salt—two key dietary components that have clear and well-demonstrated impacts on CVD risk—and then moving on to a discussion of different dietary patterns and CVD risk.

WHO and FAO reviewed the evidence on the relationship between diet, physical activity, and CVD in the context of a broader review of the impact on all chronic diseases (Joint WHO/FAO Expert Consultation, 2003). The most convincing evidence for decreasing dietary risk involves addressing the following factors: reducing saturated fat intake, maintaining low to moderate intake of alcohol, and increasing the consumption of linoleic acid, fish and fish oils, vegetables and fruits, and potassium. On the other hand, intake of myristic and palmitic acids, transfatty acids, high levels of sodium, overweight, and heavy alcohol use increase the risk of CVD (Joint WHO/FAO Expert Consultation, 2003). Recent evidence augments this list with the addition of whole grains, nuts, beans, and seeds (Danaei et al., 2009). The evidence for these dietary factors is derived from studies in developed and, increasingly, developing countries.

As described earlier, the analysis and interpretation of dietary factors has been hampered by the poor availability of high-quality data for detecting broad-based trends. Data derived from actual consumption surveys (such as the U.S. National Health and Nutrition Examination Survey [NHANES] data) are important if we are to base policy on evidence. However, few countries provide basic data on the contribution of various food groups to the total intake of calories, sodium, or other major nutrients of interest to CVD. Improved data about details of the contribution of major food groups to diets around the world are needed to better inform future agricultural policy and gain a more accurate picture of how changes in consumption affect CVD risk.

Oils[1]   As discussed earlier, the rapid rise in the production and consumption of tropical oils has worried many CVD researchers because of their adverse effects on CVD risk. Healthy oils are those that contain no commercially introduced transfatty acids, are low in saturated fatty acids, and are high in mono- and polyunsaturated fatty acids (see Figure 2.5 for a comparison of the fatty acid composition and shelf life of selected cooking oils). Nutritionally, the most important mono- and polyunsaturated fatty acids are oleic acid and linoleic acid, respectively. Olive and canola oils have high concentrations of oleic acid, whereas nonhydrogenated soybean oils and sunflower oils have high concentrations of linoleic acid. All four of these oils are also low in saturated and transfats, but their shelf lives and cooking properties (smoke point, flavor, etc.) vary. High- and mid-oleic

---

[1] This section is based in part on a paper written for the committee by Mehmood Khan and George A. Mensah.

sunflower oils both have long shelf lives, but unfortunately they remain relatively expensive and less abundant in many low and middle income countries. In order to be truly effective, low and middle income countries that have high levels of oil consumption will need to develop affordable supplies of healthy oils at prices that are competitive with tropical oils (Khan and Mensah, 2009).

Transitioning from less healthful tropical oils to more healthful oils could significantly reduce the amount of saturated and transfatty acids used in highly processed foods and daily cooking. However, such a transition is challenging because the relatively low price of palm oil drives its predominance in oil production. In order to transition away from tropical oils, there is a need to find or develop oils that are healthful and have favorable cooking properties but are also affordable and have a long shelf life. Some countries, such as Argentina, Chile, Brazil, and Turkey, have had modest success in increasing the availability and reducing the costs of healthful oils through oilseed plantation and production projects. Other initiatives have had less success, such as in Peru, where pilot programs concluded that low yields and high costs make the transition unprofitable (Khan and Mensah, 2009).

In sum, the challenge of transitioning to healthier oils highlights a critical need for agricultural policy and production to be better aligned with a heart-healthy diet. Dramatic changes in the food supply in developing countries have occurred over the past two decades. Changes in agricultural opportunities and investments have driven many of these changes, without careful consideration of the system-wide impacts on CVD. Further, the sharp increases in palm oil deserve special focus given the ubiquity of palm oil use, especially in emerging economies where its relatively low price acts as a barrier to the development and production of heart-healthier oils. The rationale for supporting transitions to more healthful oils is discussed further in Chapter 5.

Salt There is a strong and robust base of evidence that excessive sodium intake significantly increases CVD risk and that reduction in sodium intake on a population level decreases CVD burden (He and MacGregor, 2009). The most well-established mechanism by which sodium intake increases CVD risk is by increasing blood pressure. Numerous studies have found that there is a continuous and graded relationship between salt intake and blood pressure. This relationship has been confirmed in epidemiological, animal, population, migration, intervention, and genetic studies. Furthermore, population studies have established that reductions in sodium intake lead to declines in systolic and diastolic blood pressure, which in turn leads to a decrease in heart attacks and strokes (He and MacGregor, 2009). For example, since the 1970s, salt intake in Finland has been reduced by ap-

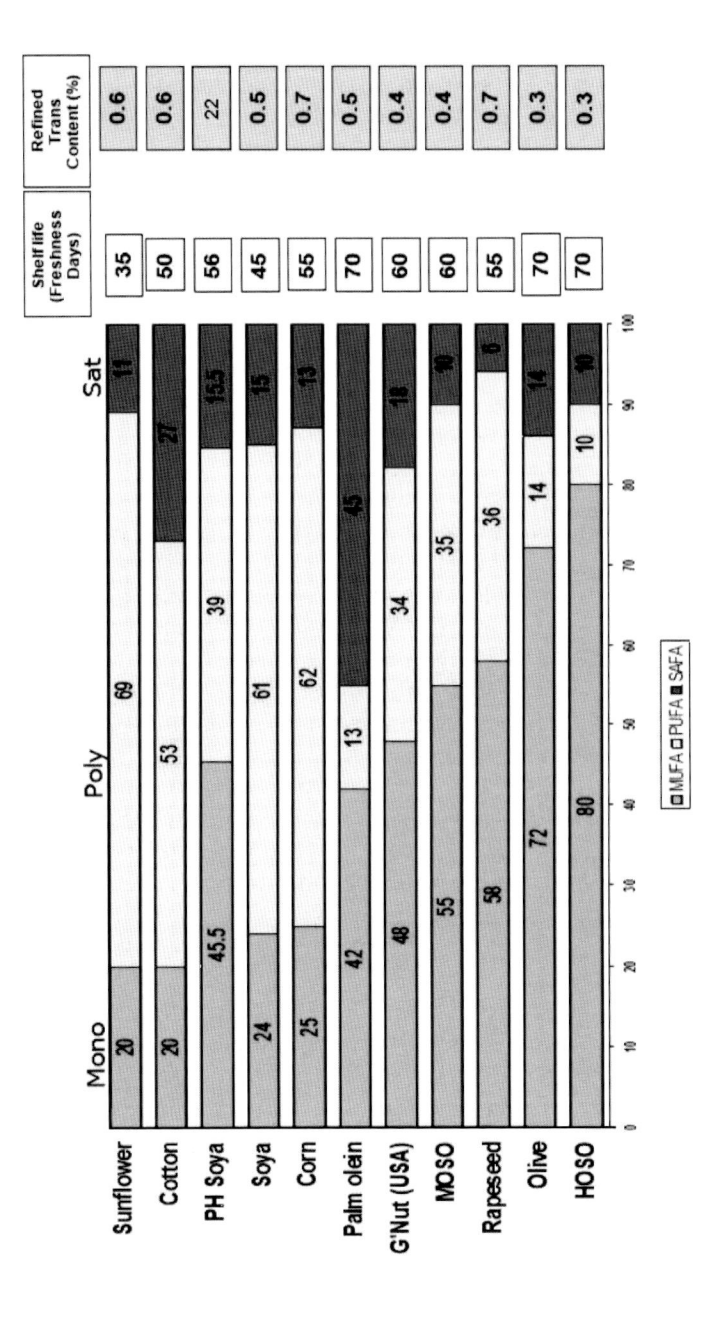

FIGURE 2.5 Fatty acid content and shelf life of selected oils used in the food industry.
SOURCE: Khan and Mensah, 2009.

proximately one-third. This has led to a reduction in systolic and diastolic blood pressure (BP) by more than 10 mmHg (Karppanen and Mervaala, 2006). In their recent major review of sodium trends and impact, He and MacGregor concluded that a reduction in salt from the current global intake of 9 to 12 g/day to the recommended levels of 5-6 g/day would have a major impact on BP and on CVD (He and MacGregor, 2009). Salt's impact on CVD, however, extends beyond blood pressure. Animal and epidemiological studies have found that a diet high in sodium may directly increase risk of stroke, which is independent and additive to salt's effect on BP (He and MacGregor, 2009).

Dietary Patterns The effect on CVD risk of diets rich in whole grains and low in processed foods that are high in fat, sodium, and sugars has been increasingly investigated in both developed and developing countries. In parallel with economic development, radical dietary shifts toward Westernized diets that are high in animal products and refined carbohydrates and low in whole grains and other plant-based foods have occurred in many developing countries (Hu, 2008). In the INTERHEART study, three major dietary patterns were identified: Oriental (high intake of tofu and soy); Western (high in fried foods, salty snacks, eggs, and meat); and prudent (high in fruits and vegetables). The Western dietary pattern was associated with an increased risk of CHD in all regions of the world, whereas the prudent pattern was associated with a lower risk (Iqbal et al., 2008).

Substantial evidence has accumulated to support the notion that the traditional Mediterranean dietary pattern is protective against CVD (Fung et al., 2009; Martinez-Gonzalez et al., 2009). This pattern is characterized by an abundance of fruits, vegetables, whole grain cereals, nuts, and legumes; olive oil as the principal source of fat; moderate consumption of fish; lower consumption of red meat; and moderate consumption of alcohol. It is important to note, however, that the dominance in research on the Mediterranean diet has come at the cost of research on other diets commonly consumed around the world that may also have heart health benefits. A review of PubMed, Google Scholar, and EBSCOhost indicated that the Mediterranean, American/Western, Japanese and prudent diets were by far the most common dietary patterns studied, while very few researchers focused on other Asian, South American, or Middle Eastern diets. Comparative studies of whole diets constitute an important neglected research area with potentially profound implications for policy development.

Alcohol

The global burden of diseases attributable to alcohol has recently been summarized, leading to the conclusion that alcohol is one the largest avoidable risk factors in low and middle income countries (Rehm et al., 2009). Indeed, WHO estimates that the harmful use of alcohol was responsible for 3.8 percent of deaths and 4.5 percent of the global burden of disease in 2004 (WHO, 2009b). In the past few decades, consumption of alcohol has increased dramatically in men in countries undergoing nutrition transition, such as India and China, and has been extremely high in Russia for many decades, where it contributes significantly to overall mortality among men (WHO Expert Committee on Problems Related to Alcohol Consumption and WHO, 2007).

It has long been known that excessive alcohol intake is associated with increased risk for hypertension, stroke, coronary artery disease, and other forms of CVD; however, there is also a robust body of evidence in a range of populations that suggests that light to moderate intake of alcohol may reduce the risk of CHD. Indeed, research suggests that the relationship between alcohol intake and CVD outcomes follows a "J" curve, with the lowest rates being associated with low to moderate intakes of alcohol (Beilin and Puddey, 2006; Lucas et al., 2005). This protective effect of low to moderate intake has been replicated in numerous studies, across populations and gender, and persists even when controlling for potential confounders such as the "sick quitter" effect (Anand et al., 2008; Mukamal and Rimm, 2001; Yusuf et al., 2004). The definition of "low to moderate" continues to be a subject of debate; however, given the totality of the evidence, a prudent recommendation appears to be no more than one drink per day for women and no more than two drinks per day for men (Beilin and Puddey, 2006; Lucas et al., 2005; Mukamal et al., 2006).

It is important to recognize that, as with any discussion of alcohol and health, the key issues are the quantity of alcohol consumed and the risk or benefit conferred by consumption. Although evidence indicates that low to moderate alcohol use can reduce the risk of CHD, excessive and harmful use clearly increases CVD risk (Beilin and Puddey, 2006; Lucas et al., 2005). Alcohol may also contribute to overweight and obesity as it is a significant source of daily calories in many countries (Foster and Marriott, 2006; Jequier, 1999). It is also important to consider the demonstrated negative health effects of excessive and harmful alcohol use on other diseases such as neuropsychiatric disorders, cirrhosis of the liver, and various cancers. Taking into account these factors, it is important that approaches to reduce the burden of CVD not neglect the importance of reducing excessive alcohol consumption. WHO has proposed interventions for alcohol that are being considered in developing a global strategy for alcohol control. These include pricing policies, restricting the sale of alcohol, drunk-driving countermeasures, restrictions on marketing, awareness and education, and access to effective treatment (WHO, 2009d).

Physical Activity

WHO and FAO highlighted the importance of physical activity as a key determinant of obesity, CVD, and diabetes (Joint WHO/FAO Expert Consultation, 2003). For decades, evidence of the relationship between physical activity and CVD, independent of effects on weight and obesity, has strengthened. Increasing physical activity—including through brisk walking—has been shown to decrease the risk of chronic diseases such as CHD, stroke, some cancers (e.g., colorectal and breast cancer), type 2 diabetes, osteoporosis, high blood pressure, and high cholesterol (Physical Activity Guidelines Advisory Committee, 2008). Physical activity is also important for weight control and maintenance. In addition, regular physical activity is associated with a decreased risk of depression and improved cognitive function. Moreover, people who are physically active have improved quality of life and reduced risk of premature death (Physical Activity Guidelines Advisory Committee, 2008). Despite this powerful evidence, measurement weaknesses have contributed to the generally poor quality and availability of data on worldwide physical activity trends and impacts.

Guthold et al. (2008) recently published new data on levels of physical inactivity in 51 countries, most of which were low or middle income, and observed several trends. Globally, with the exception of several Eastern European countries (Croatia, the Czech Republic, Hungary, Kazakhstan, the Russian Federation, Slovenia, and the Ukraine), women were more likely to be physically inactive than men. Further, adults over 50 years of age were more likely to be inactive than younger adults, and city dwellers were more likely to be inactive than those who lived in rural areas. Physical inactivity levels were, with a few exceptions, similar in Eastern European, South Asian, and Western Pacific countries. In most of these countries, between 5 and 10 percent of men and between 10 and 16 percent of women were found to be physically inactive. By contrast, there was considerable variation in the levels of physical activity in both men and women within and across African, American, and Eastern European countries. For example, while women in 7 of the 18 African countries surveyed had the lowest levels of physical inactivity (fewer than 10 percent classified as physically inactive), Guthold found that more than 40 percent of women in Namibia, Swaziland, and South Africa were physically inactive. Despite the heterogeneity of the data, the study indicated that levels of physical inactivity in a number of low and middle income countries and among certain subgroups, particularly women aged 60-69 years, are disconcertingly high.

Few studies have explored the reasons why levels of physical activity are declining in developing countries. Therefore, the recent work by Ng et al. (2009) from China is important. The authors estimate that, between 1991 and 2006, average weekly physical activity among adults fell by 32 percent. This period was associated with rapid urbanization (especially improved housing and transport infrastructure) and industrialization leading to profound shifts in how people in China eat, move, and work. Meanwhile, sedentary behaviors such as prolonged television watching have increased dramatically. Many aspects of improving quality of life (such as better educational and sanitation facilities) were strongly associated with declines in physical activity, suggesting that multisectoral approaches involving workplace, transit, school, and leisure time need to be tackled if the trends are to be reversed. For this to happen, health professionals and policy makers need to fully appreciate the value of physical activity, both as a means to address energy balance and as an important avoidable cause of the global burden of chronic diseases. Currently this is not the case in most countries.

Overweight and Obesity

Another broad trend related to physical activity and nutrition, especially excess calorie intake, is obesity and overweight. This topic was not raised as an important issue at the inception of the Framingham Study, possibly because population levels of overweight in the 1940s were relatively low. It was also only briefly mentioned in the 1998 IOM report. During the past several decades, however, there have been steady increases in levels of overweight and obesity reported from developed and developing countries (Sassi et al., 2009). Even in low and middle income countries where undernutrition is still highly prevalent, overweight and obesity—especially among women—is a bourgeoning issue (Caballero, 2005). For instance, in South Africa, 59 percent of women and 29 percent of men over age 15 are overweight or obese (South African Department of Health and Medical Research Council, 2007). In China, trend lines for obesity are going up fairly sharply among all geographic groups in communities of all sizes, from rural villages to megacities (Wang et al., 2007). As described in more detail in Chapter 6, rates of overweight and obesity in children are also rising in low and middle income countries (WHO, 2008a).

As mentioned earlier, WHO and FAO reviewed the evidence on the relationship between obesity and the risk of CVD and concluded that overweight and obesity confer a significantly elevated risk of CHD (Joint WHO/FAO Expert Consultation, 2003). Increased body mass index (BMI) is also associated with greater risk of stroke in both Asian and Western populations (WHO/FAO, 2003). The association between obesity and CVD is partly, but not completely, mediated through hypertension, high cholesterol, and diabetes. Abdominal or central obesity measured by waist-to-hip ratio or waist circumference is associated with both CHD and stroke independent of BMI and other cardiovascular risk factors. Moreover, obesity is also an independent risk factor for other cardiovascular outcomes, such as congestive heart failure and sudden cardiac death.

Excess energy intake is one of the key contributors to obesity. As highlighted earlier, the lack of data limits policy makers' abilities to focus attention on which dietary components lend themselves to effective interventions that would reduce total calorie intake. In those countries that do have data, the collection methods vary so direct comparisons are not possible; however, a review of the data does indicate that the dietary contributors to total energy intake vary by country. National surveys of calorie intake from India indicate that in urban areas, cereals account for 56 percent of intake, compared to about 9 percent each for edible oils and dairy, 1 percent for meat and fish, and 0.4 percent for all beverages (Chatterjee et al., 2007). In China, cereals also dominate and account for 58 percent of total calorie intake compared to meat (13 percent) and cooking oils (17 percent) (Wang et al., 2005). As discussed earlier, trends in consumption indicate very rapid increases in oil use and slow decline in the consumption of cereals as contributors to calories. These trends in developing countries are in contrast to data for the United Kingdom, which could indicate where trends are headed in developing countries. National data from 2003 indicate that cereals and related products account for 31 percent of calories with other major categories including meat (15 percent), milk and related products (19 percent), and beverages (10 percent) (Office of National Statistics et al., 2003).

One category that has been well studied in developed countries relates to sugar consumption, primarily in the form of sugar-sweetened beverages (including soft drinks, juice drinks, and energy and vitamin water drinks). Recent NHANES data shows that up to 5.5 percent of dietary calories come from sugar-sweetened beverages in the United States (Bosire et al., 2009), which has led the American Heart Association to recommend an upper limit of 100 calories per day for women and 150 calories per day for men from added sugars, including soft drinks (Johnson et al., 2009).

In some developing countries, consumption of sugar-sweetened beverages has increased dramatically in recent decades. In Mexico, for example, it is estimated that adolescents consume more than 20 percent of their total energy intake from caloric beverages (Barquera et al., 2008). Because of its excess caloric and sugar content, increasing consumption of sugar-sweetened beverages may have important implications for obesity and cardiometabolic risk. Maintaining the relatively low per capita consumption of sugar-sweetened beverages in countries like India and China is a potential target of prevention programs. In India, all beverages account for less than 0.5 percent of total calories (Chatterjee et al., 2007). The equivalent figure in the United Kingdom is about 16 percent for all beverages for young adult men between 19 and 24 years of age with sweetened soft drinks accounting for about a third and alcohol the remainder (Henderson et al., 2003). This indicates how critical it is to have national and even age- and gender-specific data if we are to develop effective nutrition messages and policies.

In summary, obesity has become a major global contributor to CVD incidence and mortality. It needs to be placed more centrally within future CVD policy initiatives. Better data on the sources of calorie intake and especially those calories that are high in salt, sugar, and saturated fat are also needed in order to develop science-based approaches to obesity prevention and control.

Blood Pressure

A recent review of the global burden of high blood pressure found that approximately 54 percent of stroke, 47 percent of IHD, 75 percent of hypertensive disease, and 25 percent of other CVDs were attributable to hypertension. This equates to an annual burden of approximately 7.6 million deaths, or 13.5 percent of the total number of annual global deaths, attributable to high blood pressure (Lawes et al., 2008). Furthermore, Lawes et al. (2008) found that more than 80 percent of the attributable burden of hypertension in 2001 occurred in low and middle income countries, and both another recent review and an analysis commissioned for this report found the prevalence of hypertension to be equally high in developed and developing countries (Gaziano and Kim, 2009; Pereira et al., 2009).

In China alone, it is estimated that the current age-standardized prevalence rate of hypertension is 17.7 percent, which translates into 177 million people, and that approximately 20 percent of deaths in China are attributable to high blood pressure (He et al., 2009; Yang, 2008). A significant contributor to these levels is the high average daily salt intake in China, which is estimated at 12 g per day—twice the Chinese and WHO recommended levels. Further, only 30 percent of adults with hypertension are aware of their condition, and of those only 6 percent manage their hypertension effectively (Yang et al., 2008). While antihypertensive medications have become more effective, their widespread use remains low and the number of people with uncontrolled blood pressure is increasing (Chobanian, 2009).

In Sub-Saharan Africa, hypertension is a predominant driver of CVD. Hypertensive heart disease and stroke, rather than ischemic heart disease, account for the majority of the CVD burden in the region, especially among black Africans (Mayosi et al., 2009; Mbewu and Mbanya, 2006; Muna, 1993). Prevalence of hypertension is particularly high in urban Sub-Saharan Africa, with between 8 and 25 percent of adults affected, depending on how hypertension is defined (Mbewu and Mbanya, 2006). In South Africa, the 2003 Demographic and Health Survey found that 12.5 percent of men and 17.9 percent of women were hypertensive (South African Department of Health and Medical Research Council, 2007). Unfortunately, the number of people with uncontrolled hypertension is also high in the region (Mbewu and Mbanya, 2006). Researchers found that more than 70 percent of South African hypertensive patients' blood pressure remained uncontrolled (South African Department of Health and Medical Research Council, 2007).

Among the major underlying risks for hypertension are sodium, body weight, and access to treatment (He and MacGregor, 2009; Reuser et al., 2009; Steyn, 2006; Yang et al., 2008). Primary prevention focused on sodium reduction, fruit and vegetable intake, weight control, and avoidance of excessive alcohol intake has been shown to make a difference. Finland's experience (Karppanen and Mervaala, 2006) has potential applications for low and middle income countries where treatment levels remain extremely low and health systems have yet to adapt to managing chronic diseases like hypertension.

Blood Lipids

Researchers have studied the role of blood lipids in the development of atherosclerosis and the increase of CVD risk for decades. The Framingham Study first demonstrated the link between hypercholesterolemia and increased risk of CHD in the 1960s with the finding that lower levels of high-density lipoprotein (HDL) cholesterol as well as elevated levels of low-density lipoprotein (LDL) cholesterol were associated with increased CHD risk (Kannel et al., 1961, 1971). Subsequent studies confirmed these results and further established that elevated triglycerides also increase CVD risk (Gotto, 2005; Manninen et al., 1992). Furthermore, randomized controlled trials have shown that reduction of LDL cholesterol, both in primary and secondary prevention, is associated with reduced coronary event rates (Downs et al., 1998; Sacks et al., 1996; Shepherd et al., 1995). Reductions in LDL cholesterol have also been associated with a lowered incidence of stroke, although the data are not as strong as for CHD (Collins et al., 2004). In addition, lipoprotein(a) (Lp(a)) is an LDL–like particle that was independently associated with CHD and stroke in a recent comprehensive meta-analysis (Erqou et al., 2009).

The INTERHEART study recently confirmed that there was a graded relationship between abnormal lipid levels and risk for CHD in all regions of the world. In fact, the INTERHEART study found that abnormal blood lipids were the most important risk factor for myocardial infarction by odds ratio in all global regions (Yusuf et al., 2004). Further underscoring this, the Global Burden of Disease study estimated that elevated cholesterol was the third leading risk factor for worldwide mortality in general, after hypertension and smoking (Lopez et al., 2006).

While it is clear that dyslipidemia is one of the leading risk factors for CVD, there is significant regional variation in the prevalence of hyperlipidemia. Hypercholesterolemia was found in 22 percent of subjects enrolled in the Heart of Soweto study of patients with newly diagnosed CVD in South Africa (Sliwa et al., 2008). In Mongolia, the Ministry of Health, in collaboration with WHO, performed a STEPS survey across the country and reported 7 percent prevalence of hypercholesterolemia (WHO Regional Office for the Western Pacific, 2007). In contrast, a nationally representative population-based study in Iran found the prevalence of hypercholesterolemia to be more than 45 percent (Alikhani et al., 2009). In accordance with this geographic variability in the prevalence of hypercholesterolemia, the population-attributable risk of dyslipidemia for CHD in the INTERHEART study varied widely by geographic region (Yusuf et al., 2004). Although systematic data specifically regarding Lp(a) and its relationship to CVD among different populations around the world are lacking, levels have been shown to vary among different ethnic groups; in general, Asian Indians have higher Lp(a) levels than ethnic Chinese and Caucasian populations (Anand et al., 1998, 2000; Low et al., 1996). In addition, African Americans have higher average Lp(a) levels than Caucasians (Marcovina et al., 1996; Srinivasan et al., 1991), and studies in Africa have also shown higher average Lp(a) levels than in Caucasians (Evans et al., 1997).

Successful intervention programs in a number of countries have further supported the causal link between dyslipidemia and CVD by demonstrating that reductions in cholesterol lead to decreased CVD morbidity and mortality. In Finland, a nationwide multisectoral program targeted at multiple cardiovascular risk factors decreased population mean serum cholesterol levels as well as CVD mortality between 1972 and 1992 (Puska et al., 1998; Vartiainen et al., 1994a). These reductions in cholesterol were largely credited to reductions in saturated fat intake as well as more comprehensive cholesterol monitoring and treatment (Puska et al., 2009). Further analysis showed that among men the 13 percent reduction in cholesterol levels was singlehandedly responsible for a 26 percent reduction in CVD mortality (Vartiainen et al., 1994b). The proven success of interventions to reduce cholesterol has shifted thinking on the inevitability of atherosclerosis, with researchers now realizing that it is not an unavoidable byproduct of aging, but rather that it can be prevented and largely reversed through the use of diet modification and secondary prevention with statins.

Diabetes

Around the world, diabetes is growing increasingly common and is a significant contributor to CVD risk. People with diabetes have a more than two-fold greater risk of fatal and nonfatal CVD compared to non-diabetics, with some indication that diabetes mellitus may confer an equivalent risk of having had a cardiovascular event (Asia Pacific Cohort Studies Collaboration, 2003; Haffner et al., 1998; Stamler et al., 1993). In fact, CVD is the leading cause of morbidity and mortality in people with diabetes (Booth et al., 2006a; Diabetologia, 2007; Kengne et al., 2007, 2009; Thomas et al., 2003).

The magnitude of the risk of CVD associated with diabetes is even greater in women and younger individuals. Indeed, there is substantial evidence that diabetes mellitus may erase, or substantially attenuate, the "female advantage" in the risk of CVD observed in non-diabetics, and that having diabetes may be equivalent to aging by at least 15 years with regard to the clinical manifestations of CVD (Booth et al., 2006b; Huxley et al., 2006).

Cardiovascular risk associated with blood glucose is continuous; thus, individuals without established clinical diabetes, but who are at increased risk of developing diabetes in the future, also have a higher risk of CVD (Asia Pacific Cohort Studies Collaboration, 2004). Based on this continuous association, higher-than-optimum blood glucose (fasting plasma glucose > 4.9 mmol/l) has been identified as the leading cause of cardiovascular deaths in most regions (Danaei et al., 2006). In 2001, for instance, 1.49 million deaths from IHD (21 percent of all IHD deaths) and 709,000 from stroke (13 percent of all stroke deaths) were attributable to high blood glucose in addition to the 950,000 deaths directly attributed to diabetes mellitus in the world (Danaei et al., 2006). These figures are particularly worrisome given that it is estimated that more than 344 million people around the world will have impaired glucose tolerance in 2010 (IDF, 2006).

Obesity is the single most important risk factor for type 2 diabetes, but unhealthy diet and physical inactivity also independently raise the population risk for diabetes (Schulze and Hu, 2005). According to the International Diabetes Federation's Diabetes Atlas 2010, the global estimated prevalence of diabetes for 2010 among people aged 20 to 79 years will be approximately 285 million people (6.4 percent of the global population), of which some 70 percent will be living in developing countries (International Diabetes Federation, 2010). By 2030 this figure is expected to increase by more than 50 percent to some 438 million people, or 7.7 of the world's population if preventive interventions are not put in place. The largest increases will take place in the regions dominated by developing economies (see Figure 2.6). Close to 4 million deaths in the same age group will be attributable to diabetes in 2010, representing 6.8 percent of all-cause global mortality. The highest number of deaths due to diabetes are expected to occur in countries with large populations—1,008,000 deaths in India, 575,000 in China, 231,000 in the United States, and 182,000 in the Russian Federation (Roglic and Unwin, 2010). Currently, 83 percent of all diabetes deaths occur in low and middle income countries (WHO, 2009b).

Diabetes is emerging as a particular concern in Asia, where more than 110 million individuals were living with diabetes in 2007, a large proportion of whom were young and middle aged. Asians tend to develop diabetes at a relatively young age and low BMI, and by 2025 the number of individuals with diabetes in the region is expected to rise to almost 180 million, of which approximately 70 million will be in India and almost 60 million in China (Chan et al., 2009). The reasons for this increased risk are still being fully elucidated; however, "normal weight" Asians often exhibit features of abdominal or central obesity, which is particularly detrimental to insulin resistance and glucose metabolism. Moreover, the increased risk of gestational diabetes combined with exposure to poor nutrition in utero and overnutrition in later life may contribute to increased diabetes, resulting in a situation of "diabetes begetting diabetes" (Chan et al., 2009).

The balance of risks and benefits associated with intensive glucose control has been assessed in recent clinical trials, which have convincingly demonstrated beneficial microvascular outcomes of diabetes. By contrast, these trials have individually failed to show such an effect on cardiovascular outcomes. However, the extension of the follow-up of the Diabetes Control and Complications Trial in type 1 diabetes (Nathan et al., 2005) and the United Kingdom Prospective Diabetes Study in type 2 diabetes (Holman et al., 2008) have shown that intensive glucose control substantially lowered the risk of cardiovascular outcomes, suggesting a legacy effect with still unexplained underlying mechanisms. Recently conducted meta-analyses of relevant trials in people with type 2 diabetes have also consistently shown that intensive glucose control reduces the risk of major cardiovascular events by approximately 10 percent, primarily driven by a 10 to 15 percent reduction in the risk of CHD, compared with standard treatment in people with diabetes. Interestingly, this benefit appeared to be independent of concurring cardiovascular risk factors (Kelly et al., 2009; Ray et al., 2009; Stettler et al., 2006; Turnbull et al., 2009).

In sum, as with the escalating obesity epidemic, the prevalence of diabetes has increased dramatically worldwide. It is associated with serious health consequences and is a major risk factor for CHD and stroke. As such, prevention and management of diabetes are critical in reducing the global burden of CVD.

Psychosocial Risk and Mental Health

Psychosocial factors have been consistently associated with both the onset and the progression of CVD in large prospective and epidemiologic studies in multiple populations and regions, yet they remain underrecognized when compared with more traditional CVD risk factors. The factors that have been associated with CVD include depression, anxiety, anger, hostility, acute and chronic life stressors, and lack of social support (Everson-

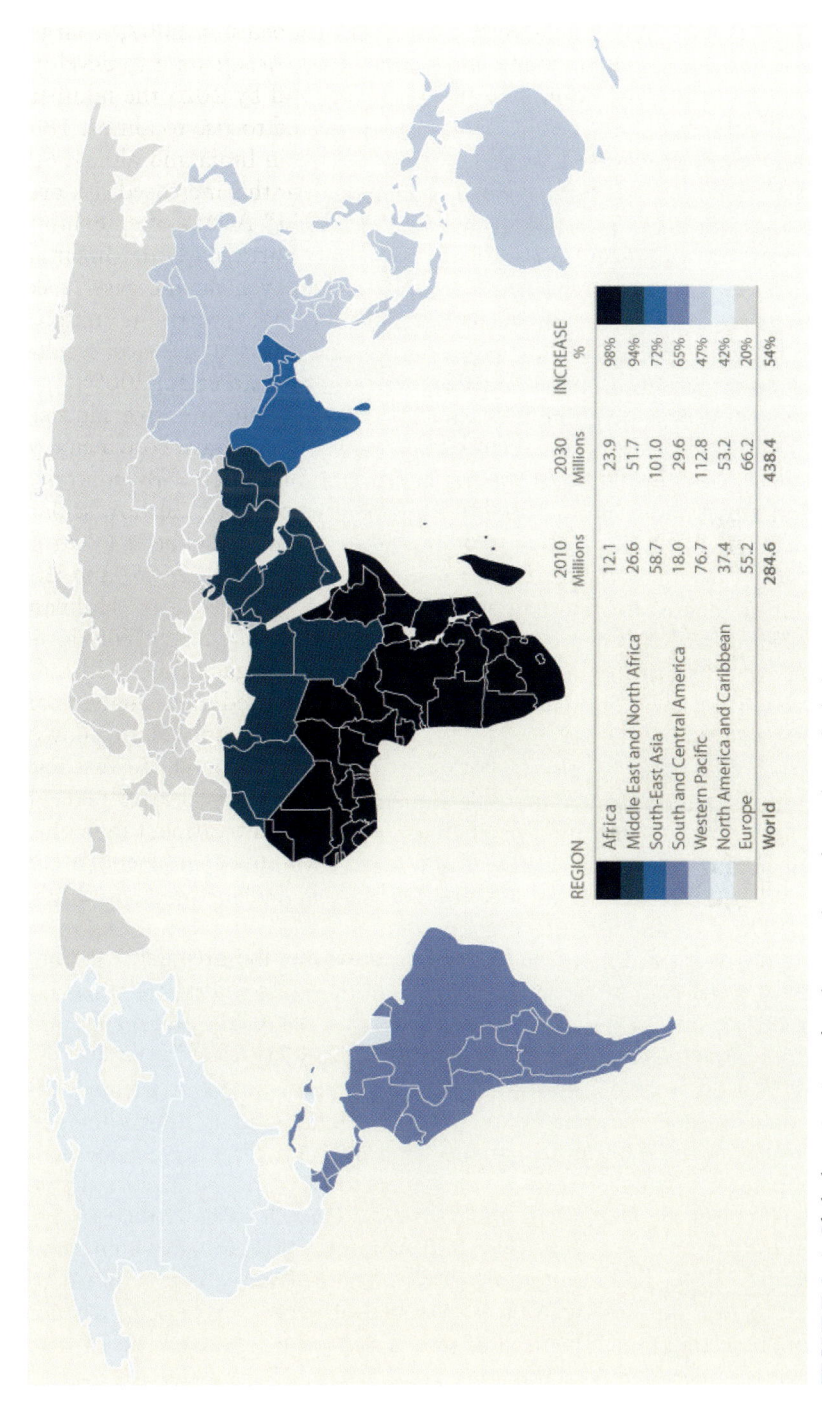

REGION	2010 Millions	2030 Millions	INCREASE %
Africa	12.1	23.9	98%
Middle East and North Africa	26.6	51.7	94%
South-East Asia	58.7	101.0	72%
South and Central America	18.0	29.6	65%
Western Pacific	76.7	112.8	47%
North America and Caribbean	37.4	53.2	42%
Europe	55.2	66.2	20%
World	284.6	438.4	54%

FIGURE 2.6 Global projections for the number of people with diabetes (20-79 years), 2010-2030.
SOURCE: International Diabetes Atlas, 4th edition, © International Diabetes Federation, 2010.

Rose and Lewis, 2005; Figueredo, 2009; Shen et al., 2008). Although the causal pathways are not as well elucidated as for other risk factors, a robust body of evidence supports the conclusion that psychosocial factors independently and significantly increase both the risk of developing CVD and CVD morbidity and mortality.

Of all the psychosocial stressors associated with CVD, the link between depression and CVD is probably the best documented. There have been more than 100 published reviews and numerous meta-analyses since the early 1990s that have consistently found that depression and depressive symptoms are associated with an increased likelihood of developing CVD, a higher incidence of CVD events, poorer outcomes after CVD treatment and prevention efforts, and increased mortality from CVD. These associations remain even after controlling for other CVD risk factors and most studies have found a dose-response relationship between severity of depression and depressive symptoms and the frequency and severity of cardiac events (Everson-Rose and Lewis, 2005; Frasure-Smith and Lesperance, 2006; Glassman et al., 2003; Lesperance and Frasure-Smith, 2007; Lichtman et al., 2008; Rugulies, 2002). In one meta-analysis, Rugulies (2002) found that clinical depression increased risk of MI or coronary death by more than 2.5-fold and that depressed mood increased the likelihood of a future cardiac event by approximately 1.5-fold.

Depression and depressive symptoms are also associated with behaviors that increase CVD risk. Depressed patients are more likely to smoke, have poor diets, and be physically inactive. Furthermore, depression has been found to significantly increase the risk of nonadherence to medical treatment regiments and lifestyle changes, making depressed patients with CVD or high CVD risk less likely to adhere to prevention efforts (Lichtman et al., 2008; Ziegelstein et al., 2000). This has significant implications as most CVD risk-reduction interventions require patients to adopt long-term lifestyle changes or remain on risk factor–lowering medications for long periods of time. Poor adherence to long-term therapies for chronic diseases significantly reduces their effectiveness, increases the cost of treatment, and leads to a higher disease burden (Sabaté et al., 2003).

Depression is also significantly more common among patients with CVD than among the general population. Depression is approximately three times more common in patients after an AMI than among the general population, and between 15 and 20 percent of hospitalized patients with CHD meet the *Diagnostic and Statistical Manual of Mental Disorders* criteria for major depression (Burg and Abrams, 2001; Frasure-Smith and Lesperance, 2006; Lichtman et al., 2008). The evidence for this link is so compelling that the American Heart Association recently released a science advisory asserting that "the need to screen and treat depression [in cardiac patients] is imperative" (Lichtman et al., 2008, p. 1769).

Anger, hostility, anxiety, chronic and acute stress, and lack of social support have all been associated with increased CVD morbidity and mortality. Numerous studies dating back to the 1950s have linked individuals with so-called type A personalities (extremely hard driving, ambitious, competitive, time-urgent, and unusually quick-tempered) with increased risk of developing CHD (Everson-Rose and Lewis, 2005; Shen et al., 2008). General anxiety has been linked to increased risk of sudden cardiac death, as well as increased CVD morbidity, especially among men. Chronic stress, most often studied by examining work-related stress, has been associated with negative behaviors such as low physical activity and poor diet, increased likelihood of recurrent CVD, as well as physiological consequences such as decreased heart rate variability. Acute stress from traumatic life events such as the death of a relative, earthquakes, or terrorist attacks have all been associated with significant temporal increases in the incidence of MI (Everson-Rose and Lewis, 2005; Figueredo, 2009).

The varied psychosocial factors that have been associated with CVD are believed to effect CVD risk through largely the same direct (physiological) and indirect (nonphysiological) mechanisms. There is also a high degree of clustering of psychosocial risk factors, with individuals often experiencing multiple psychosocial conditions at once. Although the definitive causal physiological pathways by which psychosocial factors increase CVD morbidity and mortality have not been elucidated, there is consensus within the research community around several hypotheses. Psychosocial stressors have been shown to activate several nervous system pathways, such as the hypothalamic-pituitary-adrenocortical (HPA) axis as well as alter hormonal and pro-inflammatory secretions. All these responses have been shown to contribute to atherogenesis. Furthermore, as discussed earlier, psychosocial factors have also been associated with higher prevalence of unhealthy behaviors such as smoking, alcohol abuse, poor diet, physical inactivity, and nonadherence to medical regimens, thus representing an indirect means of increasing CVD risk (Everson-Rose and Lewis, 2005; Figueredo, 2009; Lesperance and Frasure-Smith, 2007; Lichtman et al., 2008).

While the associations between psychosocial factors and CVD have been found in numerous studies in a variety of different populations, the majority of these studies were conducted in high income countries with mostly male, Caucasian samples. Women and diverse ethnic groups have been underrepresented, and limited research has been conducted in low and middle income countries. There are, however, a few examples of studies examining the association between psychosocial factors and CVD in low and middle income countries and non-Caucasian, mixed-gender samples. Sarker and Mukhopadhyay (2008) examined stress among the Bhuttia population in Sikkim, India, and found that perceived psychosocial stress significantly affected blood pressure as well as the ratio of total cholesterol over HDL cholesterol in both males and females. The INTERHEART study found that psychosocial risk factors (measured by answers to questions assessing levels of financial stress, work and home stress, major life events in the past year, and presence of depression) were significantly associated with increased risk of MI in all global regions and across gender and ethnic groups. Indeed, of the nine risk factors examined, psychosocial risk factors were the fourth most significant factor in the risk of MI globally in terms of population-attributable risk, and they appear to be particularly influential in China, North America, Western Europe, the Middle East, and Africa (Rosengren et al., 2004).

It is clear that psychosocial factors play an important role in increasing CVD risk through both direct and indirect means. Continued research is needed to further elucidate the mechanisms by which psychosocial stressors and mental illness affect CVD risk. It is also important that clinicians are made aware of the effect of psychosocial factors on CVD risk, prognosis, and adherence to prevention efforts through improved training and knowledge sharing.

Air Pollution

Over the past 20 years, there has been a growing body of evidence linking air pollution to increased CVD incidence and mortality. While many people intuitively associate air pollution with respiratory problems, research has shown that the majority of the adverse health outcomes related to air pollution are cardiovascular in nature (Brook, 2008).

Air pollution is composed of a mix of gaseous and particulate matter and is created largely as a result of fossil fuel combustion. In developing countries, cooking and wood burning are also significant contributors. Although there is evidence that gaseous components of air pollution may have an adverse effect on human health, the majority of research to date has focused on the detrimental effects of particulate matter air pollution, with the majority of this research focusing on the effects of fine particulate air pollution (particles that are 2.5 µm or less in diameter) (Brook, 2008; Brook et al., 2004).

Numerous epidemiological studies in both developed and developing regions of the world have found that both short-term (several hours to a few days) and long-term exposure to particulate matter air pollution significantly increases cardiovascular events and CVD deaths (Brook, 2008; Brook et al., 2004; Dominici et al., 2006; Gouveia et al., 2006; IOM, 2004, 2009; Langrish et al., 2008; Peng et al., 2008; Pope and Dockery, 2006; Pope et al., 2004). These studies indicate that the relative risk of CVD mortality increases by approximately 1 percent for every 10 µg/m^3 increase in daily concentration of fine particle air pollution. Although this increased risk of CVD mortality from short-term changes in particulate matter concentration translates into a fairly small increase in absolute number of deaths, evidence from long-term studies have found larger increases in risk. These studies, of which there are fewer, have found relative risk of CVD mortality increases between 9 and 95 percent for every 10 $\mu g/m^3$ increase in annual average fine particle air pollution concentration, with the majority finding increases of less than 34 percent per 10 $\mu g/m^3$ increase. It should be noted that while short-term studies have been conducted in many regions throughout the world, all the large-scale long-term studies have taken place in the United States and Europe (Pope and Dockery, 2006).

One of the reasons that this data causes concern is that concentrations of particulate matter air pollution in some cities, especially the rapidly growing mega-cities in some developing countries, reach alarmingly high levels. Although air pollution levels in most cities in the United States and Europe have been decreasing—with current concentrations between 5 and 30 $\mu g/m^3$—levels in some large cities in the developing world have been increasing, with daily particulate concentrations that may exceed 200-500 $\mu g/m^3$. At these high levels, particulate matter concentration in the air approaches that found in smoke-filled bars (Brook, 2008).

Indeed, the evidence of air pollution's negative effect on cardiovascular health is consistent and strong enough that, in 2004, the American Heart Association published a scientific statement on the link, stating, "At the very least, short-term exposure to elevated PM [particulate matter] significantly contributes to increased acute cardiovascular mortality, particularly in certain at-risk subsets of the population. . . . The evidence further implicates prolonged exposure to elevated levels of PM in reducing overall life expectancy on the order of a few years" (Brook et al., 2004, p. 2666). The Institute of Medicine has also highlighted the detrimental effects of particulate matter air pollution on CVD incidence and mortality in several studies (IOM, 2004, 2009).

Despite the robust epidemiological evidence of air pollution's negative effect on CVD incidence and mortality, the specific mechanisms by which particulate matter increases CVD risk are still unclear. A number of different mechanisms by which particulate matter air pollution could increase CVD risk have been proposed, specifically through autonomic mechanisms related to the activation of the sympathetic nervous system or the withdrawal of the parasympathetic nervous system, the release of pro-inflammatory or oxidative stress-inducing compounds from the lungs, and soluble particulate matter entering the blood-stream after inhalation that directly act on the cardiovascular system (Brook, 2008; Brook et al., 2004; Pope and Dockery, 2006). Many of these mechanisms are similar to those that have been proposed for second-hand smoke (which is, in and of itself, a component of air pollution and a significant contributor to indoor air pollution) (Brook et al., 2004; IOM, 2009). Additional research is necessary to better elucidate the biological mechanisms by which air pollution increases CVD risk.

Genetics

Researchers have recognized for decades that family history of CVD is associated with increased atherosclerotic risk of heart disease, which led to the presumption of a genetic component to CVD. There are several well-characterized single-gene disorders that contribute to CVD, such as certain forms of familial hypercholesterolemia linked to mutations of the apolipoprotein B gene, and during the past few years, there have been major advances in the identification of genetic risk factors for CHD, stroke, and CVD risk factors such as blood pressure, blood lipids, obesity, and diabetes (Arking and Chakravarti, 2009; Arnett et al., 2007). The identification of genetic loci associated with CVD, such as 9p21 (Palomaki et al., 2010), has led to major advances in understanding the pathophysiology of CVD, but genetic variants identified to date have explained only a fraction of heritability and do not appear to have substantial added value in predicting CVD beyond traditional CVD risk factors. These genetic risk factors are unlikely to have substantial clinical utility with respect to prediction, diagnosis, and treatment in the near future (Arking and Chakravarti, 2009). The prevailing view within the research community is that the genetic underpinnings of most common forms of CVD involve a complex interplay of many different genes, and much work remains to develop a more thorough understanding of the complex gene–gene and gene–environment interactions involved in the development of CVD (Arnett et al., 2007).

Indeed, in addition to the investigation of genes that influence CVD and its risk factors, there has recently been a surge in research examining how environmental factors affect gene expression. Although research indicates that gene expression is most sensitive to environmental influence from conception to early life, there is also evidence that environmentally related gene expression changes can occur throughout life (Gluckman et al., 2009). This is an important emerging area of research for CVD. Future findings could have implications to help elucidate the physiological processes by which individuals with similar CVD risk profiles have different outcomes. Future research also could conceivably help develop new prevention and treatment strategies aimed at taking advantage of exogenous mechanisms that enhance or suppress the expression of key genes that play a role in mediating the development of CVD.

Looking forward, the explosive growth in molecular genetics techniques, advanced statistical methods, high-throughput technologies, and progress in studying gene–environment interactions should provide researchers with the ability to broaden the scope and applicability of their research. Techniques such as proteomics could lead to potential biomarkers to profile CVD risk more accurately, which could, for example, improve prediction of acute vascular events (Arnett et al., 2007). In addition, there is also significant promise in the emerging field of pharmacogenetics, which could not only help researchers develop more effective medications, but also better understand why certain drugs appear to be more effective in certain people. Since the initial availability of statins in late 1980, few new CVD drugs have emerged. Advances in genomic research could prompt more effective use of existing drugs and new drug development. At this stage, however, research in these fields has only modest potential for influencing population outcomes (Arnett et al., 2007).

Gender Differences in CVD Risk

Although CVD has sometimes been considered a disease that predominantly affects men, it is the leading cause of death among both men and women globally (Blauwet and Redberg, 2007; Jackson, 2008). There are, however, a number of notable gender differences in CVD incidence, mortality, risk-factor profiles, outcomes, and clinical presentation. These differences remain consistent across populations and regions and are thus important to consider when developing CVD prevention and treatment programs.

In all but the oldest age groups, CVD prevalence, incidence, and mortality rates tend to be higher for men than for women. This finding has remained consistent historically (Lawlor et al., 2001) and across countries and regions (Allen and Szanton, 2005; Pilote et al., 2007; WHOSIS, 2009). In addition, women experience their first cardiovascular events later in life than men. The INTERHEART study found that, on average, women experience their first MI 9 years later than men (Anand et al., 2008). Similarly, a recent review of stroke epidemiology found that men have their first stroke an average of 4.3 years earlier than women (Appelros et al., 2009). These findings are supported by WHO Global Burden of Disease data, which show that the average age of MI and first stroke is consistently lower among men across countries (WHO, 2009a).

The reason most often cited for these gender differences is a protective effect of estrogen on the development of CVD risk factors, most notably hypertension and dyslipidemia (Regitz-Zagrosek, 2006; Roeters van Lennep et al., 2002). Estrogen is thought to contribute to premenopausal women's tendency to have lower systolic blood pressure, higher levels of HDL cholesterol, and lower triglyceride levels than men (Buchanan and Brister, 2001; Pilote et al., 2007; Roeters van Lennep et al., 2002). The specific mechanisms of this protection have not been fully elucidated; however, estrogen is known to affect the atherosclerotic and blood-lipid control process in a number of different ways (Roeters van Lennep et al., 2002). The erosion of this protection that occurs after menopause provides further evidence of estrogen's protective role. Indeed, by age 75, women tend to have higher rates of hypertension and CVD than men (Legato, 1998; Narkiewicz et al., 2006).

However, despite the protective effect of endogenous estrogen on CVD development, estrogen replacement therapy in postmenopausal women does not reduce CVD risk and is not recommended as a method of primary or secondary prevention. In fact, recent evidence from clinical trials indicates that hormone replacement therapy increases the risk of adverse CVD events, especially stroke (Regitz-Zagrosek, 2006; Rossouw et al., 2002; Schaefer et al., 2003; Wassertheil-Smoller et al., 2003). In addition, oral contraceptives have also been associated with an increased risk of hypertension. Early formulations of these drugs contained a higher dose of hormones and increased risk of hypertension two- to three-fold. The current generation of oral contraceptives contain less than one-seventh the amount of hormones of the original generation of drugs, and most researchers believe they increase CVD risk far less than the contraceptives of the 1960s (Schaefer et al., 2003). However, smoking while taking oral contraceptives does increase CVD risk more than smoking alone (Rao, 1998).

The lower prevalence of smoking among women is another factor that could contribute to their decreased CVD incidence and mortality rates. Around the world, the prevalence of female smoking is lower than that of men (Pilote et al., 2007). These differences are particularly marked in low and middle income countries; however, they are also apparent in high income countries (see the discussion of regional differences in CVD earlier in this chapter). Unfortunately, this trend appears to be changing, as the gap between male and female smoking prevalence among adolescents aged 13 to 15 years is much narrower (WHOSIS, 2009). Furthermore, although smoking rates among both men and women have declined in high income countries since the middle of the 20th century, this has been less pronounced among women (Jackson, 2008). These trends are particularly troubling given that smoking lowers the age of menopause and there is evidence that it may be a stronger risk factor for MI among middle-aged women than men (Roeters van Lennep et al., 2002).

Although rates of smoking, dyslipidemia, and hypertension are generally lower among women than men, women tend to have less favorable profiles for other key CVD risk factors. Worldwide, women are more likely to be sedentary than men (Guthold et al., 2008). Some researchers have suggested that women's subservient social status in many cultures and their lack of leisure time due to childcare and other familial responsibilities likely contribute to their lower levels of physical activity (Brands and Yach, 2002; Pilote et al., 2007).

Another troubling gender difference is the increased prevalence of obesity among women. WHO data indicate that although overweight (BMI ≥ 25 kg/m^2) is more common among men globally, obesity (BMI ≥ 30 kg/m^2) is more common among women. This trend of increased obesity prevalence among women is consistent around the world, including in Sub-Saharan Africa (Barnighausen et al., 2008; Steyn, 2006), but it is particularly striking in a number of Middle Eastern countries where prevalence among women is more than 40 percent (WHOSIS, 2009). The trend is of particular concern in part because of the close association between obesity and diabetes. Diabetes is currently more common in men than women; however, its prevalence is increasing in both sexes and it appears to be a much stronger risk factor for CVD in women (Jackson, 2008; Pilote et al., 2007; Rao, 1998; Regitz-Zagrosek, 2006). Indeed, the presence of diabetes appears to eliminate any premenopausal protection associated with female gender (Roeters van Lennep et al., 2002).

In addition to traditional CVD risk factors, there are also several situations unique to women that can place them at increased CVD risk. During pregnancy and the post partum period, women are at an increased risk of stroke. Indeed, some researchers have found that women in their childbearing years (aged 15-35 years) have a higher incidence of stroke than men of the same age (Turtzo and McCullough, 2008). Furthermore, preeclampsia and eclampsia increase this risk and increase the risk of hypertension later in life (Jamieson and Skliut, 2009).

Finally, research has shown that women experience poorer outcomes when they have a CVD event. Studies in North America and Western Europe have found that women delay longer before seeking medical treatment at the onset of symptoms, wait longer to receive life-saving cardiac interventions, and have poorer outcomes following MI or stroke (Allen and Szanton, 2005; Pilote et al., 2007). Indeed, after a stroke or MI, women tend to have longer hospital stays, increased prevalence of depression and anxiety, higher short-term mortality, greater long-term disability, and higher rates of reinfarction than men (Allen and Szanton, 2005; Blauwet and Redberg, 2007; Pilote et al., 2007; Polk and Naqvi, 2005; Reeves et al., 2008).

CVD researchers have proposed a number of different reasons why women might delay seeking medical attention, receive delayed treatment, and experience poorer outcomes during and after an MI or stroke. One often-cited reason that women tend to wait longer to seek treatment during an AMI or a stroke is that many do not perceive themselves as being at risk. Studies in the United States and Europe have found that many women are not aware of the signs of an MI or stroke and do not know that CVD is the number one cause of death among women (Jensen and Moser, 2008). Women are also more likely than men to present with atypical symptoms of stroke or MI, which researchers have cited as a possible reason for the delays in the administration of appropriate care (Allen and Szanton, 2005; Appelros et al., 2009; Blauwet and Redberg, 2007; Jamieson and Skliut, 2009; Pilote et al., 2007; Polk and Naqvi, 2005; Reeves et al., 2008; Turtzo and McCullough, 2008; Witt and Roger, 2003). Additionally, some researchers have postulated that much of the poorer outcomes women experience post MI or stroke might be because women tend to be older with more comorbid conditions than men when they experience a CVD event (Reeves et al., 2008). Whatever the reasons, because of the robust evidence demonstrating gender differences in CVD incidence, morbidity, and outcomes, these differences, as well as the unique needs of women, should be considered when developing CVD research priorities, policies, and health service interventions.

HEALTH SYSTEMS AND CVD

The status of health systems can have a profound impact on CVD outcomes. Significant gaps in the health care infrastructure and access to health care in many low and middle income countries contribute to CVD incidence and mortality (Yach et al., 2004). These include gaps in adequate systems for all health needs as well as specific imbalances when it comes to chronic disease needs. Mayosi et al. (2009) recently highlighted the reality of health systems in many low and middle income countries dealing with a diverse set of health problems, noting that HIV/AIDS and TB require similar approaches to disease management as CVD, yet health care systems are too often neither integrated nor adapted to tackle chronic conditions. In China, for example, the health care system has been set up for maternal and child health and controlling infectious diseases and is extremely weak for meeting the challenges of chronic diseases. Only 47 percent of people with hypertension are aware of their conditions (Gu et al., 2002). Among those who are treated, less than 10 percent have good control of their blood pressure or blood glucose (Gu et al., 2002). Because only 61 percent of urban residents and 46 percent of rural residents in China have health insurance (Liu et al., 2008), millions of people forgo medical care when they are ill because they cannot afford care for chronic diseases. Clearly, the system is too vulnerable to meet the increasing challenges of chronic diseases (Liu et al., 2008). Reports from Sub-Saharan Africa also reveal a disturbing imbalance in access to care for chronic diseases. Lack of diagnosis, drug stock-outs, ignorance and community indifference, and

TABLE 2.4 Comparison of Treatment Usage in EUROASPIRE and PREMISE Surveys of Patients with Coronary Heart Disease

Study	β Blockers (%)	Statins (%)
EUROASPIRE I (1995-1996)	56.0	18.1
EUROASPIRE II (1999-2000)	69.0	57.3
EUROASPIRE III (2006-2007)	85.5	87.0
WHO PREMISE (2002-2003)	22.1	12.2

NOTE: EUROASPIRE data summarize average treatment usage from eight countries that were included in all three EUROASPIRE surveys (Czech Republic, Finland, France, Germany, Hungary, Italy, Netherlands, and Slovenia). PREMISE data represent all CHD patients in the study.
SOURCES: Kotseva et al., 2009a; Mendis et al., 2005.

premature death are common for diabetes and hypertension patients even while a successful treatment model for chronic infectious disease is widely available (Harries et al., 2008). Poor households in South Africa trying to access care for chronic illness face a range of breakdowns in the public health system (Goudge et al., 2009).

The WHO-led Prevention of Occurrences of Myocardial Infarction and Stroke (PREMISE) study included developing countries from the Middle East, Asia, and Latin America (Mendis et al., 2005) and gives some indication of gaps in delivery of needed health care for CVD in these settings. The PREMISE study quantified the size of the treatment gap for patients with CHD and, as shown in Table 2.4, showed much lower use of beta-blockers and statins compared to data in Europe from the European Action on Secondary Prevention by Intervention to Reduce Events (EUROASPIRE), which in particular reflected improvements in access to statins over time with a concomitant 51 percent decline in blood cholesterol levels (Kotseva et al., 2009b).

Although differences in methodology prevent rigorous comparisons of these data, the relative lack of implemented use of pharmaceutical interventions in the PREMISE study is illustrative of the potential link between rising trends in risk factors, lack of availability of and access to medicines, and inadequate delivery of health care services in developing countries. Importantly, in 2007, statins were added to the WHO Essential Medicine List (WHO, 2007). Furthermore, in 2009, nicotine replacement therapy for smoking cessation was approved (WHO, 2009c). While being on the list does not guarantee improved availability and access, these decisions may help ensure that governments can increase the access of their populations to pharmaceutical products needed to tackle leading risk factors for CVD.

Developing countries experience multiple simultaneous burdens of disease in settings where health systems are generally weak and where public health infrastructure is suboptimal. It is critical that decision makers consider this reality when determining which CVD interventions to prioritize. Interventions need to be appropriate to the health development capacity of the country. Because of this similarity in approaches to disease management, there is the potential for synergy between AIDS, TB, and CVD programs to achieve better integrated chronic disease models of care in rural and urban settings. The role of improved health care delivery in reducing the burden of CVD is discussed in more detail in Chapter 5.

THE INTERFACE BETWEEN INFECTIOUS DISEASES AND CARDIOVASCULAR DISEASE

Infectious Causes of Heart Disease

Although often overlooked because of their low incidence in developed countries, heart diseases caused by infectious agents remain a significant problem in many low and middle income countries (Muna, 1993; WHO, 2003; WHO Study Group on Rheumatic Fever and Rheumatic Heart Disease and WHO, 2004). These infection-related heart diseases include rheumatic heart disease (RHD), chagas heart disease, as well as pericarditis and cardiomyopathies caused by TB and HIV.

Rheumatic Heart Disease

RHD is probably the most well-known form of heart disease caused by infection. The pathophysiology of RHD involves several stages—an initial upper respiratory infection with group A streptococcus triggers a delayed immune response leading to acute rheumatic fever (ARF), with recurrent bouts of ARF leading ultimately to RHD. Once RHD has affected a person's heart valves, the damage is permanent and can lead to heart failure, atrial fibrillation, sudden cardiac death, and embolic stroke later in life (Gaziano et al., 2006; Mackay et al., 2004). WHO estimates that an average of 1.5 percent of people living with RHD die each year (WHO Department of Child and Adolescent Health and Development, 2005).

Over the past 50 years, prevalence of RHD has declined significantly in high income countries; however, it remains common in low and middle income countries (Karthikeyan and Mayosi, 2009). A recent WHO Department of Child and Adolescent Health and Development assessment estimated that at least 15.6 million people are living with RHD and that between 200,000 and 300,000 deaths occur each year due to the disease and its sequelae (Carapetis et al., 2005; WHO Department of Child and

Adolescent Health and Development, 2005). This annual mortality is approximately the same as that of rotavirus and about half that of malaria (Watkins et al., 2009). Nearly 80 percent of the individuals with RHD live in less developed countries, making RHD—perhaps more than any other form of CVD—a disease that almost exclusively affects the poor and disenfranchised (Karthikeyan and Mayosi, 2009).

Although prevalence rates vary by region, RHD appears to be most common in Africa, Southeast Asia, and the Western Pacific with the greatest number of annual deaths in China, Indonesia, and the Indian subcontinent (Steer et al., 2002; WHO Department of Child and Adolescent Health and Development, 2005). The disease is also common among indigenous populations such as Australian Aborigines and the Maori in New Zealand (Steer et al., 2002).

Of all forms of heart disease, RHD is responsible for the greatest toll on children. The disease and its sequelae are the most common cause of cardiac problems in children in low and middle income countries, and WHO estimates that it affects nearly 2.4 million children aged 5-14 years worldwide (Steer et al., 2002; WHO Department of Child and Adolescent Health and Development, 2005). Of these, approximately 1 million live in Sub-Saharan Africa, 750,000 live in South-Central Asia (Southeast Asia and some Eastern Mediterranean countries), and more than 175,000 live in China (WHO Department of Child and Adolescent Health and Development, 2005).

The decline of RHD in developed countries has been attributed to a number of factors. One is better access to prevention of RHD through the diagnosis and treatment of streptococcal throat infections in children with penicillin and through the continuous administration of antibiotics to patients with RHD or to individuals with a previous attack of ARF in order to prevent recurrent attacks of ARF and subsequent RHD. Another factor is the reduction of risk for streptococcal infection through improved hygiene and underlying socioeconomic factors, especially with respect to living conditions and overcrowding (Steer et al., 2002; WHO Study Group on Rheumatic Fever and Rheumatic Heart Disease and WHO, 2004).

Unfortunately, many low and middle income countries have not seen such a drastic decline, and some regions, such as Sub-Saharan Africa, have experienced no significant declines. This is most likely because many in developing regions have poor access to basic primary care and living conditions that do not promote reduction of risk of initial infection. In addition, many low and middle income countries rely almost exclusively on providing prophylactic antibiotics to those already diagnosed with RHD to control the disease rather than on other prevention efforts. (Karthikeyan and Mayosi, 2009). There remains a large unmet need for a widespread strategy using all levels of preventive efforts to prevent the onset of RHD.

Targeting strategies to help avoid and treat initial infections in children has the potential for a major impact on mortality, morbidity, and quality of life, especially given the difficulties of treating and managing RHD in its advanced stages of valvular disease and heart failure (Carapetis, 2007; Steer and Carapetis, 2009).

Chagas Heart Disease

Chagas heart disease is another form of CVD caused by an infectious agent. The disease is endemic throughout Central and South America but does not exist outside of the continent. In the 1980s, countrywide surveillance found the prevalence of Chagas to be approximately 17 million cases in 18 countries, with an incidence of 700,000 to 800,000 new infections and approximately 45,000 deaths each year (Morel and Lazdins, 2003). Between 10 and 30 percent of individuals infected with the *Trypanosoma cruzi* parasite that causes Chagas develop some form of cardiac damage, although this damage does not usually occur until 10 to 20 years after the acute phase of the disease. Chagas can lead to a variety of clinical symptoms including heart failure and death, with chagistic cardiomyopathy being the deadliest form of the disease (Marin-Neto et al., 2007; Moncayo and Yanine, 2006).

Since the 1980s, Central and South America have experienced significant declines in both incidence and prevalence of Chagas as a result of widescale prevention efforts, with the transmission of the disease successfully interrupted in Chile, Uruguay, and Brazil. These have primarily consisted of widespread spraying of insecticides to prevent the parasite's insect hosts from entering homes and careful screening of the blood supply. The current estimated prevalence of Chagas is 13 million cases in 15 countries, with an annual incidence of 200,000 new infections and 21,000 annual deaths from Chagas heart disease (Moncayo and Yanine, 2006; Morel and Lazdins, 2003; WHO Expert Committee on the Control of Chagas Disease and WHO, 2002).

Infectious Pericarditis and Cardiomyopathies

Certain infections, most notably HIV and TB, can lead to pericarditis and cardiomyopathies. Autopsy studies indicate that tuberculosis pericarditis occurs in approximately 1 percent of TB cases and 1 to 2 percent of pulmonary TB cases. It is the most common cause of pericarditis in Africa and other regions with high TB prevalence. Because of the HIV/AIDS epidemic, incidence of TB pericarditis is increasing in Africa (Mayosi et al., 2005). HIV infection itself, especially in its later stages, has also been associated with inflammation of the endothelium, pericarditis, pericardial effusion, myocarditis, cardiomyopathy, pulmonary hypertension, and a number of different types of vascular lesions (Aberg, 2009; Kamin and Grinspoon, 2005; Krishnaswamy et al., 2000). As the prevalence of TB, HIV, and TB/HIV co-infection continue to increase, it is likely that such TB- and HIV-related cardiovascular complications will also become more common (Mayosi et al., 2005). This poses major treatment and diagnostic challenges for the future especially as noninfectious causes increasingly occur in conjunction with infectious causes of heart disease.

***Conclusion 2.4:** Rheumatic heart disease, Chagas, and infectious pericarditis and cardiomyopathies continue to cause a substantial burden of disease and death in some low and middle income countries despite having been nearly eliminated in high income countries. Their ongoing prevalence in developing countries further widens the gap between the rich and poor, yet they are easily prevented through basic primary health care screenings or proven interventions. Additional surveillance is necessary to obtain a better epidemiological picture of these infectious forms of CVD in developing countries, and efforts to improve health care delivery are needed to facilitate the widespread delivery of existing interventions to prevent and treat these diseases.*

CVD Risk and Other Chronic Infectious Diseases

The past 15 years have produced considerable research investigating the associations among HIV infection, antiretroviral therapy, and cardiovascular disease and between CVD risks and TB, and to a lesser extent, the similarities from a health systems perspective of HIV/AIDS, TB, and CVD. Here the focus lies on the first two aspects.

HIV/AIDS and CVD Risks and Diseases

Studies among middle-aged patients in developed countries have found that there is a high prevalence of CVD risk factors among the HIV-infected population, and both HIV infection and highly active antiretroviral treatment (HAART) are associated with an increased risk of CVD. This increased risk is mostly mediated through HIV and HAART's effects on traditional CVD risk factors such as dyslipidemia and insulin resistance; however, there is also evidence that HIV infection and HAART themselves contribute an additional risk beyond what can be explained by other factors (Aberg, 2009; Boccara, 2008; Martinez et al., 2009).

By contrast, in Sub-Saharan Africa, where many HIV patients are younger, access to HAART is more limited, and tuberculosis is endemic, the predominant forms of heart disease associated with HIV/AIDS are pericarditis, cardiomyopathy, and pulmonary hypertension. Indeed, coronary artery disease, lipodystrophy, and metabolic syndrome are still not significant clinical problems among HIV patients in Sub-Saharan Africa (Ntsekhe and Mayosi, 2009).

CVD Prevalence Among HIV Patients While there are limited data on the prevalence of clinical CVD events among HIV patients worldwide, estimation can be extrapolated from the prevalence rates of CVD events from some of the major studies. The Data Collection on Adverse Events of Anti-HIV Drugs (D:A:D) study, one of the largest prospective studies of CVD risk among HIV-infected patients in 21 mostly high income countries in North America, Europe, and Australia, found that the incidence rate of a patient's first cardio or cerebrovascular event was 5.7 per 1000 person-years. From this data set, the authors concluded that although HIV and HAART do increase the risk of CVD, the absolute prevalence is still quite low, although it should be noted that the cohort is relatively young (The Writing Committee, 2004).

Data are generally lacking on the prevalence and characteristics of CVD among the HIV-infected population in most developing regions, although there have been several reviews of CVD in HIV-infected populations in Africa. In Sub-Saharan Africa, studies have found that the prevalence of cardiac abnormalities among African with HIV (most commonly involving the pericardium or myocardium as discussed in the previous section) is up to 60 percent, although patients are often asymptomatic and the profile of these cardiac abnormalities can be quite different from developed countries, as described above (Ntsekhe and Mayosi, 2009).

HIV's Direct Effects on CVD Risk Factors There is a growing body of evidence that HIV infection itself may result in metabolic and inflammatory events that increase cardiovascular risk. Uncontrolled HIV infection has been associated with lowered HDL cholesterol, increased triglyceride levels, and increased insulin resistance (Aberg, 2009; Boccara, 2008; Kamin and Grinspoon, 2005). Currently, data are lacking to quantify the exact magnitude of the increased CVD risk conferred by HIV disease itself.

HAART Effects on CVD HAART, especially those regimens containing protease inhibitors, has been the focus of extensive research regarding its effects on cardiovascular risk. Certain HAART regimens have been associated with dyslipidemia (increased LDL cholesterol, increased triglycerides, increased total cholesterol, and decreased HDL cholesterol), increased insulin resistance, body fat redistribution, and diabetes (Aberg, 2009; Boccara, 2008; Pao et al., 2008). These associations between HAART and CVD risk factors have also been demonstrated in HIV-infected children (Miller et al.,

2008). HAART regimens have also been associated with increased rates of myocardial infarction and other cardio- and cerebrovascular events, an association that appears to get stronger the longer a patient is on HAART (Law et al., 2006).

It is important to note that while the increase in risk of CVD caused by HIV and HAART is significant, the absolute risk of having a CVD event remains low, and there is universal agreement that the life-saving benefits of HAART outweigh the added CVD risks (Aberg, 2009; Adeyemi, 2007; Friis-Moller et al., 2007). In addition, a large prospective study found that intermittent use of HAART (stopping treatment once patients had stabilized CD4+ cell counts and then restarting when cell counts dropped below threshold) resulted in significantly poorer CVD outcomes (Strategies for Management of Antiretroviral Therapy Study Group et al., 2006).

HIV and Tobacco Smoking One of the consistent findings in many of the studies on the link between CVD and HIV is the high prevalence of tobacco smoking among HIV-infected individuals, which is often significantly higher than that of the general population (De Socio et al., 2008; Furber et al., 2007; Gritz et al., 2007). In the D:A:D study, more than 50 percent of the HIV-infected participants were smokers (Friis-Moller et al., 2003), and other studies have recorded that up to two-thirds of their HIV-positive participants smoked (Burkhalter et al., 2005). One study suggested that tobacco smoking could be an independent risk factor for acquiring HIV infection, although a causal relationship has not been established (Furber et al., 2007).

These high rates of smoking are worrisome because in addition to being a significant contributor to cardiovascular risk, there is evidence that smoking is also associated with poorer outcomes in HIV. In HIV-infected patients, smoking has been associated with an increased risk of tuberculosis and other opportunistic infections (Arcavi and Benowitz, 2004; Burkhalter et al., 2005; Furber et al., 2007), a lower adherence to HAART (Shuter and Bernstein, 2008), and a reduction in the efficacy of HAART (Miguez-Burbano et al., 2003).

CVD Risk Factors and TB

Recently WHO reviewed the relationship between major risk factors for CVD and TB. They concluded that both tobacco use and diabetes were important TB risk factors in the 22 high-burden TB countries in the world (Dye et al., 2009). The evidence is strongest for the links between smoking tobacco and tuberculosis. Taken together, there is sufficient evidence to conclude a causal link between tobacco use and TB (Chiang et al., 2007; Lin et al., 2007; Slama et al., 2007). In various studies, tobacco use has been associated with significantly increased risk of TB infection, increased conversion from latent to active TB, poorer treatment outcomes (Bates et al., 2007; Dhamgaye, 2008), increased mortality (Gajalakshmi et al., 2003; Hassmiller, 2006; Lin et al., 2007; Slama et al., 2007), increased drug resistance (Chiang et al., 2007), and increased rate of relapse (d'Arc Lyra Batista et al., 2008). One large study in India found that the mortality rate from TB was four times greater for ever smokers than for never smokers (Gajalakshmi et al., 2003a). There is a strong dose-response association between both the quantity of tobacco smoked and duration of smoking and risk of TB infection, disease, and mortality (Chiang et al., 2007; Dhamgaye, 2008; Slama et al., 2007). Unfortunately, smoking cessation is not actively supported in most TB treatment settings (Schneidera and Novotnya, 2007).

These associations have been found to be consistent across populations (both developing and industrialized), geographical regions, socioeconomic statuses, and cultures. Furthermore, studies have found these associations to be independent of confounding factors often associated with smoking such as alcohol use (Chiang et al., 2007; Hassmiller, 2006; Slama et al., 2007). Because smoking is generally more prevalent in men than in women, the majority of studies have focused on risk to male smokers. Indeed, Watkins and Plant (2006) proposed that smoking might explain some of the sex difference in the global TB epidemic, although this was based on an ecological study and needs to be assessed with individual-level data.

Recent major reviews of the relationship between diabetes and TB (Jeon and Murray, 2008; Young et al., 2009a, 2009b) suggest that there is a bi-directional relationship between the diseases. Diabetes is associated with a three-fold increased risk of TB, and TB contributes to the risk of developing diabetes (Young, 2009a). This relationship becomes critical to understand in countries where the burden of TB infection is already high (as in South Africa, India, China, and other developing countries) and where overweight and obesity are drivers of increased prevalence of diabetes.

In sum, TB and HIV/AIDS are common in many countries where CVD incidence is increasing. Furthermore, they share common risk factors, which suggests opportunities for integrated approaches to prevention and disease management at the health service and broader policy levels. As the HIV and TB epidemics continue to spread and more people get placed on long-term treatment, these opportunities for integrated approaches will likely increase.

CONCLUSION

Large parts of the world today are at moderate or high levels of risk for CVD, and cumulative behavioral, biological, and social risks will increase the global impact of chronic diseases in the future. CVDs (mainly IHD and stroke) are, and will remain for decades, the major causes of death in the world. This chapter has presented evidence on the determinants of CVD, establishing a rationale for intervention approaches that will be discussed later in this report.

The breadth of determinants that contribute to CVD points to the need for lifelong and multisectoral approaches. Because unhealthful diet, tobacco use, and decreased physical activity levels are among the major drivers of the CVD epidemic, prevention through promoting healthful diet and lifestyle should remain one of the cornerstones of global CVD reduction efforts. This does not exclude the importance of the potential to reduce CVD burden through better health care delivery, including better integration and development of chronic disease care models. Together, these approaches have the potential to address the burden of disease and overlapping determinants that are common in most emerging economies.

Prevention efforts need to start early in life and continue through the life course. A new and far greater emphasis on early childhood development is warranted, including greater attention to chronic disease risk in maternal and child health programs. However, trends in major risks will continue to influence incidence for many decades even if childhood prevention is rapidly implemented. Therefore, concerted and combined primary and secondary prevention efforts are also needed to reduce death rates in middle age and beyond.

Finally, although the epidemiological data described in this chapter provide a clear rationale for the proximal risk factors and broader determinants that need to be targeted in prevention efforts as well as compelling evidence that if these factors can be reduced, the burden of CVD will decrease. However, the epidemiological data does not detail how specifically to design and implement programs that will effectively achieve these goals, nor does it provide sufficient guidance on how to tailor such interventions to work in disparate settings with different cultural, structural, and epidemiological backdrops. The complex, interrelated determinants of global CVD and the variation in both risk profiles and capacity among low and middle income countries means that prevention efforts will only be effective if they are adapted to account for the specific needs of the settings in which they will be applied. To achieve this, additional surveillance and implementation research in all global regions, but especially in low and middle income countries, is required. These important issues are the subject of the remaining chapters of this report.

REFERENCES

Aberg, J. A. 2009. Cardiovascular complications in HIV management: Past, present, and future. *Journal of Acquired Immune Deficiency Syndromes* 50(1):54-64.
Aboderin, I., A. Kalache, Y. Ben-Shlomo, J. W. Lynch, C. S. Yajnik, D. Kuh, and D. Yach. 2002. *Life course perspectives on coronary heart disease, stroke and diabetes: Key issues and implications for policy and research.* Geneva: World Health Organization.
Adeyemi, O. 2007. Cardiovascular risk and risk management in HIV-infected patients. *Topics in HIV Medicine* 15(5):159-162.
Adeyi, O., O. Smith, and S. Robles. 2007. *Public policy and the challenge of chronic noncommunicable diseases.* Washington, DC: The World Bank.
Al-Hamdan, N., A. Kutbi, A. J. Choudhry, R. Nooh, M. Shoukri, and S. Mujib. 2005. *WHO stepwise approach to NCD surveillance country-specific standard report Saudi Arabia.* Geneva: World Health Organization.
Alikhani, S., A. Delavari, F. Alaedini, R. Kelishadi, S. Rohbani, and A. Safaei. 2009. A province-based surveillance system for the risk factors of non-communicable diseases: A prototype for integration of risk factor surveillance into primary healthcare systems of developing countries. *Public Health* 123(5):358-364.
Allen, J., and S. Szanton. 2005. Gender, ethnicity, and cardiovascular disease. *Journal of Cardiovascular Nursing* 20(1):1-6; quiz 7-8.
Anand, S. S., E. A. Enas, J. Pogue, S. Haffner, T. Pearson, and S. Yusuf. 1998. Elevated lipoprotein(a) levels in South Asians in North America. *Metabolism* 47(2):182-184.
Anand, S. S., S. Yusuf, V. Vuksan, S. Devanesen, K. K. Teo, P. A. Montague, L. Kelemen, C. Yi, E. Lonn, H. Gerstein, R. A. Hegele, and M. McQueen. 2000. Differences in risk factors, atherosclerosis, and cardiovascular disease between ethnic groups in Canada: The Study of Health Assessment and Risk in Ethnic groups (SHARE). *Lancet* 356(9226):279-284.
Anand, S. S., S. Islam, A. Rosengren, M. G. Franzosi, K. Steyn, A. H. Yusufali, M. Keltai, R. Diaz, S. Rangarajan, and S. Yusuf. 2008. Risk factors for myocardial infarction in women and men: Insights from the INTERHEART study. *European Heart Journal* 29(7):932-940.
Appelros, P., B. Stegmayr, and A. Terent. 2009. Sex differences in stroke epidemiology: A systematic review. *Stroke* 40(4):1082-1090.
Arcavi, L. M. D., and N. L. M. D. Benowitz. 2004. Cigarette smoking and infection. *Archives of Internal Medicine* 164(20):2206-2216.
Arking, D. E., and A. Chakravarti. 2009. Understanding cardiovascular disease through the lens of genome-wide association studies. *Trends in Genetics* 25(9):387-394.
Arnett, D. K., A. E. Baird, R. A. Barkley, C. T. Basson, E. Boerwinkle, S. K. Ganesh, D. M. Herrington, Y. Hong, C. Jaquish, D. A. McDermott, and C. J. O'Donnell. 2007. Relevance of genetics and genomics for prevention and treatment of cardiovascular disease: A scientific statement from the American Heart Association Council on Epidemiology and Prevention, the Stroke Council, and the Functional Genomics and Translational Biology Interdisciplinary Working Group. *Circulation* 115(22):2878-2901.
Asia Pacific Cohort Studies Collaboration. 2003. The effects of diabetes on the risks of major cardiovascular diseases and death in the Asia Pacific region. *Diabetes Care* 26(2):360-366.
Asia Pacific Cohort Studies Collaboration. 2004. Blood glucose and risk of cardiovascular disease in the Asia Pacific region. *Diabetes Care* 27(12):2836-2842.
Asia Pacific Cohort Studies Collaboration. 2007. Cholesterol, diabetes and major cardiovascular diseases in the Asia-Pacific region. *Diabetologia* 50(11):2289-2297.
Barker, D. J., C. N. Martyn, C. Osmond, C. N. Hales, and C. H. Fall. 1993. Growth in utero and serum cholesterol concentrations in adult life. *British Medical Journal* 307(6918):1524-1527.

Barker, D. J. P., C. Osmond, T. J. Forsen, E. Kajantie, and J. G. Eriksson. 2005. Trajectories of growth among children who have coronary events as adults.[see comment]. *New England Journal of Medicine* 353(17):1802-1809.

Barnighausen, T., T. Welz, V. Hosegood, J. Batzing-Feigenbaum, F. Tanser, K. Herbst, C. Hill, and M. L. Newell. 2008. Hiding in the shadows of the HIV epidemic: Obesity and hypertension in a rural population with very high HIV prevalence in South Africa. *Journal of Human Hypertension* 22(3):236-239.

Barquera, S., L. Hernandez-Barrera, M. L. Tolentino, J. Espinosa, W. N. Shu, J. A. Rivera, and B. M. Popkin. 2008. Energy intake from beverages is increasing among Mexican adolescents and adults. *Journal of Nutrition* 138(12):2454-2461.

Bates, M. N., A. Khalakdina, M. Pai, L. Chang, F. Lessa, and K. R. Smith. 2007. Risk of tuberculosis from exposure to tobacco smoke: A systematic review and meta-analysis. *Archives of Internal Medicine* 167(4):335-342.

Beaglehole, R. 1999. International trends in coronary heart disease mortality and incidence rates. *Journal of Cardiovascular Risk* 6(2):63-68.

Beaglehole, R., and R. Bonita. 2008. Global public health: A scorecard. *Lancet* 372(9654): 1988-1996.

Beilin, L. J., and I. B. Puddey. 2006. Alcohol and hypertension: An update. *Hypertension* 47(6):1035-1038.

Bhardwaj, S., A. Misra, L. Khurana, S. Gulati, P. Shah, and N. K. Vikram. 2008. Childhood obesity in Asian Indians: A burgeoning cause of insulin resistance, diabetes and subclinical inflammation. *Asia Pacific Journal of Clinical Nutrition* 17(Suppl 1):172-175.

Blauwet, L. A., and R. F. Redberg. 2007. The role of sex-specific results reporting in cardiovascular disease. *Cardiology in Review* 15(6):275-278.

Boccara, F. 2008. Cardiovascular complications and atherosclerotic manifestations in the HIV-infected population: Type, incidence and associated risk factors. *AIDS* 22 (Suppl 3):S19-S26.

Booth, G. L., M. K. Kapral, K. Fung, and J. V. Tu. 2006a. Recent trends in cardiovascular complications among men and women with and without diabetes. *Diabetes Care* 29(1):32-37.

Booth, G. L., M. K. Kapral, K. Fung, and J. V. Tu. 2006b. Relation between age and cardiovascular disease in men and women with diabetes compared with non-diabetic people: A population-based retrospective cohort study. *Lancet* 368(9529):29-36.

Bosire, C., J. Reedy, and S. M. Krebs-Smith. 2009. *Sources of energy and selected nutrient intakes among the US population, 2005-06: A report prepared for the 2010 dietary guidelines advisory committee.* Bethesda, MD: National Cancer Institute.

Brands, A., and D. Yach. 2002. Women and the rapid rise of noncommunicable diseases. *World Health Organization NMH Reader* (1):1-22.

Brook, R. D. 2008. Cardiovascular effects of air pollution. *Clinical Science* 115(5-6): 175-187.

Brook, R. D., B. Franklin, W. Cascio, Y. Hong, G. Howard, M. Lipsett, R. Luepker, M. Mittleman, J. Samet, S. C. Smith Jr., and I. Tager. 2004. Air pollution and cardiovascular disease: A statement for healthcare professionals from the expert panel on population and prevention science of the American Heart Association. *Circulation* 109(21):2655-2671.

Buchanan, M. R., and S. J. Brister. 2001. Sex-related differences in the pathophysiology of cardiovascular disease: Is there a rationale for sex-related treatments? *Canadian Journal of Cardiology* 17(Suppl D):7D-13D.

Bump, J. B., M. R. Reich, O. Adeyi, and S. Khetrapal. 2009. *Towards a political economy of tobacco control in low- and middle-income countries.* Washington, DC: The World Bank.

Burg, M. M., and D. Abrams. 2001. Depression in chronic medical illness: The case of coronary heart disease. *Journal of Clinical Psychology* 57(11):1323-1337.

Burkhalter, J. E., C. M. Springer, R. Chhabra, J. S. Ostroff, and B. D. Rapkin. 2005. Tobacco use and readiness to quit smoking in low-income HIV-infected persons. *Nicotine & Tobacco Research* 7(4):511-522.

Caballero, B. 2005. A nutrition paradox—underweight and obesity in developing countries. *New England Journal of Medicine* 352(15):1514-1516.

Caballero, B. 2009. Early undernutrition and risk of CVD in the adult. Presentation at Public Information Gathering Session for the Institute of Medicine Committee on Preventing the Global Epidemic of Cardiovascular Disease, Washington, DC.

Capewell, S., C. E. Morrison, and J. J. McMurray. 1999. Contribution of modern cardiovascular treatment and risk factor changes to the decline in coronary heart disease mortality in Scotland between 1975 and 1994. *Heart* 81(4):380-386.

Capewell, S., R. Beaglehole, M. Seddon, and J. McMurray. 2000. Explanation for the decline in coronary heart disease mortality rates in Auckland, New Zealand, between 1982 and 1993. *Circulation* 102(13):1511-1516.

Carapetis, J. R. 2007. Rheumatic heart disease in developing countries. *New England Journal of Medicine* 357(5):439-441.

Carapetis, J. R., A. C. Steer, E. K. Mulholland, and M. Weber. 2005. The global burden of group a streptococcal diseases. *Lancet Infectious Diseases* 5(11):685-694.

Celermajer, D. S., and J. G. Ayer. 2006. Childhood risk factors for adult cardiovascular disease and primary prevention in childhood. *Heart* 92(11):1701-1706.

Chan, J. C., V. Malik, W. Jia, T. Kadowaki, C. S. Yajnik, K. H. Yoon, F. B. Hu. 2009. Diabetes in Asia: Epidemiology, risk factors, and pathophysiology. *Journal of the American Medical Association* 301(20):2129-2140.

Chatterjee, S., R. Allan, and R. Ranjan. 2007. *Discussion paper no. 07.05: Food consumption and calorie intake in contemorary India*. Palmerston North, New Zealand: Massey University Department of Applied and International Economics.

Chelala, C. 1998. Tobacco corporations step up invasion of developing countries. *Lancet* 351(9106):889.

Chiang, C. Y., K. Slama, and D. A. Enarson. 2007. Associations between tobacco and tuberculosis. *International Journal of Tuberculosis and Lung Disease* 11(3):258-262; Erratum. 11(8):936.

Chiuve, S. E., K. M. Rexrode, D. Spiegelman, G. Logroscino, J. E. Manson, E. B. Rimm. 2008. Primary prevention of stroke by healthy lifestyle. *Circulation* 118(9):947-954.

Chobanian, A. V. 2009. Shattuck lecture. The hypertension paradox—more uncontrolled disease despite improved therapy. *New England Journal of Medicine* 361(9):878-887.

Christensen, K., G. Doblhammer, R. Rau, and J. W. Vaupel. 2009. Ageing populations: The challenges ahead. *Lancet* 374(9696):1196-1208.

Clarke, R., J. Emberson, A. Fletcher, E. Breeze, M. Marmot, M. J. Shipley. 2009. Life expectancy in relation to cardiovascular risk factors: 38 year follow-up of 19,000 men in the Whitehall study. *British Medical Journal* 339:b3513.

Collins, R., J. Armitage, S. Parish, P. Sleight, and R. Peto. 2004. Effects of cholesterol-lowering with simvastatin on stroke and other major vascular events in 20536 people with cerebrovascular disease or other high-risk conditions. *Lancet* 363(9411):757-767.

Connolly, G. N. 1992. Worldwide expansion of transnational tobacco industry. *Journal of the National Cancer Institute Monographs* (12):29-35.

Critchley, J. A., and S. Capewell. 2003. Mortality risk reduction associated with smoking cessation in patients with coronary heart disease: A systematic review. *Journal of the American Medical Association 2003* 290:1.

Critchley, J., J. Liu, D. Zhao, W. Wei, and S. Capewell. 2004. Explaining the increase in coronary heart disease mortality in Beijing between 1984 and 1999. *Circulation* 110(10):1236-1244.

d'Arc Lyra Batista, J., M. de Fatima Pessoa Militao de Albuquerque, R. A. de Alencar Ximenes, and L. C. Rodrigues. 2008. Smoking increases the risk of relapse after successful tuberculosis treatment. *International Journal of Epidemiology* 37(4):841-851.

Danaei, G., C. M. Lawes, S. Vander Hoorn, C. J. Murray, and M. Ezzati. 2006. Global and regional mortality from ischaemic heart disease and stroke attributable to higher-than-optimum blood glucose concentration: Comparative risk assessment. *Lancet* 368(9548):1651-1659.

Dangour, A. D., and R. Uauy. 2006. Nutrition challenges for the twenty-first century. *British Journal of Nutrition* 96 (Suppl 1)S5-S7.

Davey Smith, G., P. McCarron, M. Okasha, and J. McEwen. 2001. Social circumstances in childhood and cardiovascular disease mortality: Prospective observational study of Glasgow University students. *Journal of Epidemiology and Community Health* 55(5): 340-341.

Davies, A. R., L. Smeeth, and E. M. Grundy. 2007. Contribution of changes in incidence and mortality to trends in the prevalence of coronary heart disease in the UK: 1996-2005. *European Heart Journal* 28(17):2142-2147.

Dawber, T. R., and W. B. Kannel. 1958. An epidemiologic study of heart disease: The Framingham Study. *Nutrition Reviews* 16(1):1-4.

Dawber, T. R., G. F. Meadors, and F. E. Moore, Jr. 1951. Epidemiological approaches to heart disease: The Framingham Study. *American Journal of Public Health and the Nations Health* 41(3):279-281.

Dawber, T. R., F. E. Moore, and G. V. Mann. 1957. Coronary heart disease in the Framingham Study. *American Journal of Public Health and the Nations Health* 47(4 Pt 2):4-24.

De Socio, G. V. L., G. Parruti, T. Quirino, E. Ricci, G. Schillaci, B. Adriani, P. Marconi, M. Franzetti, C. Martinelli, F. Vichi, G. Penco, C. Sfara, G. Madeddu, and P. Bonfanti. 2008. Identifying HIV patients with an unfavorable cardiovascular risk profile in the clinical practice: Results from the Simone study. *Journal of Infection* 57(1):33-40.

Dhamgaye, T. M. 2008. Tobacco smoking and pulmonary tuberculosis: A case-control study. *Journal of the Indian Medical Association* 106(4):216-219.

Dominici, F., R. D. Peng, M. L. Bell, L. Pham, A. McDermott, S. L. Zeger, and J. M. Samet. 2006. Fine particulate air pollution and hospital admission for cardiovascular and respiratory diseases. *Journal of the American Medical Association* 295(10):1127-1134.

Dong, M., W. H. Giles, V. J. Felitti, S. R. Dube, J. E. Williams, D. P. Chapman, and R. F. Anda. 2004. Insights into causal pathways for ischemic heart disease: Adverse childhood experiences study. *Circulation* 110(13):1761-1766.

Downs, J. R., M. Clearfield, S. Weis, E. Whitney, D. R. Shapiro, P. A. Beere, A. Langendorfer, E. A. Stein, W. Kruyer, and A. M. Gotto, Jr. 1998. Primary prevention of acute coronary events with lovastatin in men and women with average cholesterol levels: Results of AFCAPS/TEXCAPS. Air Force/Texas Coronary Atherosclerosis Prevention Study. *Journal of the American Medical Association* 279(20):1615-1622.

Dye, C., K. Lönnroth, E. Jaramillo, B. G. Williams, and M. Raviglione. 2009. Trends in tuberculosis incidence and their determinants in 134 countries. In *Bulletin of the World Health Organization*. Geneva: World Health Organization.

Ellis, L. B. 1948. Underlying causes of heart disease. *The American Journal of Nursing* 48(11):697-698.

ERC. 2007. *World cigarettes 1: The 2007 report*. Suffolk, England: ERC Statistics Intl Plc.

Erqou, S., S. Kaptoge, P. L. Perry, E. Di Angelantonio, A. Thompson, I. R. White, S. M. Marcovina, R. Collins, S. G. Thompson, J. Danesh. 2009. Lipoprotein(a) concentration and the risk of coronary heart disease, stroke, and nonvascular mortality. *Journal of the American Medical Association* 302(4):412-423.

Evans, R. W., C. H. Bunker, F. A. Ukoli, and L. H. Kuller. 1997. Lipoprotein (a) distribution in a Nigerian population. *Ethnicity Health* 2(1-2):47-58.

Everson-Rose, S. A., and T. T. Lewis. 2005. Psychosocial factors and cardiovascular diseases. In *Annual Review of Public Health* 26(1):469-500

Ezzati, M., S. J. Henley, M. J. Thun, and A. D. Lopez. 2005. Role of smoking in global and regional cardiovascular mortality. *Circulation* 112(4):489-497.

Fernald, L. C., and L. M. Neufeld. 2007. Overweight with concurrent stunting in very young children from rural Mexico: Prevalence and associated factors. *European Journal of Clinical Nutrition* 61(5):623-632.

Figueredo, V. M. 2009. The time has come for physicians to take notice: The impact of psychosocial stressors on the heart. *American Journal of Medicine* 122(8):704-712.

Flegal, K. M., B. I. Graubard, D. F. Williamson, M. H. Gail, K. M. Flegal, B. I. Graubard, D. F. Williamson, and M. H. Gail. 2007. Cause-specific excess deaths associated with underweight, overweight, and obesity. *Journal of the American Medical Association* 298(17):2028-2037.

Ford, E. S., U. A. Ajani, J. B. Croft, J. A. Critchley, D. R. Labarthe, T. E. Kottke, W. H. Giles, and S. Capewell. 2007. Explaining the decrease in U.S. deaths from coronary disease, 1980-2000. *New England Journal of Medicine* 356(23):2388-2398.

Foster, R. K., and H. E. Marriott. 2006. Alcohol consumption in the new millennium—weighing up the risks and benefits for our health. *Nutrition Bulletin* 31(4):286-331.

Fox, C. S., J. C. Evans, M. G. Larson, W. B. Kannel, and D. Levy. 2004. Temporal trends in coronary heart disease mortality and sudden cardiac death from 1950 to 1999: The Framingham Heart Study. *Circulation* 110(5):522-527.

Frasure-Smith, N., and F. Lesperance. 2006. Recent evidence linking coronary heart disease and depression. *Canadian Journal of Psychiatry—Revue Canadienne de Psychiatrie* 51(12):730-737.

Freedman, D. S., L. K. Khan, W. H. Dietz, S. R. Srinivasan, and G. S. Berenson. 2001. Relationship of childhood obesity to coronary heart disease risk factors in adulthood: The Bogalusa Heart Study. *Pediatrics* 108(3):712-718.

Fries, J. F. 1980. Aging, natural death, and the compression of morbidity. *New England Journal of Medicine* 303(3):130-135.

Friis-Moller, N., R. Weber, P. Reiss, R. Thiébaut, O. Kirk, A. D'Arminio Monforte, C. Pradier, L. Morfeldt, S. Mateu, M. Law, W. El-Sadr, S. De Wit, C. A. Sabin, A. N. Phillips, and J. D. Lundgren. 2003. Cardiovascular disease risk factors in HIV patients—association with antiretroviral therapy. Results from the DAD study. *AIDS* 17(8):1179-1193.

Friis-Moller, N., P. Reiss, C. A. Sabin, R. Weber, A. d'Arminio Monforte, W. El-Sadr, R. Thiebaut, S. De Wit, O. Kirk, E. Fontas, M. G. Law, A. Phillips, and J. D. Lundgren. 2007. Class of antiretroviral drugs and the risk of myocardial infarction. *New England Journal of Medicine* 356(17):1723-1735.

Fung, T. T., K. M. Rexrode, C. S. Mantzoros, J. E. Manson, W. C. Willett, and F. B. Hu. 2009. Mediterranean diet and incidence of and mortality from coronary heart disease and stroke in women. *Circulation* 119(8):1093-1100.

Furber, A. S., R. Maheswaran, J. N. Newell, and C. Carroll. 2007. Is smoking tobacco an independent risk factor for HIV infection and progression to AIDS? A systemic review. *Sexually Transmitted Infections* 83(1):41-46.

Gager, L. T. 1931. Heart disease: Its nature, study, and prevention. *American Journal of Nursing* 31(4):397-406.

Gajalakshmi, V., R. Peto, T. S. Kanaka, and P. Jha. 2003a. Smoking and mortality from tuberculosis and other diseases in India: Retrospective study of 43 000 adult male deaths and 35 000 controls. *Lancet* 362(9383):507-515.

Galobardes, B., G. D. Smith, and J. W. Lynch. 2006. Systematic review of the influence of childhood socioeconomic circumstances on risk for cardiovascular disease in adulthood. *Annals of Epidemiology* 16(2):91-104.

Gaziano, T., and G. I. Kim. 2009. *Cost of treating non-optimal blood pressure in select low and middle income countries in comparison to the United States.* Background paper commissioned by the Committee on Preventing the Global Epidemic of Cardiovascular Disease.

Gaziano, T. A., K. S. Reddy, F. Paccaud, S. Horton, and V. Chaturvedi. 2006. Cardiovascular disease. In *Disease control priorities in developing countries.* 2nd ed, Edited by D. T. Jamison, J. G. Breman, A. R. Measham, G. Alleyne, M. Claeson, D. B. Evans, P. Jha, A. Mills and P. Musgrove. New York: Oxford University Press. Pp. 645-662.

Glassman, A., P. A. Shapiro, D. E. Ford, L. Culpepper, M. S. Finkel, J. R. Swenson, J. T. Bigger, B. L. Rollman, and T. N. Wise. 2003. Cardiovascular health and depression. *Journal of Psychiatric Practice* 9(6):409-421.

Gluckman, P. D., and M. A. Hanson. 2008. Developmental and epigenetic pathways to obesity: An evolutionary-developmental perspective. *International Journal of Obesity* 32(Suppl 7):S62-S71.

Gluckman, P. D., M. A. Hanson, T. Buklijas, F. M. Low, and A. S. Beedle. 2009. Epigenetic mechanisms that underpin metabolic and cardiovascular diseases. *Nature Reviews Endocrinology* 5(7):401-408.

Goldman, D. P., Y. Zheng, F. Girosi, P.-C. Michaud, S. J. Olshansky, D. Cutler, and J. W. Rowe. 2009. The benefits of risk factor prevention in Americans aged 51 years and older. *American Journal of Public Health* 99(11):2096-2101.

Goraya, T. Y., S. J. Jacobsen, T. E. Kottke, R. L. Frye, S. A. Weston, and V. L. Roger. 2003. Coronary heart disease death and sudden cardiac death: A 20-year population-based study. *American Journal of Epidemiology* 157(9):763-770.

Gotto, A. M., Jr. 2005. Evolving concepts of dyslipidemia, atherosclerosis, and cardiovascular disease: The Louis F. Bishop lecture. *Journal of the American College of Cardiology* 46(7):1219-1224.

Goudge, J., L. Gilson, S. Russell, T. Gumede, and A. Mills. 2009. Affordability, availability and acceptability barriers to health care for the chronically ill: Longitudinal case studies from South Africa. *Biomed Central Health Services Research* 9:75.

Gouveia, N., C. U. De Freitas, L. C. Martins, and I. O. Marcilio. 2006. Respiratory and cardiovascular hospitalizations associated with air pollution in the city of Sao Paulo, Brazil. Hospitalizacoes por causas respiratorias e cardiovasculares associadas a contaminacao atmosferica no Municipio de Sao Paulo, Brasil. *Cadernos de Saúde Pública* 22(12):2669-2677.

Goyal, A., and S. Yusuf. 2006. The burden of cardiovascular disease in the Indian subcontinent. *Indian Journal of Medical Research* 124(3):235-244.

Gritz, E. R., D. J. Vidrine, and M. Cororve Fingeret. 2007. Smoking cessation. A critical component of medical management in chronic disease populations. *American Journal of Preventive Medicine* 33(6 Suppl):S414-S422.

Gu, D., K. Reynolds, X. Wu, J. Chen, X. Duan, P. Muntner, G. Huang, R. F. Reynolds, S. Su, P. K. Whelton, J. He, and InterAsia Collaborative Group. The International Collaborative Study of Cardiovascular Disease in Asia. 2002. Prevalence, awareness, treatment, and control of hypertension in China. *Hypertension* 40(6):920-927.

Guindon, E. G., and D. Boisclair. 2003. *Current and future trends in tobacco use.* Geneva: World Health Organization Tobacco Free Initiative.

Guthold, R., T. Ono, K. L. Strong, S. Chatterji, and A. Morabia. 2008. Worldwide variability in physical inactivity—a 51-country survey. *American Journal of Preventive Medicine* 34(6):486-494.

Haffner, S. M., S. Lehto, T. Ronnemaa, K. Pyorala, and M. Laakso. 1998. Mortality from coronary heart disease in subjects with type 2 diabetes and in nondiabetic subjects with and without prior myocardial infarction. *New England Journal of Medicine* 339(4): 229-234.

Hardoon, S. L., P. H. Whincup, L. T. Lennon, S. G. Wannamethee, S. Capewell, and R. W. Morris. 2008. How much of the recent decline in the incidence of myocardial infarction in British men can be explained by changes in cardiovascular risk factors? Evidence from a prospective population-based study. *Circulation* 117(5):598-604.

Harries, A. D., A. Jahn, R. Zachariah, and D. Enarson. 2008. Adapting the DOTS framework for tuberculosis control to the management of non-communicable diseases in Sub-Saharan Africa. *PLoS Med* 5(6):e124.

Hassmiller, K. M. 2006. The association between smoking and tuberculosis. *Salud Publica de Mexico* 48(Suppl 1):S201-S216.

He, F. J., and G. A. MacGregor. 2009. A comprehensive review on salt and health and current experience of worldwide salt reduction programmes. *Journal of Human Hypertension* 23(6):363-384.

He, J., D. Gu, J. Chen, X. Wu, T. N. Kelly, J.-F. Huang, J.-C. Chen, C.-S. Chen, L. A. Bazzano, K. Reynolds, P. K. Whelton, and M. J. Klag. 2009. Premature deaths attributable to blood pressure in China: A prospective cohort study. *Lancet* 374(9703):1765-1772.

Heart disease likely fate of young men in big cities. 1937. *The Science News-Letter* 32(847): 10-11.

HEM Project Team. 2008. *Closing the health gap in the European union.* Warsaw, Poland: Maria Skłodowska-Curie Cancer Memorial Cancer Center and Institute of Oncology, Epidemiology and Prevention Division.

Henderson, L., J. Gregory, K. Irving, and G. Swan. 2003. *National diet & nutrition survey: Adults aged 19 to 64: Energy, protein, carbohydrate, fat, and alcohol intake.* London: Office of National Statistics.

Holman, R. R., S. K. Paul, M. A. Bethel, D. R. Matthews, and H. A. Neil. 2008. 10-year follow-up of intensive glucose control in type 2 diabetes. *New England Journal of Medicine* 359(15):1577-1589.

Holzman, D. 1997. Tobacco abroad: Infiltrating foreign markets. *Environmental Health Perspectives* 105(2):178-183.

Hu, F. B. 2008. Globalization of food patterns and cardiovascular disease risk. *Circulation* 118(19):1913-1914.

Hu, F. B., M. J. Stampfer, J. E. Manson, F. Grodstein, G. A. Colditz, F. E. Speizer, and W. C. Willett. 2000. Trends in the incidence of coronary heart disease and changes in diet and lifestyle in women. *New England Journal of Medicine* 343(8):530-537.

Hu, F. B., J. E. Manson, M. J. Stampfer, G. Colditz, S. Liu, C. G. Solomon, and W. C. Willett. 2001. Diet, lifestyle, and the risk of type 2 diabetes mellitus in women. *New England Journal of Medicine* 345(11):790-797.

Hunink, M. G., L. Goldman, A. N. Tosteson, M. A. Mittleman, P. A. Goldman, L. W. Williams, J. Tsevat, and M. C. Weinstein. 1997. The recent decline in mortality from coronary heart disease, 1980-1990. The effect of secular trends in risk factors and treatment. *Journal of the American Medical Association* 277(7):535-542.

Huxley, R., F. Barzi, and M. Woodward. 2006. Excess risk of fatal coronary heart disease associated with diabetes in men and women: Meta-analysis of 37 prospective cohort studies. *British Medical Journal* 332(7533):73-78.

IDF (International Diabetes Federation). 2006. The diabetes atlas. Brussels: IDF.

IDF. 2010. *The diabetes atlas.* Brussels: IDF.

IOM (Institute of Medicine). 1998. *Control of cardiovascular diseases in developing countries.* Washington, DC: National Academy Press.
IOM. 2004. *Research priorities for airborne particulate matter: IV. Continuing research progress.* Washington, DC: The National Academies Press.
IOM. 2009. *Secondhand smoke exposure and cardiovascular effects: Making sense of the evidence.* Washington, DC: The National Academies Press.
Iqbal, R., S. Anand, S. Ounpuu, S. Islam, X. Zhang, S. Rangarajan, J. Chifamba, A. Al-Hinai, M. Keltai, and S. Yusuf. 2008. Dietary patterns and the risk of acute myocardial infarction in 52 countries: Results of the INTERHEART study. *Circulation* 118(19):1929-1937.
Jackson, G. 2008. Gender differences in cardiovascular disease prevention. *Menopause International* 14(1):13-17.
Jamieson, D. G., and M. Skliut. 2009. Gender considerations in stroke management. *Neurologist* 15(3):132-141.
Jensen, L. A., and D. K. Moser. 2008. Gender differences in knowledge, attitudes, and beliefs about heart disease. *Nursing Clinics of North America* 43(1):77-104; vi-vii.
Jeon, C. Y., and M. B. Murray. 2008. Diabetes mellitus increases the risk of active tuberculosis: A systematic review of 13 observational studies. *PLoS Med* 5(7):e152.
Jequier, E. 1999. Alcohol intake and body weight: A paradox. *American Journal of Clinical Nutrition* 69(2):173-174.
Jha, P., and F. J. Chaloupka. 1999. *Curbing the epidemic: Governments and the economics of tobacco control.* Washington, DC: World Bank.
Johnson, R. K., L. J. Appel, M. Brands, B. V. Howard, M. Lefevre, R. H. Lustig, F. Sacks, L. M. Steffen, J. Wylie-Rosett, P. A. American Heart Association Nutrition Committee of the Council on Nutrition, Physical Activity, and Metabolism, and the the Council on Epidemiology and Prevention. 2009. Dietary sugars intake and cardiovascular health: A scientific statement from the American Heart Association. *Circulation* 120(11):1011-1020.
Joint WHO/FAO Expert Consultation on Diet Nutrition and the Prevention of Chronic Diseases and World Health Organization Department of Nutrition for Health and Development. 2003. *Diet, nutrition and the prevention of chronic diseases: Report of a joint WHO/FAO expert consultation, Geneva, 28 January-1 February 2002, WHO technical report series.* Geneva: World Health Organization.
Kalache, A. 1999. Active ageing makes the difference: Editorial. *Bulletin of the World Health Organization* 77(4):299.
Kalache, A., I. Aboderin, and I. Hoskins. 2002. Compression of morbidity and active ageing: Key priorities for public health policy in the 21st century: Public health classics. *Bulletin of the World Health Organization* 80(3):243-244.
Kamin, D. S., and S. K. Grinspoon. 2005. Cardiovascular disease in HIV-positive patients. *AIDS* 19(7):641-652.
Kannel, W. B., T. R. Dawber, A. Kagan, N. Revotskie, and J. Stokes, 3rd. 1961. Factors of risk in the development of coronary heart disease—six year follow-up experience. The Framingham Study. *Annals of Internal Medicine* 55:33-50.
Kannel, W. B., W. P. Castelli, T. Gordon, and P. M. McNamara. 1971. Serum cholesterol, lipoproteins, and the risk of coronary heart disease. The Framingham Study. *Annals of Internal Medicine* 74(1):1-12.
Karppanen, H., and E. Mervaala. 2006. Sodium intake and hypertension. *Progress in Cardiovascular Diseases* 49(2):59-75.
Karthikeyan, G., and B. M. Mayosi. 2009. Is primary prevention of rheumatic fever the missing link in the control of rheumatic heart disease in Africa? *Circulation* 120(8):709-713.
Kelishadi, R. 2007. Childhood overweight, obesity, and the metabolic syndrome in developing countries. *Epidemiologic Reviews* 29:62-76.

Kelly, T. N., L. A. Bazzano, V. A. Fonseca, T. K. Thethi, K. Reynolds, and J. He. 2009. Glucose control and cardiovascular disease in type 2 diabetes. *Annals of Internal Medicine* 151(6):1-10.

Kengne, A. P., A. Patel, F. Barzi, K. Jamrozik, T. H. Lam, H. Ueshima, D. F. Gu, I. Suh, and M. Woodward. 2007. Systolic blood pressure, diabetes and the risk of cardiovascular diseases in the Asia-Pacific region. *Journal of Hypertension* 25(6):1205-1213.

Kengne, A. P., K. Nakamura, F. Barzi, T. H. Lam, R. Huxley, D. Gu, A. Patel, H. C. Kim, and M. Woodward. 2009. Smoking, diabetes and cardiovascular diseases in men in the Asia Pacific region. *Journal of Diabetes* 1(3):173-181.

Khan, M., and G. Mensah. 2009. *Changing practices to improve dietary outcomes and reduce cardiovascular risk: A food company's perspective*. Purchase, NY: Background Paper Commissioned by the Committee.

Kotseva, K., D. Wood, G. De Backer, D. De Bacquer, K. Pyorala, and U. Keil. 2009a. Cardiovascular prevention guidelines in daily practice: A comparison of EUROASPIRE I, II, and III surveys in eight European countries. *Lancet* 373(9667):929-940.

Kotseva, K., D. Wood, G. De Backer, D. De Bacquer, K. Pyorala, U. Keil, and EUROASPIRE Study Group. 2009b. EUROASPIRE iii: A survey on the lifestyle, risk factors and use of cardioprotective drug therapies in coronary patients from 22 European countries. *European Journal of Cardiovascular Prevention & Rehabilitation* 16(2):121-137.

Krishnaswamy, G. M., D. S. P. Chi, J. I. M. L. P. Kelley, F. M. Sarubbi, K. J. M. Smith, and A. M. Peiris. 2000. The cardiovascular and metabolic complications of HIV infection. *Cardiology in Review* 8(5):260-268.

Laatikainen, T., J. Critchley, E. Vartiainen, V. Salomaa, M. Ketonen, and S. Capewell. 2005. Explaining the decline in coronary heart disease mortality in Finland between 1982 and 1997. *American Journal of Epidemiology* 162(8):764-773.

Langrish, J. P., N. L. Mills, and D. E. Newby. 2008. Air pollution: The new cardiovascular risk factor. *Internal Medicine Journal* 38(12):875-878.

Law, M. G., N. Friis-Moller, W. M. El-Sadr, R. Weber, P. Reiss, A. D'Arminio Monforte, R. Thiebaut, L. Morfeldt, S. De Wit, C. Pradier, G. Calvo, O. Kirk, C. A. Sabin, A. N. Phillips, J. D. Lundgren, and D. A. D. Study Group. 2006. The use of the Framingham equation to predict myocardial infarctions in HIV-infected patients: Comparison with observed events in the D:A:D study. *HIV Medicine* 7(4):218-230.

Lawes, C. M. M., S. Vander Hoorn, A. Rodgers, and International Society of Hypertension. 2008. Global burden of blood-pressure-related disease, 2001. *Lancet* 371(9623):1513-1518.

Lawlor, D. A., S. Ebrahim, and G. Davey Smith. 2001. Sex matters: Secular and geographical trends in sex differences in coronary heart disease mortality. *British Medical Journal* 323(7312):541-545: Erratum 325(7364):580.

Leeder, S., S. Raymond, and H. Greenberg. 2004. *A race against time: The challenge of cardiovascular disease in developing economics*. New York: Columbia University.

Legato, M. J. 1998. Cardiovascular disease in women: Gender-specific aspects of hypertension and the consequences of treatment. *Journal of Women's Health* 7(2):199-209.

Lesperance, F., and N. Frasure-Smith. 2007. Depression and heart disease. *Cleveland Clinic Journal of Medicine* 74(Suppl 1):S63-S66.

Lichtman, J. H., J. T. Bigger Jr., J. A. Blumenthal, N. Frasure-Smith, P. G. Kaufmann, F. Lesperance, D. B. Mark, D. S. Sheps, C. B. Taylor, and E. S. Froelicher. 2008. Depression and coronary heart disease: Recommendations for screening, referral, and treatment—a science advisory from the American Heart Association Prevention Committee of the Council on Cardiovascular Nursing, Council on Clinical Cardiology, Council on Epidemiology and Prevention, and Interdisciplinary Council on Quality of Care and Outcomes Research. *Circulation* 118(17):1768-1775.

Lin, H. H., M. Ezzati, and M. Murray. 2007. Tobacco smoke, indoor air pollution and tuberculosis: A systematic review and meta-analysis. *PLoS Medicine* 4(1).

Liu, G. G., W. H. Dow, A. Z. Fu, J. Akin, and P. Lance. 2008. Income productivity in China: On the role of health. *Journal of Health Economics* 27(1):27-44.

Lopez, A. D., C. D. Mathers, M. Eszati, D. T. Jamison, and C. J. L. Murray. 2006. *Global burden of disease and risk factors*. Washington, DC: World Bank.

Lopez-Jaramillo, P., S. Y. Silva, N. Rodriguez-Salamanca, A. Duran, W. Mosquera, and V. Castillo. 2008. Are nutrition-induced epigenetic changes the link between socio-economic pathology and cardiovascular diseases? *American Journal of Therapeutics* 15(4):362-372.

Low, P. S., C. K. Heng, N. Saha, and J. S. Tay. 1996. Racial variation of cord plasma lipoprotein(a) levels in relation to coronary risk level: A study in three ethnic groups in Singapore. *Pediatric Research* 40(5):718-722.

Lucas, D. L., R. A. Brown, M. Wassef, and T. D. Giles. 2005. Alcohol and the cardiovascular system research challenges and opportunities. *Journal of the American College of Cardiology* 45(12):1916-1924.

Mackay, J. 1992. US tobacco export to third world: Third world war. *Journal of the National Cancer Institute Monographs* (12):25-28.

Mackay, J., and M. Eriksen. 2002. *The tobacco atlas*. Geneva: World Health Organization.

Mackay, J., G. Mensah, S. Mendis, K. Greenlund, and World Health Organization Department of Management of Noncommunicable Diseases. 2004. *The atlas of heart disease and stroke*. Geneva: World Health Organization.

Manninen, V., L. Tenkanen, P. Koskinen, J. K. Huttunen, M. Manttari, O. P. Heinonen, and M. H. Frick. 1992. Joint effects of serum triglyceride and LDL cholesterol and HDL cholesterol concentrations on coronary heart disease risk in the Helsinki Heart Study. Implications for treatment. *Circulation* 85(1):37-45.

Marcovina, S. M., J. J. Albers, E. Wijsman, Z. Zhang, N. H. Chapman, and H. Kennedy. 1996. Differences in Lp[a] concentrations and apo[a] polymorphs between black and white Americans. *Journal of Lipid Research* 37(12):2569-2585.

Marin-Neto, J. A., E. Cunha-Neto, B. C. Maciel, and M. V. Simões. 2007. Pathogenesis of chronic Chagas heart disease. *Circulation* 115(9):1109-1123.

Martinez, D., and V. Grise. 1990. With U.S. sale down, tobacco industry looks abroad. *Farmline US Department of Agriculture Economic Research Service* 11(3):18-20.

Martinez, E., M. Larrousse, and J. M. Gatell. 2009. Cardiovascular disease and HIV infection: Host, virus, or drugs? *Current Opinion in Infectious Diseases* 22(1):28-34.

Martinez-Gonzalez, M. A., M. Bes-Rastrollo, L. Serra-Majem, D. Lairon, R. Estruch, A. Trichopoulou, M. A. Martinez-Gonzalez, M. Bes-Rastrollo, L. Serra-Majem, D. Lairon, R. Estruch, and A. Trichopoulou. 2009. Mediterranean food pattern and the primary prevention of chronic disease: Recent developments. *Nutrition Reviews* 67(Suppl 1):S111-S116.

Mathers, C. D., and D. Loncar. 2006. Projections of global mortality and burden of disease from 2002 to 2030. *PLoS Med* 3(11):e442.

Mathers, C. D., C. Bernard, K. M. Iburg, M. Inoue, D. M. Fat, K. Shibuya, N. Timijuma, and H. Xu. 2003. *Global burden of disease in 2002: Data sources, methods, and results*. Global Programme on Evidence for Health Policy Discussion Paper No. 54. Geneva: World Health Organization.

Mathers, C. D., D. Ma Fat, M. Inoue, C. Rao, and A. D. Lopez. 2005. Counting the dead and what they died from: An assessment of the global status of cause of death data. *Bulletin of the World Health Organization* 83:171-177c.

Mayosi, B. M., L. J. Burgess, and A. F. Doubell. 2005. Tuberculous pericarditis. *Circulation* 112(23):3608-3616.

Mayosi, B. M., A. J. Flisher, U. G. Lalloo, F. Sitas, S. M. Tollman, and D. Bradshaw. 2009. The burden of non-communicable diseases in South Africa. *Lancet* 374(9693):934-947.

Mbewu, A., and J. Mbanya. 2006. Cardiovascular disease. In *Disease and mortality in Sub-Saharan Africa*. Edited by D. Jamison, R. G. Feachem, M. W. Makgoba, E. R. Bos, F. K. Baingana, K. J. Hofman and K. O. Rogo. Washington, DC: World Bank Group. Pp. 305-328.

Mendis, S., D. Abegunde, S. Yusuf, S. Ebrahim, G. Shaper, H. Ghannem, and B. Shengelia. 2005. WHO study on prevention of recurrences of myocardial infarction and stroke (WHO-PREMISE). *Bulletin of the World Health Organization* 83(11):820-828.

Miguez-Burbano, M. J., X. Burbano, D. Ashkin, A. Pitchenik, R. Allan, L. Pineda, N. Rodriguez, and G. Shor-Posner. 2003. Impact of tobacco use on the development of opportunistic respiratory infections in HIV seropositive patients on antiretroviral therapy. *Addiction Biology* 8(1):39-43.

Miller, T. L., E. J. Orav, S. E. Lipshultz, K. L. Arheart, C. Duggan, G. A. Weinberg, L. Bechard, L. Furuta, J. Nicchitta, S. L. Gorbach, and A. Shevitz. 2008. Risk factors for cardiovascular disease in children infected with human immunodeficiency virus-1. *Journal of Pediatrics* 153(4):491-497.

Mirzaei, M., A. S. Truswell, R. Taylor, and S. R. Leeder. 2009. Coronary heart disease epidemics: Not all the same. *Heart* 95(9):740-746.

Misra, A., and L. Khurana. 2008. Obesity and the metabolic syndrome in developing countries. *Journal of Clinical Endocrinology and Metabolism* 93(11 Suppl 1):S9-S30.

Moncayo, A., and M. I. O. Yanine. 2006. An update on Chagas disease (human American trypanosomiasis). In *Annals of Tropical Medicine and Parasitology*: Maney Publishing. 100(8):663-677.

Morel, C. M., and J. Lazdins. 2003. Chagas disease. *Nature Reviews Microbiology* 1(1): 14-15.

Mukamal, K. J., and E. B. Rimm. 2001. Alcohol's effects on the risk for coronary heart disease. *Alcohol Research and Health* 25(4):255-261.

Mukamal, K. J., S. E. Chiuve, E. B. Rimm, K. J. Mukamal, S. E. Chiuve, and E. B. Rimm. 2006. Alcohol consumption and risk for coronary heart disease in men with healthy lifestyles. *Archives of Internal Medicine* 166(19):2145-2150.

Muna, W. F. T. 1993. Cardiovascular disorders in Africa. *World Health Statistics Quarterly* 46(2):125-133.

Myint, P. K., R. N. Luben, N. J. Wareham, S. A. Bingham, and K. T. Khaw. 2009. Combined effect of health behaviours and risk of first ever stroke in 20,040 men and women over 11 years' follow-up in Norfolk cohort of European prospective investigation of cancer (EPIC Norfolk): Prospective population study. *British Medical Journal* 338:b349.

Narkiewicz, K., S. E. Kjeldsen, and T. Hedner. 2006. Hypertension and cardiovascular disease in women: Progress towards better understanding of gender-specific differences? *Blood Pressure* 15(2):68-70.

Nathan, D. M., P. A. Cleary, J. Y. Backlund, S. M. Genuth, J. M. Lachin, T. J. Orchard, P. Raskin, and B. Zinman. 2005. Intensive diabetes treatment and cardiovascular disease in patients with type 1 diabetes. *New England Journal of Medicine* 353(25):2643-2653.

Ng, N. 2006. *Chronic disease risk factors in a transitional country: The case of rural Indonesia*, Folkhälsa och klinisk medicin, Umeå.

Ng, N., H. Stenlund, R. Bonita, M. Hakimi, S. Wall, and L. Weinehall. 2006. Preventable risk factors for noncommunicable diseases in rural Indonesia: Prevalence study using WHO STEPS approach. *Bulletin of the World Health Organization* 84(4):305-313.

Ng, S. W., E. C. Norton, and B. M. Popkin. 2009. Why have physical activity levels declined among Chinese adults? Findings from the 1991-2006 China health and nutrition surveys. *Social Science and Medicine* 68(7):1305-1314.

Nishtar, S., A. M. A. Faruqui, M. A. Mattu, K. B. Mohamud, and A. Ahmed. 2004. The national action plan for the prevention and control of non-communicable diseases and health promotion in Pakistan—cardiovascular diseases. *Journal of the Pakistan Medical Association* 54(12 Suppl 3):S14-S25.

Ntsekhe, M., and B. M. Mayosi. 2009. Cardiac manifestations of HIV infection: An African perspective. *Nature Clinical Practice Cardiovascular Medicine* 6(2):120-127.

Office of National Statistics, L. Henderson, K. Irving, and J. Gregory. 2003. *The national diet & nutrition survey: Adults aged 19 to 64 years*. London: Office of National Statistics.

Olshansky, S. J. 2006. Commentary: Prescient visions of public health from Cornaro to Breslow. *International Journal of Epidemiology* 35(1):22-23.

Olshansky, S. J., and A. B. Ault. 1986. The fourth stage of the epidemiologic transition: The age of delayed degenerative diseases. *Milbank Quarterly* 64(3):355-391.

Omran, A. R. 1971. The epidemiologic transition. A theory of the epidemiology of population change. *The Milbank Memorial Fund Quarterly* 49(4):509-538.

Palomaki, G. E., S. Melillo, and L. A. Bradley. 2010. Association between 9p21 genomic markers and heart disease: A meta-analysis. *Journal of the American Medical Association* 303(7):648-656.

Pao, V., G. A. Lee, and C. Grunfeld. 2008. HIV therapy, metabolic syndrome, and cardiovascular risk. *Current Atherosclerosis Reports* 10(1):61-70.

Pencina, M. J., R. B. D'Agostino, M. G. Larson, J. M. Massaro, and R. S. Vasan. 2009. Predicting the 30-year risk of cardiovascular disease: The Framingham Heart Study. *Circulation* 119(24):3078-3084.

Peng, R. D., H. H. Chang, M. L. Bell, A. McDermott, S. L. Zeger, J. M. Samet, and F. Dominici. 2008. Coarse particulate matter air pollution and hospital admissions for cardiovascular and respiratory diseases among medicare patients. *Journal of the American Medical Association* 299(18):2172-2179.

Pereira, M., N. Lunet, A. Azevedo, and H. Barros. 2009. Differences in prevalence, awareness, treatment and control of hypertension between developing and developed countries. *Journal of Hypertension* 27(5):963-975.

Physical Activity Guidelines Advisory Committee. 2008. *Physical activity guidelines advisory committee report, 2008*. Washington, DC: U.S. Department of Health and Human Services.

Pietinen, P., E. Vartiainen, R. Seppanen, A. Aro, and P. Puska. 1996. Changes in diet in Finland from 1972 to 1992: Impact on coronary heart disease risk. *Preventive Medicine* 25(3):243-250.

Pilote, L., K. Dasgupta, V. Guru, K. H. Humphries, J. McGrath, C. Norris, D. Rabi, J. Tremblay, A. Alamian, T. Barnett, J. Cox, W. A. Ghali, S. Grace, P. Hamet, T. Ho, S. Kirkland, M. Lambert, D. Libersan, J. O'Loughlin, G. Paradis, M. Petrovich, and V. Tagalakis. 2007. A comprehensive view of sex-specific issues related to cardiovascular disease. *Canadian Medical Association Journal* 176(6):S1-S44: Erratum 176(9):1310.

Polk, D. M., and T. Z. Naqvi. 2005. Cardiovascular disease in women: Sex differences in presentation, risk factors, and evaluation. *Current Cardiology Reports* 7(3):166-172.

Pope, C. A., and D. W. Dockery. 2006. Health effects of fine particulate air pollution: Lines that connect. *EM: Air and Waste Management Association's Magazine for Environmental Managers* (JUN).

Pope, C. A., R. T. Burnett, G. D. Thurston, M. J. Thun, E. E. Calle, D. Krewski, and J. J. Godleski. 2004. Cardiovascular mortality and long-term exposure to particulate air pollution: Epidemiological evidence of general pathophysiological pathways of disease. *Circulation* 109(1):71-77.

Prentice, A. M., and S. E. Moore. 2005. Early programming of adult diseases in resource poor countries. *Archives of Disease in Childhood* 90(4):429-432.

Puska, P., E. Vartiainen, J. Tuomilehto, V. Salomaa, and A. Nissinen. 1998. Changes in premature deaths in Finland: Successful long-term prevention of cardiovascular diseases. *Bulletin of the World Health Organization* 76(4):419-425.

Puska, P., E. Vartiainen, T. Laatinkainen, P. Jousilahti, and M. Paavola, eds. 2009. *The North Karelia project: From North Karelia to national action.* Helsinki: Helsinki University Printing House.

Rao, A. V. 1998. Coronary heart disease risk factors in women: Focus on gender differences. *Journal of the Louisiana State Medical Society* 150(2):67-72.

Rao, C., A. D. Lopez, G. Yang, S. Begg, and J. Ma. 2005. Evaluating national cause-of-death statistics: Principles and application to the case of China. *Bulletin of the World Health Organization* 83:618-625.

Ray, K. K., S. R. K. Seshasai, S. Wijesuriya, R. Sivakumaran, S. Nethercott, D. Preiss, S. Erqou, and N. Sattar. 2009. Effect of intensive control of glucose on cardiovascular outcomes and death in patients with diabetes mellitus: A meta-analysis of randomised controlled trials. *Lancet* 373(9677):1765-1772.

Reddy, K. S. 2007. India wakes up to the threat of cardiovascular diseases. *Journal of the American College of Cardiology* 50(14):1370-1372.

Reddy, S. P., S. Panday, D. Swart, C. C. Jinabhai, S. L. Amosun, S. James, K. D. Monyeki, G. Stevens, N. Morejele, N. S. Kambaran, R. G. Omardien, and H. W. Van den Borne. 2003. *Umthenthe uhlaba usamila: The South African Youth Risk Behavior Survey 2002.* Cape Town: South African Medical Research Council.

Reeves, M. J., C. D. Bushnell, G. Howard, J. W. Gargano, P. W. Duncan, G. Lynch, A. Khatiwoda, and L. Lisabeth. 2008. Sex differences in stroke: Epidemiology, clinical presentation, medical care, and outcomes. *Lancet Neurology* 7(10):915-926.

Regitz-Zagrosek, V. 2006. Therapeutic implications of the gender-specific aspects of cardiovascular disease. *Nature Reviews Drug Discovery* 5(5):425-438.

Rehm, J., C. Mathers, S. Popova, M. Thavorncharoensap, Y. Teerawattananon, and J. Patra. 2009. Global burden of disease and injury and economic cost attributable to alcohol use and alcohol-use disorders. *Lancet* 373(9682):2223-2233.

Reuser, M., L. G. Bonneux, and F. J. Willekens. 2009. Smoking kills, obesity disables: A multistate approach of the US Health and Retirement Survey. *Obesity* 17(4):783-789.

Rich, M. W., and G. A. Mensah. 2009. Fifth pivotal research in cardiology in the elderly (price-v) symposium: Preventive cardiology in the elderly—executive summary. Part I: Morning session. *Preventive Cardiology* 12(4):198-204.

Rich, M. W., and G. A. Mensah. 2010. Fifth pivotal research in cardiology in the elderly (price-v) symposium: Preventive cardiology in the elderly—executive summary. Part II: Afternoon session. *Preventive Cardiology* 13(1):42-47.

Rodriguez, T., M. Malvezzi, L. Chatenoud, C. Bosetti, F. Levi, E. Negri, and C. La Vecchia. 2006. Trends in mortality from coronary heart and cerebrovascular diseases in the Americas: 1970-2000. *Heart* 92(4):453-460.

Roeters van Lennep, J. E., H. T. Westerveld, D. W. Erkelens, and E. E. van der Wall. 2002. Risk factors for coronary heart disease: Implications of gender. *Cardiovascular Research* 53(3):538-549.

Roglic, G., and N. Unwin. 2009. Mortality attributable to diabetes: Estimates for the year 2010. *Diabetes Research and Clinical Practice* 87(1):15-19.

Rosengren, A., S. Hawken, S. Ounpuu, K. Sliwa, M. Zubaid, W. A. Almahmeed, K. N. Blackett, C. Sitthi-amorn, H. Sato, and S. Yusuf. 2004. Association of psychosocial risk factors with risk of acute myocardial infarction in 11119 cases and 13648 controls from 52 countries (the INTERHEART study): Case-control study. *Lancet* 364(9438):953-962.

Rossouw, J. E., G. L. Anderson, R. L. Prentice, A. Z. LaCroix, C. Kooperberg, M. L. Stefanick, R. D. Jackson, S. A. Beresford, B. V. Howard, K. C. Johnson, J. M. Kotchen, J. Ockene, and Writing Group for the Women's Health Initiative. 2002. Risks and benefits of estrogen plus progestin in healthy postmenopausal women: Principal results from the Women's Health Initiative randomized controlled trial. *Journal of the American Medical Association* 288(3):321-333.

Rugulies, R. 2002. Depression as a predictor for coronary heart disease: A review and meta-analysis. *American Journal of Preventive Medicine* 23(1):51-61.

Sabaté, E., WHO Adherence to Long Term Therapies Project, Global Adherence Interdisciplinary Network, and World Health Organization Deptartment of Management of Noncommunicable Diseases. 2003. *Adherence to long-term therapies: Evidence for action.* Geneva: World Health Organization.

Sacks, F. M., M. A. Pfeffer, L. A. Moye, J. L. Rouleau, J. D. Rutherford, T. G. Cole, L. Brown, J. W. Warnica, J. M. Arnold, C. C. Wun, B. R. Davis, and E. Braunwald. 1996. The effect of pravastatin on coronary events after myocardial infarction in patients with average cholesterol levels. Cholesterol and recurrent events trial investigators. *New England Journal of Medicine* 335(14):1001-1009.

Sarkar, S., and B. Mukhopadhyay. 2008. Perceived psychosocial stress and cardiovascular risk: Observations among the Bhutias of Sikkim, India. *Stress and Health* 24(1):23-34.

Sassi, F., M. Cecchini, J. Lauer, and D. Chisholm. 2009. *Improving lifestyles, tackling obesity: The health and economic impact of prevention strategies.* Paris: OECD.

Sattelmair, J. R., J. H. Pertman, and D. E. Forman. 2009. Effects of physical activity on cardiovascular and noncardiovascular outcomes in older adults. *Clinics in Geriatric Medicine* 25(4):677-702.

Schaefer, B. M., V. Caracciolo, W. H. Frishman, and P. Charney. 2003. Gender, ethnicity, and genes in cardiovascular disease. Part 2: Implications for pharmacotherapy. *Heart Disease* 5(3):202-214.

Schneidera, N. K., and T. E. Novotnya. 2007. Addressing smoking cessation in tuberculosis control. *Bulletin of the World Health Organization* 85(10):820.

Schulze, M. B., F. B. Hu. 2005. Primary prevention of diabetes: What can be done and how much can be prevented? *Annual Review of Public Health* 26:445-467.

Shafey, O., M. Eriksen, H. Ross, and J. Mackay. 2009. *The tobacco atlas.* 3rd ed. Atlanta: American Cancer Society.

Shen, B. J., Y. E. Avivi, J. F. Todaro, A. Spiro III, J. P. Laurenceau, K. D. Ward, and R. Niaura. 2008. Anxiety characteristics independently and prospectively predict myocardial infarction in men. The unique contribution of anxiety among psychologic factors. *Journal of the American College of Cardiology* 51(2):113-119.

Shepherd, J., S. M. Cobbe, I. Ford, C. G. Isles, A. R. Lorimer, P. W. MacFarlane, J. H. McKillop, and C. J. Packard. 1995. Prevention of coronary heart disease with pravastatin in men with hypercholesterolemia. West of Scotland coronary prevention study group. *New England Journal of Medicine* 333(20):1301-1307.

Shopland, D. R. 1995. Tobacco use and its contribution to early cancer mortality with a special emphasis on cigarette smoking. *Environmental Health Perspectives* 103(Suppl 8):131-142.

Shuter, J., and S. Bernstein. 2008. Cigarette smoking is an independent predictor of nonadherence in HIV-infected individuals receiving highly active antiretroviral therapy. *Nicotine and Tobacco Research* 10(4):731-736.

Slama, K., C. Y. Chiang, D. A. Enarson, K. Hassmiller, A. Fanning, P. Gupta, and C. Ray. 2007. Tobacco and tuberculosis: A qualitative systematic review and meta-analysis. *International Journal of Tuberculosis and Lung Disease* 11(10):1049-1061.

Slattery, M. L., and D. E. Randall. 1988. Trends in coronary heart disease mortality and food consumption in the united states between 1909 and 1980. *American Journal of Clinical Nutrition* 47(6):1060-1067.

Sliwa, K., D. Wilkinson, C. Hansen, L. Ntyintyane, K. Tibazarwa, A. Becker, and S. Stewart. 2008. Spectrum of heart disease and risk factors in a black urban population in South Africa (the Heart of Soweto study): A cohort study. *Lancet* 371(9616):915-922.

South African Department of Health and Medical Research Council. 2007. *South Africa Demographic and Health Survey 2003*. Pretoria, South Africa: South African Department of Health.

Srinivasan, S. R., G. H. Dahlen, R. A. Jarpa, L. S. Webber, and G. S. Berenson. 1991. Racial (black-white) differences in serum lipoprotein (a) distribution and its relation to parental myocardial infarction in children. Bogalusa Heart Study. *Circulation* 84(1):160-167.

Stamler, J., R. Stamler, and J. D. Neaton. 1993. Blood pressure, systolic and diastolic, and cardiovascular risks: US population data. *Archives of Internal Medicine* 153(5):598-615.

Steer, A. C., and J. R. Carapetis. 2009. Prevention and treatment of rheumatic heart disease in the developing world. *Nature Reviews Cardiology* 6(11):689-698.

Steer, A. C., J. R. Carapetis, T. M. Nolan, and F. Shann. 2002. Systematic review of rheumatic heart disease prevalence in children in developing countries: The role of environmental factors. *Journal of Paediatrics and Child Health* 38(3):229-234.

Stein, A. D., A. M. Thompson, and A. Waters. 2005. Childhood growth and chronic disease: Evidence from countries undergoing the nutrition transition. *Maternal & Child Nutrition* 1(3):177-184.

Stettler, C., S. Allemann, P. Juni, C. A. Cull, R. R. Holman, M. Egger, S. Krahenbuhl, and P. Diem. 2006. Glycemic control and macrovascular disease in types 1 and 2 diabetes mellitus: Meta-analysis of randomized trials. *American Heart Journal* 152(1):27-38.

Steyn, N. P., D. Bradshaw, R. Norman, J. Joubert, M. Schneider, and K. Steyn. 2006. *Dietary changes and the health transition in South Africa: Implications for health policy*. Cape Town: South African Medical Research Council.

Strong, J. P., G. T. Malcom, C. A. McMahan, R. E. Tracy, W. P. Newman, 3rd, E. E. Herderick, and J. F. Cornhill. 1999. Prevalence and extent of atherosclerosis in adolescents and young adults: Implications for prevention from the pathobiological determinants of atherosclerosis in youth study. *Journal of the American Medical Association* 281(8):727-735.

Thomas, R. J., P. J. Palumbo, L. J. Melton Iii, V. L. Roger, J. Ransom, P. C. O'Brien, and C. L. Leibson. 2003. Trends in the mortality burden associated with diabetes mellitus: A population-based study in Rochester, Minn, 1970-1994. *Archives of Internal Medicine* 163(4):445-451.

Turnbull, F. M., C. Abraira, R. J. Anderson, R. P. Byington, J. P. Chalmers, W. C. Duckworth, G. W. Evans, H. C. Gerstein, R. R. Holman, T. E. Moritz, B. C. Neal, T. Ninomiya, A. A. Patel, S. K. Paul, F. Travert, and M. Woodward. 2009. Intensive glucose control and macrovascular outcomes in type 2 diabetes. *Diabetologia*. DOI 10.1007/s00125-00009-01470-00120.

Turtzo, L. C., and L. D. McCullough. 2008. Sex differences in stroke. *Cerebrovascular Diseases* 26(5):462-474.

Unal, B., J. A. Critchley, and S. Capewell. 2004. Explaining the decline in coronary heart disease mortality in England and Wales between 1981 and 2000. *Circulation* 109(9):1101-1107.

United Nations Development Program. 2007. *Human development report 2007/2008: Fighting climate change: Human solidarity in a divided world*. New York: United Nations Development Program.

van Cappelle, F. 2009. StatPlanet: Interactive Data Visualization and Mapping Software, Southern and Eastern Africa Consortium for Monitoring Educational Quality, Paris. http://www.sacmeq.org/statplanet (accessed January 21, 2010).

van Dam, R. M., T. Li, D. Spiegelman, O. H. Franco, F. B. Hu, R. M. van Dam, T. Li, D. Spiegelman, O. H. Franco, and F. B. Hu. 2008. Combined impact of lifestyle factors on mortality: Prospective cohort study in US women. *British Medical Journal* 337:a1440.

Vartiainen, E., P. Puska, P. Jousilahti, H. J. Korhonen, J. Tuomilehto, and A. Nissinen. 1994a. Twenty-year trends in coronary risk factors in North Karelia and in other areas of Finland. *International Journal of Epidemiology* 23(3):495-504.

Vartiainen, E., P. Puska, J. Pekkanen, J. Tuomilehto, and P. Jousilahti. 1994b. Changes in risk factors explain changes in mortality from ischaemic heart disease in Finland. *British Medical Journal* 309(6946):23-27.

Victora, C. G., L. Adair, C. Fall, P. C. Hallal, R. Martorell, L. Richter, and H. S. Sachdev. 2008. Maternal and child undernutrition: Consequences for adult health and human capital. *Lancet* 371(9609):340-357.

Wagner, S., and R. M. Romano. 1994. Tobacco and the developing world: An old threat poses even bigger problems. *Journal of the National Cancer Institute* 86(23):1752.

Walker, S., and S. George. 2007. Young@heart. USA: Fox Searchlight Pictures.

Wang, L., X. Qi, C. Chen, J. Ma, L. Li, K. Rao, L. Kong, G. Ma, H. Xiang, J. Pu, J. Chen, Y. Chen, C. Chen, Y. He, J. Zhang, S. Jin, Y. Wu, X. Yang, J. Hu, C. Yao, W. Zhao, K. Ge, and F. Zai, eds. 2005. *Survey and report on the status of nutrition and health of the Chinese people: A comprehensive report for 2002*. Beijing: People's Medical Publishing House.

Wang, Y., J. Mi, X. Y. Shan, Q. J. Wang, and K. Y. Ge. 2007. Is China facing an obesity epidemic and the consequences? The trends in obesity and chronic disease in China. *International Journal of Obesity* 31(1):177-188.

Warren, C. W. 2003. Differences in worldwide tobacco use by gender: Findings from the global youth tobacco survey global. *Journal of School Health* 73(6):207-215.

Warren, C. W., N. R. Jones, A. Peruga, J. Chauvin, J. P. Baptiste, V. Costa de Silva, F. el Awa, A. Tsouros, K. Rahman, B. Fishburn, D. W. Bettcher, and S. Asma. 2008. Global youth tobacco surveillance, 2000-2007. *MMWR Surveillance Summaries* 57(1):1-28.

Wassertheil-Smoller, S., S. L. Hendrix, M. Limacher, G. Heiss, C. Kooperberg, A. Baird, T. Kotchen, J. D. Curb, H. Black, J. E. Rossouw, A. Aragaki, M. Safford, E. Stein, S. Laowattana, and W. J. Mysiw. 2003. Effect of estrogen plus progestin on stroke in postmenopausal women: The Women's Health Initiative: A randomized trial. *Journal of the American Medical Association* 289(20):2673-2684.

Watkins, D. A., L. J. Zuhlke, M. E. Engel, and B. M. Mayosi. 2009. Rheumatic fever: Neglected again. *Science* 324(5923):37.

Watkins, R. E., and A. J. Plant. 2006. Does smoking explain sex differences in the global tuberculosis epidemic? *Epidemiology and Infection* 134(2):333-339.

WHO (World Health Organization). 1999. *The world health report: 1999: Making a difference*. Geneva: World Health Organization.

WHO. 2002. *The world health report 2002—reducing risks, promoting healthy life*. Geneva: World Health Organization.

WHO. 2003. *The world health report: 2003: Shaping the future*. Geneva: World Health Organization.

WHO. 2005. *Preventing chronic diseases: A vital investment*. http://www.who.int/chp/chronic_disease_report/full_report.pdf (accessed April 23, 2009).

WHO. 2007. *WHO model list of essential medicines: 15th edition, revised March 2007*. Geneva: World Health Organization.

WHO. 2008a. Childhood overweight and obesity. http://www.who.int/dietphysicalactivity/childhood/en/ (accessed December 12, 2008).

WHO. 2008b. *The global burden of disease: 2004 update*. Geneva: World Health Organization.

WHO. 2008c. *WHO report on the global tobacco epidemic, 2008: The MPOWER package.* Geneva: World Health Organization.
WHO. 2009a. Global burden of disease 2004 data. Geneva, provided by Colin Mathers.
WHO. 2009b. *Global health risks: Mortality and burden of disease attributable to selected major risks.* Geneva: World Health Organization.
WHO. 2009c. *WHO model list of essential medicines: 16th edition, revised March 2009.* Geneva: World Health Organization.
WHO. 2009d. *Working document for developing a draft global strategy to reduce harmful use of alcohol.* Geneva: World Health Organization.
WHO. 2009e. *World health statistics 2009.* Geneva: World Health Organization.
WHO Department of Child and Adolescent Health and Development. 2005. *The current evidence for the burden of group a streptococcal diseases, Discussion papers on child health.* Geneva: World Health Organization.
WHO Expert Committee on Problems Related to Alcohol Consumption and WHO. 2007. *Second report, World Health Organization technical report series.* Geneva: World Health Organization.
WHO Expert Committee on the Control of Chagas Disease and WHO. 2002. *Control of Chagas disease: Second report of the WHO Expert Committee, WHO technical report series.* Geneva: World Health Organization.
WHO Regional Office for the Western Pacific. 2007. *Mongolian STEPS survey on the prevalence of noncommunicable disease risk factors 2006.* Manila, Philippines: WHO Regional Office for the Western Pacific.
WHO Study Group on Rheumatic Fever and Rheumatic Heart Disease and WHO. 2004. *Rheumatic fever and rheumatic heart disease: Report of a WHO expert consultation, Geneva, 20 October–1 November 2001, World Health Organization technical report series.* Geneva: World Health Organization.
WHOSIS (World Health Organization Statistical Information System). 2009. World Health Organization.
Witt, B. J., and V. L. Roger. 2003. Sex differences in heart disease incidence and prevalence: Implications for intervention. *Expert Opinion on Pharmacotherapy* 4(5):675-683.
The Writing Committee. 2004. Cardio- and cerebrovascular events in HIV-infected persons. *AIDS* 18(13):1811-1817.
Yach, D., C. Hawkes, C. L. Gould, and K. J. Hofman. 2004. The global burden of chronic diseases: Overcoming impediments to prevention and control. *Journal of the American Medical Association* 291(21):2616-2622.
Yach, D., S. R. Leeder, J. Bell, and B. Kistnasamy. 2005. Global chronic diseases. *Science* 307(5708):317.
Yang, G., L. Kong, W. Zhao, X. Wan, Y. Zhai, L. C. Chen, and J. P. Koplan. 2008. Emergence of chronic non-communicable diseases in China. *Lancet* 372(9650):1697-1705.
Young, F., J. Critchley, and N. Unwin. 2009a. Diabetes & tuberculosis: A dangerous liaison & no white tiger. *Indian Journal of Medical Research* 130(1):1-4.
Young, F., J. A. Critchley, L. K. Johnstone, and N. C. Unwin. 2009b. A review of co-morbidity between infectious and chronic disease in Sub Saharan Africa: TB and diabetes mellitus, HIV and metabolic syndrome, and the impact of globalization. *Global Health* 5:9.
Yusuf, P. S., S. Hawken, S. Ounpuu, T. Dans, A. Avezum, F. Lanas, M. McQueen, A. Budaj, P. Pais, J. Varigos, and L. Lisheng. 2004. Effect of potentially modifiable risk factors associated with myocardial infarction in 52 countries (the INTERHEART study): Case-control study. *Lancet* 364(9438):937-952.

Ziegelstein, R. C., J. A. Fauerbach, S. S. Stevens, J. Romanelli, D. P. Richter, and D. E. Bush. 2000. Patients with depression are less likely to follow recommendations to reduce cardiac risk during recovery from a myocardial infarction. *Archives of Internal Medicine* 160(12):1818-1823.

3

Development and Cardiovascular Disease

Chapter 2 reviewed the extent and nature of the burden of cardiovascular disease (CVD) and focused primarily on classically defined individual risk factors that contribute to the global burden of disease. To build on this epidemiological information, it is equally important to understand the relationship of CVD to economic growth and development, including related systemic drivers that contribute to the global burden of CVD, such as demographic change, urbanization, globalization, technological development, and social and cultural norms. This chapter presents conclusions from available evidence and analysis to help further understand the nature and consequences of the problem in low and middle income countries from this broad perspective.

This chapter first offers a discussion of the available evidence on the relationship between stage of economic development and CVD across countries. This is then expanded to a general overview of broad systemic drivers of health that affect trends in CVD and are closely related to economic growth and development—Chapter 5 will describe the drivers with the strongest rationale and evidence for targeted intervention approaches in more detail. The chapter then concludes with a review of the evidence documenting economic impacts of CVD in low and middle income countries, both for countries and for households, highlighting the finding that the burden falls disproportionately on the poor.

ECONOMIC DEVELOPMENT AND CARDIOVASCULAR DISEASE

Unfortunately, the economics of CVD in low and middle income countries is not heavily studied and methods and data are not uniform; as a result, there is a scattering of estimates that are not comparable. Although more work is needed to truly understand the economics of this pressing global health issue, the totality of the existing evidence makes it clear that now, and increasingly over time, the economic consequences of CVD are significant.

It is widely accepted that health and income are interdependent, but the magnitude of the interaction is more difficult to discern. This is probably because each country has its own unique circumstances that determine how much health it can buy for a given expenditure. The point at which poor health slows economic growth sufficiently to impede development depends on the specific economic conditions. It is therefore difficult to derive general rules. In theory, the health–wealth relationship should be improved if health promotion and disease prevention policies and programs are able to start earlier in a country's development trajectory. The relationship between health and economic development was carefully reexamined by the Commission on Growth and Development (World Bank Commission on Growth and Development, 2008), which concluded that despite considerable efforts through historical research, cross-sectional analysis, and innovative ways of integrating household factors into cross-country studies that have pushed the methodological envelope, the effects of health investments on economic performance remain inconclusive. The commission also concluded that chronic illness undermines current productivity and is likely to lead to future losses in economic output; however, it did not indicate the magnitude of that economic loss. Thus, not only will economic development alone be insufficient to improve chronic disease outcomes in developing countries, but also the widespread appearance of chronic disease also threatens to deter the economic growth needed in many low income countries.

Historical experience in and across countries illustrates how increased wealth and development can be expected to affect cardiovascular health. Two conclusions emerge from the empirical analysis. First, there is no single pattern that characterizes the relationship between economic development and CVD. Indeed, as described in Chapter 2, there is wide variation in age-standardized mortality rates from CVD even among countries in the same income category (WHOSIS, 2009). Second, despite the variability, a general pattern does emerge in which the prevalence of CVD and its risk factors appear to increase and then to decline as countries progress through phases of development. Cross-country evidence suggests that CVD and other chronic disease incidence rises as countries move from lowest income to low-middle income, driven by exposure to lifestyle risks and low access to health services. As countries move further up the income scale to upper-middle and high income status, risks and prevalence decline (Ezzati et al., 2005). As described in Chapter 2, these declines stem from both behavioral changes and better health care. Figure 3.1 shows that with increasing gross domestic product (GDP) there is an increase and then a decline in the major biological risks for CVD for both men and women.

Economic development is a major factor driving the epidemiological transition. For example, differences in GDP per capita explain almost two-thirds of the differences in female obesity among 37 developing countries (Monteiro et al., 2004). Within countries, CVD is also closely related to income level. CVD and its risks are concentrated among the lowest socioeconomic groups of the more developed (upper-middle and high income) countries, and among middle and high income populations of low-middle income countries (McLaren, 2007; Monteiro et al., 2004). However, even in some countries that have seen little economic progress, a transition to chronic disease can be observed. In part of rural Bangladesh, for example, estimated chronic disease-related mortality went from 8 to 68 percent, while estimated communicable disease mortality dropped from 52 to 11 percent (Ahsan Karar et al., 2009). Because CVD is rising in low and middle income countries and among the lowest socioeconomic groups in high income countries while falling among the wealthy, CVD is one of the few diseases that increases global health inequalities (Becker et al., 2005). Indeed, CVD and its related risks are gradually becoming diseases of the poor, and these divergences are pushing life expectancy in opposite directions in high income and low and middle income countries.

Not only can economic development influence trends in CVD risk, but also CVD can affect economic development. High CVD prevalence has likely depressed economic growth in high income countries in the past. This effect has lessened with recent declines in CVD in high income countries (Becker et al., 2005). CVD and other chronic diseases already have an economic impact in low and middle income countries, as described later in this chapter. The potential to result in a brake on economic growth may emerge as CVD risk rises (Suhrcke and Urban, 2006). Therefore, serious economic concerns remain for developing countries; however, the diminishing negative economic effects of CVD with decreasing prevalence in high income countries suggests that there is potential for risk and disease prevention to protect those countries from more serious economic ramifications.

Conclusion 3.1: In general, CVD risks are rising among low income countries, are highest for middle income developing countries, and then fall off for countries at a more advanced stage of development. This pattern reflects a complex interaction among average per capita income in a country, trends in lifestyle, and other risk factors, and health systems capacity to control CVD. Thus, the challenge facing low income developing countries is to continue to bring down prevalence of infectious diseases while avoiding an overwhelming rise in CVD, especially under conditions of resource limitations. This will require balancing

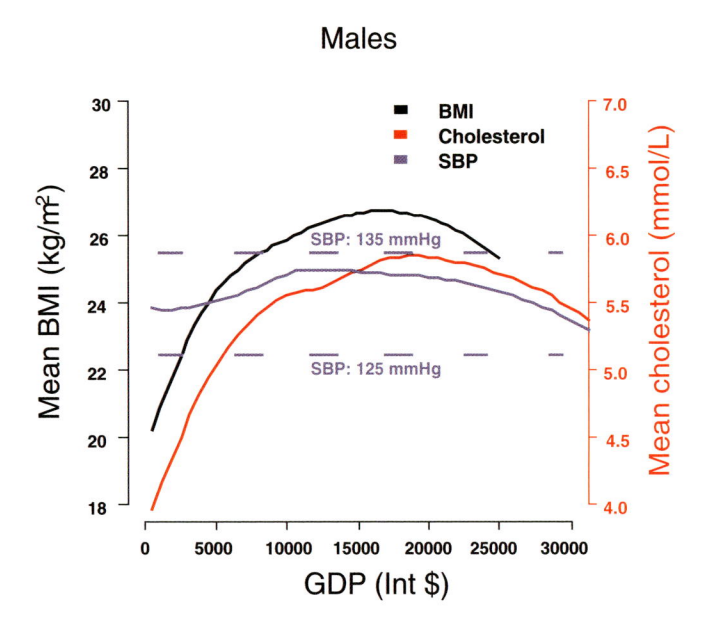

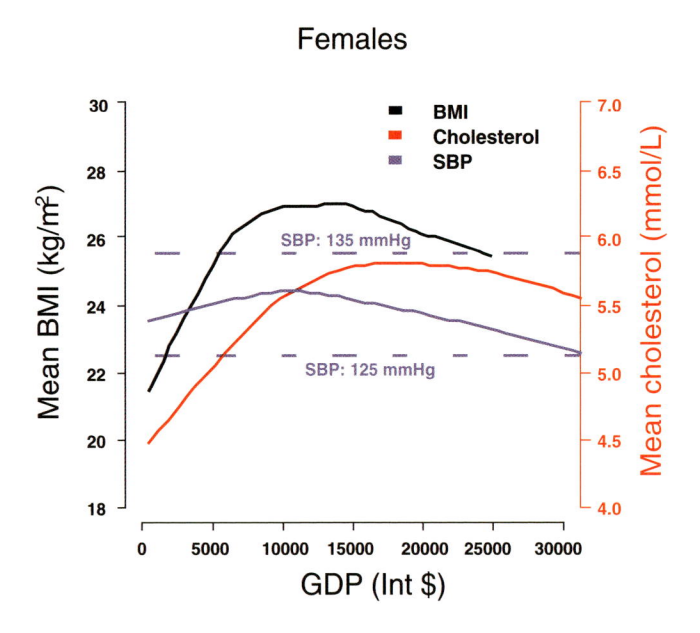

FIGURE 3.1 CVD risks in relation to national income.
NOTE: SBP = systolic blood pressure.
SOURCE: Ezzati et al., 2005.

competing population-level health demands while maintaining relatively low overall health expenditures. Investments in health will also need to be balanced with pressing needs to invest in other social needs and industrial development to produce a positive health–wealth trajectory. The challenge facing middle income developing countries is to reverse or slow the rise in CVD in an affordable and cost-effective manner.

DEVELOPMENT AND SYSTEMIC DRIVERS OF HEALTH

Most of the countries that are now considered developed went through an economic transformation in the early to mid-20th century that was accompanied by major advances in health and longer life expectancy. The catalysts for advances in economic production included the expansion of public sanitation systems, new medical technology, and improved nutrition. Today, however, the relationship between health and economic development is more complex. Key historic indicators of development progress—a relative decline in agrarian society and rise in urban lifestyles, a dominance of manufacturing and service-sector employment, and greater diversity in food and agriculture—also pose risks that threaten to undermine or thwart economic development and negatively affect health, including shifts that increase chronic disease risk.

Therefore, related to the strong role that economic development and economic conditions exert on CVD, key systemic drivers—both distal and proximate—have emerged. Systemic drivers here refer to broad processes that ultimately have an effect on classically defined individual risk factors. Distal drivers have long-term impacts across many populations and can be thought of as underlying causes; while proximate drivers are closely tied to specific conditions and periods. Both are influenced by country-specific social, political, and economic factors; yet they may present opportunities to modify the factors leading to increased CVD incidence. These opportunities are discussed in Chapter 5. The broad distal drivers that influence CVD include dynamic demographic conditions such as population aging and urbanization; shifts in agriculture; technology development and adoption; education; cultural and social norms; and the multifarious influences of globalization and increasingly open world markets. These are accompanied by more proximate drivers such as health financing structures, the built environment, and ideology diffusion. This section briefly describes the expected relationship between these drivers and CVD, summarized in Figure 3.2. The drivers with the strongest rationale and evidence for targeted intervention approaches are described in more detail in Chapter 5. The relationships between CVD and other economic conditions—such as inequality and poverty—are described in greater detail later in this chapter.

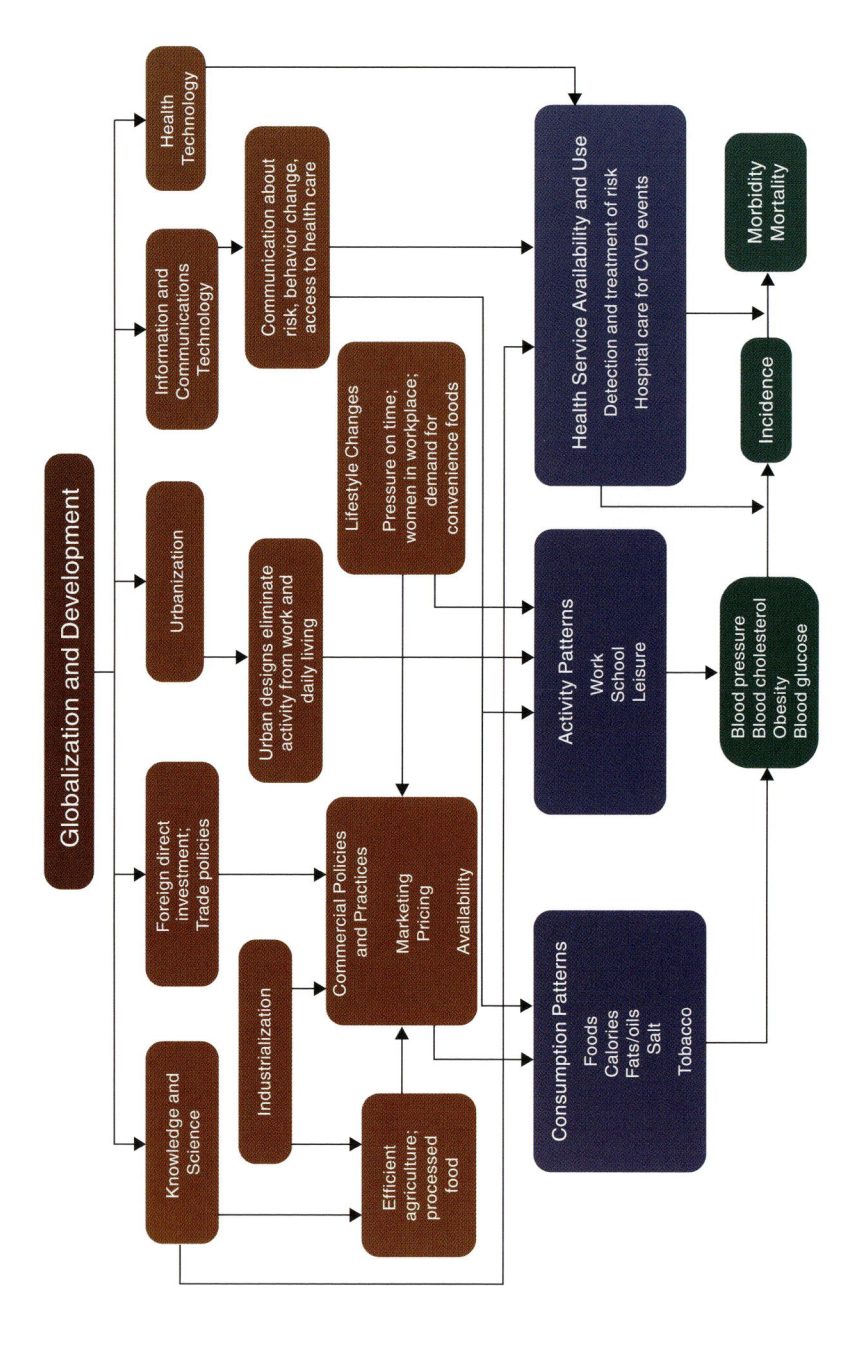

FIGURE 3.2 Systemic drivers of global CVD.

Dynamic Demographic Conditions

Population Aging

A younger population is generally at lower risk of CVD, and most developing countries have younger populations than developed countries. However, the population median age in developing countries is catching up to that of developed countries. The number of persons worldwide aged 65 years or older is projected to reach more than 690 million by 2012, with 460 million in developing countries (Reddy, 2009). The decline in infectious diseases and nutritional disorders contributes to this transition and enhances the proportional burden of CVD (Reddy and Yusuf, 1998).

Although it is often assumed that age is a risk factor for CVD, in reality, this may be overstated. As discussed in Chapter 2, with age comes cumulative exposure to specific CVD risks as well as to the impact of negative social, educational, and economic factors. For example, the relationship between increasing risk and age with respect to blood pressure has been well described in various populations as they move from low-salt and low-stress environments to cities (Danaei et al., 2009; He and MacGregor, 2009; Iqbal et al., 2008). It may be the accumulation of these risks over time that contributes to increases in CVD rather than age per se (Darnton-Hill et al., 2004). This suggests that aging need not necessarily lead to a greater burden of ill health in the future but rather that by preventing and removing the risks, a significant part of the relationship between CVD and aging may be reduced. In fact, work done by Fries (2005) shows convincingly that in the United States there is evidence that lifelong prevention can yield lower age-specific disease and disability rates.

Urbanization

While many countries still lack those basic amenities that contribute to a large proportion of the infectious disease burden, such as clean water and sanitation, many more people also inhabit urban environments that inhibit human-propelled movement or punish it with soaring rates of road traffic accidents, expose people to highly polluted air, and introduce severe limitations on access to healthy food choices, especially for the poor. The nature of economic production has also changed with the rise of technology-based and other forms of employment that accelerate the transition from rural lifestyles. Occupational health risks—including sedentariness—add to a shift toward chronic disease risk exposures.

Urbanization is perhaps the second most powerful demographic change underway worldwide, second only to population aging in terms of its impact on CVD. The world has recently passed the point where there are more people living in the urban environment than in rural areas

(UNFPA, 2007). The pace of urbanization in the developing world will not slow for decades, and will be concentrated in the poorest—currently the most rural—regions (UNDESA, 2008; Yusuf et al., 2001a). Indeed, it is estimated that developing country populations will be largely urban by 2050 (UNDESA, 2008). In China, for example, the pace of urbanization has been staggering, with more than 170 cities with a population greater than 1 million people and more than 920 million people expected to be living in cities by 2025 (Agence-France Presse, 2008). The consequences of urban living for health in general and CVD more specifically demand far greater attention.

A very simplistic summary of the trends shows that urbanization is generally associated with an increase in tobacco use, obesity, some aspects of an unhealthy diet, and a decline in physical activity (Gajalakshmi et al., 2003; Goyal and Yusuf, 2006; Steyn, 2006; Yang et al., 2008; Yusuf et al., 2001a). These relationships have profound implications for CVD risk. However, concomitant with increased risks come greater access to health care and education—both factors that are associated with reduced CVD risk. On the whole, urban populations are both healthier and wealthier than rural populations. Latin America may be the best example of these dual trends as it has almost completed the journey through the demographic and epidemiological transitions as a consequence of economic growth and urbanization, but displays increasing inequalities in both income and level of education, with adverse impacts on lifestyle and nutritional risks (PAHO, 2007).

As will be discussed in Chapter 5, there are potential opportunities to avoid the negative impacts of urbanization, and possibly to use the growing investment in new city development for health gains, including gains for CVD. However, these opportunities need to be fully grasped, which requires urban designers to be more aware of the need to consider and incorporate CVD prevention and to be more willing to plan accordingly. In this context, recent proposals by Collins and Koplan (2009) about the value of health impact assessments prior to urban development initiatives being undertaken deserves attention. There are examples in the United States and Europe where this approach has been done successfully.

Immigration and Acculturation

Part of demographic change is population migration and acculturation into new social and cultural contexts. Since the 1970s evidence has grown that immigrants to western countries have higher rates of coronary heart disease (CHD) than the rates found in their country of origin. Early studies found that Japanese immigrants to the United States had higher rates of CHD and higher prevalence of several risk factors including dyslipidemia and hypertension (Kato et al., 1973; Marmot et al., 1975). Subsequent research has found similar increases in CHD compared to that of the population of origin among immigrants from China and South Asia to western countries as well as among migrants who move from rural to urban settings within countries and adopt more "western" lifestyles (Yusuf et al., 2001a, 2001b). Research on indigenous populations within western countries has also found significant increases in rates of CVD and its associated risk factors when they abandon their traditional diets and ways of life (Yusuf et al., 2001b).

When compared to the general population in their new country, research has found that some immigrant groups exhibit higher rates of CVD, while other groups experience lower rates. For example, South Asian immigrants in the United Kingdom and Canada have higher rates of CHD compared to other ethnic groups; however, Chinese immigrants in Canada have markedly lower rates (Yusuf et al., 2001b). In general, research on immigration and acculturation supports the conclusion that the same risk factors are the main drivers of CVD across populations and countries and that it is differences in the exposure to these risks factors that influence rates of CVD in immigrant groups.

Shifts in Agriculture

In the past century, people were just beginning to move off the farms and away from small-scale food production. People were cognizant of what they were eating: if they hadn't grown it themselves, they knew where it came from. Now, food is a globalized commodity—food exports accounted for 7.1 percent of all merchandise exports globally in 2008 (World Trade Organization, 2009). Food production and consumption have become separated, and governments exert greater influence over what is produced and what it costs, driven in part by a strong agricultural lobby. Consumers in developing as well as developed countries have far greater food choices along some dimensions, but far fewer along others. Food is more often prepared and eaten outside the home. As discussed in Chapter 2, high income country patterns of eating are increasingly available everywhere in the world to those who can afford it. However, developing country populations experience these dietary patterns without the educational levels, medical care, and public health systems that, in developed countries, can somewhat mitigate the risks they pose.

Technology Development and Adoption

Sparked by the discovery of penicillin, which quickly and cheaply cured many of the infectious diseases that formerly led to death at a young age, a new era in health care and medicine since the past century has focused on devising new treatments and technologies to reduce disease. Indeed, developed countries have benefited relatively more than developing countries from reductions in mortality that required new technological developments, relatively costly change of habits, and expensive surgical interventions. In developing countries, it is transfers of previously available and less expensive health technology and knowledge from developed to developing countries that have reduced mortality from infectious, respiratory, and digestive diseases, congenital anomalies, and perinatal period conditions and helped bring life expectancy closer to the developed country average (Becker et al., 2005). It is not clear to what extent new technologies and expensive interventions of the kind that have been responsible for declines in CVD mortality in rich countries will provide feasible solutions in developing countries. Despite the technological advances being made and the market potential seen in many middle income countries, in many developing country settings there are cost-prohibitive challenges across all types of treatment options, from diagnostic technologies to provision of medication to advanced surgical interventions. It will be necessary to address the obstacles and opportunities associated with each aspect in order to ensure the continued development of affordable, sustainable solutions in low and middle income countries.

Cultural and Social Norms

Health is universally affected by cultural and social norms and behaviors, with wide variation across countries. Cultural food preferences, societal norms for body shape, cultural practices around use of leisure time and physical activity, and gender norms can interact with other risk factors to contribute to high rates of obesity and CVD risk. In Mexico, for example, high levels of consumption of traditional fruit-based sugary drinks contribute to obesity as the population has shifted from rural to urban lifestyles (Barquera et al., 2008). Cultural and social norms are embedded in society but not immutable. Greater globalization of the food supply, from agricultural production techniques to marketing, have altered consumer preferences and behaviors over a relatively brief period. Fiscal and other policies have also been used to rapidly change consumer choices for fats (Zatonski et al., 1998) and tobacco (Jha et al., 2006). Therefore, although CVD risk must be considered in view of cultural and social norms, it is not predetermined by them.

Globalization and CVD

Globalization has been associated with the spread of knowledge and science, telecommunications and other information technologies, and cultural and behavioral adaptations. Globalization is a broad term that sometimes encompasses less regulated domestic and international markets; themselves associated with increased foreign direct investment, expansion of marketing, and wider and more homogeneous consumer choices. Although still a topic that arouses vigorous debate, globalization is generally accepted as having led to substantial improvement in quality of life for millions of people by advancing social and economic modernization. Yet, at the same time, there is legitimate concern and circumstantial evidence that globalization's unintended consequences can fuel unhealthy consumption and lifestyle behaviors. Striking examples are presented by the spreading ubiquity of a "western" diet (Iqbal et al., 2008) and greater use of tobacco (Shafey et al., 2009), both of which are closely related to higher disposable incomes. While the latter phenomenon unambiguously contributes to CVD and should be addressed by aggressive public policies across agriculture, industrial, and consumer sectors, the former is more complicated. Globalization of food not only provides greater consumer choice, but also it has improved diets for large numbers of previously undernourished people. Thus, in these and other ways, globalization and its related impacts both reduce and create CVD risks. Policy action is required at the global level and through international channels such as trade discussions to, for example, address the expansion of transnational tobacco companies into low and middle income countries. Policy recommendations in international trade are generally beyond the Committee's technical expertise and therefore, although acknowledged for their potential role in addressing the global epidemic of CVD, are not fully explored in the section on intersectoral policies in this report.

In conclusion, the "healthy growth" of the past in which development was synonymous with better health is now not as easily achieved. Development brings the benefits of higher incomes including, in most countries, higher life expectancy as childhood infectious disease deaths fall. But the modern development process also confronts populations with serious and long-lasting health risks, challenging societies to find alternative organizational, technological, and policy choices. Still-developing countries have the advantage that they have not fully adopted the behaviors and conditions that raise CVD risks, and countries all along the development spectrum have opportunities to use policy tools to create strong economic incentives to reverse the course that was established only very recently, and thereby implement healthier growth. Chapter 5 enumerates a wide range of policy actions that could lead to reduced CVD risks across multiple sectors and spells out health interventions that can achieve better CVD outcomes. However, the effectiveness and cost-effectiveness evidence about the broader steps societies can take to achieve a health-promoting environment remains patchy.

Conclusion 3.2: *The drivers of CVD extend beyond the realm of the health sector, and a coordinated approach is required so that policies in non-health sectors of government, especially those involved in agriculture, urban development, transportation, education, and in the private sector can be developed synergistically to promote, or at least not adversely affect, cardiovascular health.*

ECONOMIC IMPACTS FROM CVD

Evidence from historical experience in already-developed countries and cross-country analysis of aggregate trends such as that presented earlier in this chapter can be highly informative. However, it is far from predictive, and the rapidity and variability of the emergence of CVD in developing countries discourages excess reliance on general historical patterns. This section synthesizes evidence from a different source of analysis to better understand the relationship between CVD and economics, namely country studies that demonstrate the economic consequences of CVD and CVD risk factors for individuals, households, and countries.

Due to methodological and data disparities, these estimates from country studies are not comparable across studies, but those that include multiple countries do allow differences to be noted in the degree to which CVD affects entire economies. CVD also affects the economic well-being of households and individuals in ways that vary by socioeconomic status, occupation, and other individual characteristics. Households incur several types of economic costs from CVD. Direct costs are both tangible (expenses due to health care costs) and intangible (foregone productivity and earnings). Indirect losses derive from lower savings, less investment in assets, and reduced educational attainment, all due to financial adjustments forced on families from the burden of chronic diseases.

This section begins with a discussion of estimates of macroeconomic effects based on country studies, which will be followed by a synthesis of the available evidence of the microeconomic impacts of CVD. As a guide, Box 3.1 provides a short summary of terms and data conventions from the economics literature as well as issues regarding comparisons across studies and countries.

Macroeconomic Measures of CVD Impacts

Cost-of-Illness Measures of Macroeconomic Impacts

Cost-of-illness analysis considers the loss of national income due to medical expenditures and decreased productivity, otherwise called direct economic costs. In developing countries, a large proportion (more than half) of direct costs stems from lost productivity. However, as explained in Box 3.1, estimates of lost productivity or earnings may be exaggerated depending on the underlying assumptions about economic conditions (Abegunde et al., 2007).

Estimates of macroeconomic losses due to CVD and other chronic diseases are listed in Table 3.1, with details of the key assumptions. These cost-of-illness studies indicate that CVD and other chronic diseases impose substantial economic costs, even on relatively poor countries in Africa (Kirigia et al., 2009).

Economic Growth Estimates of Macroeconomic Effects

The economic growth method incorporates a broader set of impacts of CVD on the economy compared to the cost-of-illness measures (Abegunde et al., 2007). It models the impact of reduced productivity and earnings due to death and disability on channels of economic activity that create growth, such as savings and investment. Reduced investment shifts the economy to a lower growth path over the long term, resulting in an accumulation of lost economic output. In economic terms, these studies attempt to measure general equilibrium impacts of CVD.

Estimates of macroeconomic losses from the effects of chronic diseases in developing countries range from 0.02 to 6.77 percent of a country's GDP on an annual basis (Suhrcke et al., 2006). The wide range of estimates is due to both different CVD burdens and different economic conditions. Recently, Abegunde et al. (2007) estimated the effects of four chronic diseases on the economies of 23 countries using an economic growth model. These 23 countries account for approximately 80 percent of the total burden of chronic disease mortality in developing countries. They concluded that $84 billion of economic production will be lost due to heart disease, stroke, and diabetes in 23 high-burden developing countries between 2006 and 2015. Estimates of cumulative GDP loss over 10 years range from $0.15 billion in the Democratic Republic of Congo to $16.68 billion in India. A recent World Bank study of chronic disease in Russia using a dynamic model estimates "massive and growing" economic gains could be achieved if current trends in ill health from chronic diseases and injury are stemmed. The study shows relatively small economic gains from reduced chronic diseases and injuries in 2005 of $105-$324 in GDP per capita; however the economic toll rises to between $2856 and $9243 per capita by 2025 (World Bank Europe and Central Asia Human Development Department, 2005). This starkly illustrates the significant cumulative burden that CVD can have on a country's development prospects.

> **BOX 3.1**
> **Interpreting Economic Data**
>
> - Economic results are obtained from both **empirically measured** studies and from **modeling exercises** drawing on a variety of data sources. Both have strengths and weaknesses. Studies that measure actual economic costs are credible, but not always generalizable. They are also subject to data quality problems. Modeling or econometric studies rely on assumptions, which are usually made based on data sources such as systematic reviews of empirical research, and are valuable in cases where impacts are difficult or impossible to measure directly, such as projections or policy scenarios. Interpreting economic studies of CVD impact requires comparing results from both types of studies for logical consistency and understanding when differences in assumptions account for differences in outcomes.
> - Measuring economic impact involves counting up the **costs** created by CVD. Economists divide the costs of illness and death into three categories: direct costs, indirect costs, and welfare costs. These are generally measured at the individual and household level (and, hence, are **microeconomic costs**) and sometimes aggregated to the whole economy (becoming **macroeconomic costs**).
> - **Direct costs** are expenditures on health services, nonmedical expenditures such as transportation, and the value of lost work or earnings. The sum of these is called the "cost of illness," and most economic studies of CVD and other diseases use this approach. Cost-of-illness studies to measure the economic burden of CVD have been done for a broad range of developing countries; however, there is substantial variation in which health endpoints are being measured and which costs are included. Thus there is little comparability.
> - **Indirect costs** account for the time spent by family members and other caregivers in caring for a CVD patient. In some studies lost work or earnings are considered indirect costs rather than direct costs.
> - **Other costs**, sometimes mentioned but rarely measured, are the effects on individual and national savings from reduced productivity and income, and the effects

Social Welfare Measures of Macroeconomic Impacts

Going beyond the effects of CVD on economic flows, the social welfare (or "full-income") method includes an economic valuation for lives lost due to CVD. Studies using this method typically use a rule of thumb that values human life equivalent to 100 to 200 times average annual wages (Abegunde et al., 2007). This figure is intended to account for a person's full worth, beyond simply one's role as a worker. This method arrives at an economic cost of CVD of a larger magnitude than the studies described previously. One recent example (WHO, 2005) estimated 10-year cumulative GDP losses of $2.5 billion for Tanzania and $7.6 billion for Nigeria from major chronic diseases.

on investments, both financial and human capital (such as education for children), caused by reduced income and earnings. Methods to measure or estimate these economic impacts from CVD come from **economic growth** models. They generally compare an estimate of GDP with CVD impacts to an estimate of GDP without CVD, and the difference is considered the "costs" of CVD or foregone economic output.
- The broadest economic studies of illness use **social welfare** (or **social capital** or **full-income**) methods that impute a monetary value to a person's life, much the same way that "years of life lost" and "disability-adjusted life years" (DALYs) measure the human effects of a disease. This method estimates the economic costs of disease expansively by valuing human life at 100 to 200 times a person's annual earnings. Such calculations imply economic losses in the billions from chronic diseases, even for very low income countries. Welfare cost studies are, by definition, modeling exercises, and the results should not be confused with actual expenditures on CVD.
- The primary outcome measures for economic studies of CVD impacts are expressed in monetary terms. Study authors choose a currency and base year to express results, and it is preferable that these be easily comparable across studies. Ideally, studies use **international dollars** or **purchasing power parity (PPP) dollars** to measure costs and report results. These adjust for differences in prices across countries and, thus, can be compared from one place to another. Economic costs are often presented as a proportion of a relevant denominator, such as GDP or total health expenditures.
- Economic studies employ a wide range of **assumptions about economic conditions** prevailing in the populations studied and about local health care costs. These assumptions affect the conclusions in significant, but not always transparent, ways. For instance, a common assumption is that reduced productivity from having a chronic disease will reduce a country's labor supply and thus have macroeconomic impacts. This is a tenuous assumption under conditions of less than full employment, and it can inflate the estimated economic loss from chronic disease.

Conclusion 3.3: The economic impacts of CVD are detrimental at national levels. Foregone economic output stemming from lower productivity and savings can reach several percent of GDP each year, with a significant cumulative effect. The toll is most severely felt in low and low-middle income countries, which can ill afford the lost economic output in light of already insufficient health resources.

Microeconomic Measures of CVD Impacts

The immediate impacts of CVD on households could derive both from expenditures incurred in preventing or treating disease and from lost earnings when work is reduced because of illness or premature mortality. The

TABLE 3.1 Macroeconomic Impacts from CVD and Chronic Diseases, Various Cost-of-Illness Studies

Country or Region	Economic Costs Included	Health Outcome Measured	Year	Currency	Economic Impact
China Zhao et al., 2008	Direct medical costs plus transport	Diabetes, CHD, hypertension, stroke	2003	RMB Yuan and % health costs	$2.74 billion; 3.7% of national medical expenditures
Brazil World Bank, 2005a	Direct medical, Social capital	IHD, CVD, diabetes, COPD, cancer	2000	U.S. dollars	$34 billion; $72 billion (social capital approach)
African countries Kirigia et al., 2009	Direct and indirect for 33 low-middle income countries	Diabetes	2005	PPP dollars (2000 base year)	$6.7 billion direct; $5 billion indirect
African countries Kirigia et al., 2009	Direct and indirect for 6 low- and upper-middle income countries	Diabetes	2005	PPP dollars (2000 base year)	$523 million direct; $2 billion indirect
U.S. (for comparison) Finkelstein et al., 2005	Direct medical costs	Obesity and overweight	2003	U.S. dollars and % of health care expenditures	$100 billion; 5-7% of national health care expenditures

NOTE: COPD = chronic obstructive pulmonary disease; ISD = ischemic heart disease.

fact that CVD affects people in developing countries at a younger age than in developed countries implies the potential not only for a more widespread national effect on productivity and earnings in developing countries, but also for potentially more dire effects on the long-term welfare of households. Longer-term economic effects on households and individuals can occur when savings are reduced or less is invested in building the earnings potential of adults or children in the family.

Unfortunately, there is little information that measures how CVD affects household-level economic output in developing countries. Based on a review of studies primarily in high income countries, barriers to employment for people with chronic diseases and risk factors are likely to arise from productivity limitations, costs of disability, and in some cases, stigma (Suhrcke et al., 2006). In addition, Suhrcke et al. (2007) reviewed the available literature for Central and Eastern Europe and the Commonwealth of Independent states and found that, generally speaking, the presence of chronic illness had a negative impact on individual labor productivity (as measured by the wage rate), the likelihood of labor force participation, and in some cases contributed to a significant loss of household income. Chronic illnesses also increased the likelihood that individuals would retire early.

A growing body of evidence from the employer side also demonstrates that productivity is strongly and adversely affected by chronic diseases. Global corporations monitoring the bottom line impacts of worker ill-health, particularly from chronic diseases, are showing dramatic returns on investment of up to $6 in greater productivity for every $1 spent on health promotion for their employees. Their results also show the indirect losses from absenteeism and "presenteeism" far outweigh the direct costs of health care (WEF, 2009). However, all these estimates are derived from particular labor market and economic conditions in different countries and cannot be generalized.

There is more information about how households are affected by and cope with health care expenses in developing countries, although very little is specific to chronic disease. Because poor households are rarely covered by insurance, there are often severe consequences for the entire household when sudden and significant health expenditures, or "health shocks," occur. Surveys covering 89 percent of the world's population suggest that 150 million people experience financial disaster due to health care expenses, and 100 million are pushed into poverty (Xu et al., 2007). Much of the burden imparted by these "health shocks" is from the suddenness of payment requirements (McIntyre et al., 2006).

It is less clear how households are affected specifically by CVD health care expenses, which is largely comprised of the long-term costs of drugs, routine doctors' visits, and preplanned procedures rather than acute, short-term spending. In Vietnam, where out-of-pocket expenditures constituted 84 percent of all health care spending in 1998, catastrophic spending (defined as an expenditure that exceeds 10 to 40 percent of a household's capacity to pay) was dominated by communicable disease needs. One reason may be that high costs of chronic disease care prevent lower-income groups from accessing treatment (Thuan et al., 2006). However, CVD events can also result in "catastrophic" health costs. Seventy-one percent of hospitalized Chinese stroke survivors experienced catastrophic financial impacts (defined as out-of-pocket health expenses in the 3 months after stroke that meet or exceed 30 percent of reported household income). Those without health insurance were hit particularly hard. Out-of-pocket expenses from stroke pushed 37 percent of patients and their families below the poverty line; 62 percent of those without insurance were pushed into poverty (Heeley et al., 2009).

Households employ a variety of methods to cope with these expenses, from dipping into savings accounts, to increasing the number of earners in the family, to selling assets. In general, however, poor families have little flexibility to draw on savings to finance health needs. More often, they reduce basic consumption, sell assets that form the basis of their livelihood, and go into debt (McIntyre et al., 2006). Across 15 countries in Africa, 50 percent of households that had a hospitalized family member turned to borrowing and selling assets to pay for health expenditures. In most of the countries, inpatient expenses were more likely to cause distress selling of assets and borrowing than outpatient and routine health care by both rich and poor households, although the behavior was more predominant among the poor (Leive et al., 2008). In India, the risk of distress borrowing and distress selling increases significantly for hospitalized patients if they are smokers or even just belong to households with a member who smokes or drinks (Bonu et al., 2005; Suhrcke et al., 2006). In Burkina Faso, when a household member has a chronic illness, the probability of catastrophic consequences increased by 3.3- to 7.8-fold (Su et al., 2006; Suhrcke et al., 2006).

A further household burden is the direct expense of harmful lifestyle behaviors related to CVD risk. Many households experience dramatic shifts in spending and forgo other expenditures in order to buy tobacco and alcohol, two major risk factors for CVD. In India, for example, households that consumed tobacco had lower consumption of milk, education, clean fuel, and entertainment. These households also had lower per capita nutritional intake compared to tobacco-free households (Bump et al., 2009; John, 2008). In a sample of low income workers in Eastern China, smokers spent an average 11 percent of personal monthly income on tobacco and reported foregone savings and foregone consumption of health care and major household goods compared to non-smokers (Bump et al., 2009; Hesketh et al., 2007). In another study in rural China, tobacco spending negatively affected spending on health, education, farming equipment, seeds, savings, and insurance. For every 100 yuan spent on tobacco there was an associated decline in spending on education by 30 yuan, medical care by 15 yuan, farming by 14 yuan, and food by 10 yuan (Suhrcke et al., 2006; Wang et al., 2006). Frequently, alcohol expenditures increase hand-in-hand with tobacco expenditures. Families in Delhi, India, that had at least one member that consumed three or more drinks per week spent almost 14 times more on alcohol each month (resulting in fewer financial resources for food, education, and daily consumables) and more were in debt, when compared to families with no member consuming more than one drink (Saxena et al., 2003; Suhrcke et al., 2006).

In conclusion, the economic burden of CVD in developing countries is currently borne most directly by patients and their families, either through out-of-pocket expenses that reduce their provision of basic needs, or through reduced productivity and earnings. By contrast, in middle income and high income countries where social and private insurance is available to finance health expenses, the financial costs of CVD are spread more widely.

Social Inequalities and CVD

In addition to the effects of CVD on household-level economic status, there is strong evidence that social inequalities contribute to CVD mortality and incidence. Thus, poverty plays a role both as a risk factor and as a consequence of CVD. Poverty, as a contributing factor to CVD, is related to the lack of access to health care and health information among the poor as well as exposure to multiple risk factors that increase CVD risk. Further, several studies have highlighted the effects of social and economic factors on health even when those factors are not directly related to major risks and specific treatments (CSDH, 2008).

In Brazil, for instance, the prevalence of hypertension was consistently and dramatically higher (30 to 130 percent higher) among the less educated, those with lowest income, and Afro-Brazilians. The poor had a 1.2 relative risk of dying from CVD compared to the wealthy (World Bank, 2005a). Demographic and Health Surveys from seven African countries show a 35 percent average increase in overweight and obesity between the early 1990s and 2000s, with the largest increase among the poor. The almost 50 percent rise in overweight and obesity among poor women is attributed to changing nutritional habits and urban lifestyles (Ziraba et al., 2009).

The income gradient of CVD in low and middle income countries mirrors that which has already taken place in developed countries. For example, in Scotland, a six-fold differential in CHD mortality is seen between the poorest and most affluent groups aged 35 to 44 years (O'Flaherty et al., 2009). The major causes for the social class differentials were related to unfavorable trends in risk factors, mainly related to tobacco use and poor diet. Similar findings have been reported for the United States, United Kingdom, Australia, and across Western Europe, where racial and ethnic differences in prevalence are also apparent (Mackenbach et al., 2003; Wang and Beydoun, 2007).

These factors of tobacco use, poor diet, and unequal access to care can explain the tendency for CVD to become more concentrated among the poor and near-poor within low and middle income countries. One reason worth highlighting is the transition to a more energy-dense diet. In addition to the trends in production and consumption related to the nutrition transition that were described in Chapter 2, global prices of edible oils, animal-based products, and sweeteners have declined for the past 20 years. But even while improving overall caloric and protein intake, the poor are now more likely to consume diets heavy in fats, salt, and sugar. In middle income countries, the poor are also reducing physical activity while consuming additional calories (Drewnowski and Darmon, 2005; Popkin, 2003). Government policies often play a role, directly and indirectly, in subsidizing overconsumption of energy-dense foods. In Egypt, where more than two-thirds of women and half of men are overweight or obese, food subsidies encourage consumption of energy-dense foods (Asfaw, 2006). However, both government food policies and nutrition conditions among the poor are highly country-specific and should be examined on that basis.

Conclusion 3.4: There is growing evidence that CVD and its risk factors affect the poor within and across countries, both as a cause and as a consequence of poverty. In most countries, CVD hits hardest among the poor, who have greater risk-factor exposure, tend to be uninsured, and have less financial resilience to cope with the costs of disease management.

One promising way to stem this increasing burden on the poor in low and middle income countries may be through programs that are specifically tailored and targeted to reach the poor (Gwatkin et al., 2005). Programs already targeted to the lowest income population, such as those to reduce undernutrition in children and for the chronic management of infectious diseases, offer opportunities to ensure an early healthy nutritional start for children and to integrate cardiovascular health promotion and disease prevention.

CONCLUSION

CVD risks arise on the path to an advanced stage of economic development, driven in part by a range of development-related factors such as population aging and urbanization; shifts in agriculture; and the multifarious influences of globalization. CVD can affect the entire economy of a developing nation. Disability, early mortality, and direct health expenditures can divert resources from savings, investment, and other productive uses, affecting economic well-being at the household level and growth potential at the national level. Therefore, developing countries need to maneuver diligently and carefully to avoid cementing in place long-term roadblocks to healthy economic progress.

The pattern of rising CVD risks with development reflects a complex interaction among average per capita income in a country, trends in lifestyle and other risk factors, and health systems capacity to control CVD. Developing countries at different stages of development face different challenges in choosing public health strategies to reduce the burden of CVD. The challenge facing low income developing countries is to continue to bring down prevalence of infectious diseases while avoiding an overwhelming rise in CVD, especially under conditions of resource limitations. This will require balancing competing population-level health demands while maintaining relatively low overall health expenditures. Investments in health will also need to be balanced with pressing needs to invest in other social needs and industrial development. The challenge facing middle income developing countries is to reverse or slow the rise in CVD in an affordable and cost-effective manner.

Although still not fully understood, the complex interrelationships in which economic development can contribute to and also be affected by the accelerating rates of inadequately addressed CVD and related chronic diseases in low and middle income countries supports the need for both urgent and carefully planned actions.

REFERENCES

Abegunde, D. O., C. D. Mathers, T. Adam, M. Ortegon, and K. Strong. 2007. The burden and costs of chronic diseases in low-income and middle-income countries. *Lancet* 370(9603):1929-1938.

Agence-France Presse. 2008. *China's urban problem.* http://news.asiaone.com/News/Latest%2BNews/Asia/Story/A1Story20081218-108758.html (accessed December 9, 2009).

Ahsan Karar, Z., N. Alam, and P. Kim Streatfield. 2009. Epidemiological transition in rural Bangladesh, 1986-2006. *Global Health Action* June 2009(2).

Asfaw, A. 2006. Do government food prices affect the prevalence of obesity? Empirical evidence from Egypt. *World Development* 35(4):687-701.

Barquera, S., L. Hernandez-Barrera, M. L. Tolentino, J. Espinosa, S. W. Ng, J. A. Rivera, and B. M. Popkin. 2008. Energy intake from beverages is increasing among Mexican adolescents and adults. *Journal of Nutrition* 138(12):2454-2461.

Becker, G. S., T. J. Philipson, and R. R. Soares. 2005. The quantity and quality of life and the evolution of world inequality. *American Economic Review* 95(1):277-291.

Bonu, S., M. Rani, D. H. Peters, P. Jha, and S. N. Nguyen. 2005. Does use of tobacco or alcohol contribute to impoverishment from hospitalization costs in India? *Health Policy and Planning* 20(1):41-49.

Bump, J. B., M. R. Reich, O. Adeyi, and S. Khetrapal. 2009. *Towards a political economy of tobacco control in low- and middle-income countries.* Washington, DC: World Bank.

Collins, J., and J. P. Koplan. 2009. Health impact assessment: A step toward health in all policies. *Journal of the American Medical Association* 302(3):315-317.

CSDH (WHO Commission on Social Determinants of Health). 2008. *Closing the gap in a generation: Health equity through action on the social determinants of health.* Final report of the commission on social determinants of health. Geneva: World Health Organization.

Danaei, G., E. L. Ding, D. Mozaffarian, B. Taylor, J. R. Rehm, C. J. L. Murray, and M. Ezzati. 2009. The preventable causes of death in the United States: Comparative risk assessment of dietary, lifestyle, and metabolic risk factors. *PLoS Med* 6(4):e1000058.

Darnton-Hill, I., C. Nishida, and W. P. T. James. 2004. A life course approach to diet, nutrition and the prevention of chronic diseases. *Public Health Nutrition* 7(1 A):101-121.

Drewnowski, A., and N. Darmon. 2005. Food choices and diet costs: An economic analysis. *Journal of Nutrition* 135(4):900-904.

Ezzati, M., S. Vander Hoorn, C. M. Lawes, R. Leach, W. P. James, A. D. Lopez, A. Rodgers, and C. J. Murray. 2005. Rethinking the "Diseases of affluence" paradigm: Global patterns of nutritional risks in relation to economic development. *PLoS Medicine* 2(5): e133.

Finkelstein, E. A., C. J. Ruhm, and K. M. Kosa. 2005. Economic causes and consequences of obesity. *Annual Review of Public Health* 26:239-257.

Fries, J. F. 2005. Frailty, heart disease, and stroke: The compression of morbidity paradigm. *American Journal of Preventive Medicine* 29(5 Suppl 1):164-168.

Gajalakshmi, V., R. Peto, T. S. Kanaka, P. Jha. 2003. Smoking and mortality from tuberculosis and other diseases in India: Retrospective study of 43000 adult male deaths and 35000 controls. *Lancet* 362(9383):507-515.

Goyal, A., and S. Yusuf. 2006. The burden of cardiovascular disease in the Indian subcontinent. *Indian Journal of Medical Research* 124(3):235-244.

Gwatkin, D. R., A. Wagstaff, A. Yazbeck, J. Qamruddin, H. Waters, M. Grabowsky, N. Farrell, J. Chimumbwa, T. Nobiya, A. Wolkon, J. Selanikio, D. Montagu, N. Prata, M. Campbell, J. Walsh, S. Orero, M. Thiede, N. Palmer, S. Mbatsha, A. T. M. I. Anwar, J. Killewo, M. Chowdhury, S. Dasgupta, J. B. Schwartz, I. Bhushan, M. K. Ranson, P. Joshi, M. Shah, Y. Shaikh, D. Peters, K. Rao, G. N. V. Ramana, A. Malhotra, S. Mathur, R. Pande, E. Roca, L. Gasparini, M. Panadeiros, A. Barros, C. Victora, J. Cesar, N. Neumann, A. Bertoldi, and M. Valdivia. 2005. *Reaching the poor with health, nutrition, and population services: What works, what doesn't, and why.* Washington, DC: World Bank.

He, F. J., and G. A. MacGregor. 2009. A comprehensive review on salt and health and current experience of worldwide salt reduction programmes. *Journal of Human Hypertension* 23(6):363-384.

Heeley, E., C. S. Anderson, Y. Huang, S. Jan, Y. Li, M. Liu, J. Sun, E. Xu, Y. Wu, Q. Yang, J. Zhang, S. Zhang, and J. Wang. 2009. Role of health insurance in averting economic hardship in families after acute stroke in China. *Stroke* 40(6):2149-256.

Hesketh, T., L. Lu, Y. X. Jun, and W. H. Mei. 2007. Smoking, cessation and expenditure in low income Chinese: Cross sectional survey. *BMC Public Health* 7:29.

IOM (Institute of Medicine). 2010. *Mitigating the nutritional impacts of the global food price crisis*. Washington, DC: The National Academies Press.

Iqbal, R., S. Anand, S. Ounpuu, S. Islam, X. Zhang, S. Rangarajan, J. Chifamba, A. Al-Hinai, M. Keltai, and S. Yusuf. 2008. Dietary patterns and the risk of acute myocardial infarction in 52 countries: Results of the INTERHEART study. *Circulation* 118(19):1929-1937.

Jha, P., F. J. Chaloupka, M. Corrao, and B. Jacob. 2006. Reducing the burden of smoking world-wide: Effectiveness of interventions and their coverage. *Drug and Alcohol Review* 25(6):597-609.

John, R. M. 2008. Crowding out effect of tobacco expenditure and its implications on household resource allocation in India. *Social Science and Medicine* 66(6):1356-1367.

Kato, H., J. Tillotson, and M. Z. Nichaman. 1973. Epidemiologic studies of coronary heart disease and stroke in Japanese men living in Japan, Hawaii and California: Serum lipids and diet. *American Journal of Epidemiology* 97(6):372-385.

Kirigia, J. M., H. B. Sambo, L. G. Sambo, and S. P. Barry. 2009. Economic burden of diabetes mellitus in the WHO African region. *BMC International Health and Human Rights* 9(1):6.

Leive, A., K. Xu, A. Leive, and K. Xu. 2008. Coping with out-of-pocket health payments: Empirical evidence from 15 African countries. *Bulletin of the World Health Organization* 86(11):849-856.

Mackenbach, J. P., V. Bos, O. Andersen, M. Cardano, G. Costa, S. Harding, A. Reid, O. Hemstrom, T. Valkonen, and A. E. Kunst. 2003. Widening socioeconomic inequalities in mortality in six Western European countries. *International Journal of Epidemiology* 32:830-837.

Marmot, M. G., S. L. Syme, and A. Kagan. 1975. Epidemiologic studies of coronary heart disease and stroke in Japanese men living in Japan, Hawaii and California: Prevalence of coronary and hypertensive heart disease and associated risk factors. *American Journal of Epidemiology* 102(6):514-525.

McIntyre, D., M. Thiede, G. Dahlgren, M. Whitehead, 2006. What are the economic consequences for households of illness and of paying for health care in low- and middle-income country contexts? *Social Science and Medicine* 62(4):858-865.

McLaren, L. 2007. Socioeconomic status and obesity. *Epidemiologic Reviews* 29:29-48.

Monteiro, C. A., W. L. Conde, B. Lu, and B. M. Popkin. 2004. Obesity and inequities in health in the developing world. *International Journal of Obesity* 28(9):1181-1186.

O'Flaherty, M., J. Bishop, A. Redpath, T. McLaughlin, D. Murphy, J. Chalmers, S. Capewell. 2009. Coronary heart disease mortality among young adults in Scotland in relation to social inequalities: Time trend study. *British Medical Journal* 339:b2613.

PAHO (Pan American Health Organization). 2007. *Regional strategy and plan of action on an integrated approach to the prevention and control of chronic diseases*. Washington, DC: Pan American Health Organization.

Popkin, B. M. 2003. Dynamics of the nutrition transition and its implications for the developing world. *Forum Nutrition* 56:262-264.

Reddy, K. S. 2009. Global perspectives on cardiovascular diseases. In *Evidence based cardiology*. 2nd ed. Edited by S. Yusuf, J. A. Caitns, A. J. Camm, E. L. Fallen and B. J. Gersh. London: BMJ Books.

Reddy, K. S., and S. Yusuf. 1998. Emerging epidemic of cardiovascular disease in developing countries. *Circulation* 97(6):596-601.

Saxena, S., R. Sharma, and P. K. Maulik. 2003. Impact of alcohol use on poor families: A study from north India. *Journal of Substance Use* 8:78-84.

Shafey, O., M. Eriksen, H. Ross, and J. Mackay. 2009. *The tobacco atlas*. 3rd ed. Atlanta: American Cancer Society.

Steyn, N. P., D. Bradshaw, R. Norman, J. Joubert, M. Schneider, K. Steyn. 2006. *Dietary changes and the health transition in South Africa: Implications for health policy*. Cape Town: South African Medical Research Council.

Su, T. T., B. Kouyate, and S. Flessa. 2006. Catastrophic household expenditure for health care in a low-income society: A study from Nouna district, Burkina Faso. *Bulletin of the World Health Organization* 84(1):21-27.

Suhrcke, M., and D. M. Urban. 2006. Are cardiovascular diseases bad for economic growth? http:/ssrn.com/paper=949412 (accessed February 5, 2010).

Suhrcke, M., and L. Rocco. 2008 (unpublished). *Macroeconomics consequences of noncommunicable diseases at the individual or household level, with a focus on labor market outcomes*.

Suhrcke, M., R. A. Nugent, D. Stuckler, and L. Rocco. 2006. *Chronic disease: An economic perspective*. London: Oxford Health Alliance.

Suhrcke, M., L. Rocco, M. McKee, WHO Regional Office for Europe, and European Observatory on Health Systems and Policies. 2007. *Health: A vital investment for economic development in Eastern Europe and central Asia*. Copenhagen: WHO Regional Office for Europe.

Thuan, N. T., C. Lofgren, N. T. Chuc, U. Janlert, L. Lindholm. 2006. Household out-of-pocket payments for illness: Evidence from Vietnam. *BMC Public Health* 6:283.

UNDESA (United Nations Department of Economic and Social Affairs). 2008. *World urbanization prospects: The 2007 update.* Geneva: United Nations.

UNFPA (United Nations Fund for Population Activities). 2007. *State of world population 2007.* New York: UNFPA.

Wang, H., J. L. Sindelar, and S. H. Busch. 2006. The impact of tobacco expenditure on household consumption patterns in rural China. *Social Science and Medicine* 62(6):1414-1426.

Wang, Y., and M. A. Beydoun. 2007. The obesity epidemic in the United States—gender, age, socioeconomic, racial/ethnic, and geographic characteristics: A systematic review and meta-regression analysis. *Epidemiologic Reviews* 29:6-28.

WEF (World Economic Forum). 2009. *Employee health as a strategic imperative: Report of the governors meeting of the consumer industries.* Geneva: World Economic Forum.

WHO (World Health Organization). 2005. *Preventing chronic diseases: A vital investment.* Geneva: World Health Organization.

WHOSIS (World Health Organization Statistical Information System). *World Health Statistics.* 2009. Geneva: World Health Organization.

World Bank. 2005a. *Brazil: Addressing the challenge of non-communicable diseases in Brazil.* Washington, DC: World Bank.

World Bank. 2005b. *World development report overview 2006: Equity and development.* Washington, DC: World Bank.

World Bank Commission on Growth and Development. 2008. *The growth report: Strategies for sustained growth and inclusive development.* Washington, DC: World Bank.

World Bank Europe and Central Asia Human Development Department. 2005. *Dying too young: Addressing premature mortality and ill health due to non-communicable diseases and injuries in the Russian Federation.* Washington, DC: World Bank.

World Trade Organization. 2009. *International trade statistics 2009.* Geneva: World Trade Organization.

Xu, K., D. B. Evans, G. Carrin, A. M. Aguilar-Rivera, P. Musgrove, T. Evans. 2007. Protecting households from catastrophic health spending. *Health Affairs* 26(4):972-983.

Yang, G., L. Kong, W. Zhao, X. Wan, Y. Zhai, L. C. Chen, and J. P. Koplan. 2008. Emergence of chronic non-communicable diseases in China. *Lancet* 372(9650):1697-1705.

Yusuf, S., S. Reddy, S. Ounpuu, and S. Anand. 2001a. Global burden of cardiovascular diseases: Part I: General considerations, the epidemiologic transition, risk factors, and impact of urbanization. *Circulation* 104(22):2746-2753.

Yusuf, S., S. Reddy, S. Ounpuu, and S. Anand. 2001b. Global burden of cardiovascular diseases: Part II: Variations in cardiovascular disease by specific ethnic groups and geographic regions and prevention strategies. *Circulation* 104(23):2855-2864.

Zatonski, W. A., A. J. McMichael, and J. W. Powles. 1998. Ecological study of reasons for sharp decline in mortality from ischaemic heart disease in Poland since 1991. *British Medical Journal* 316(7137):1047-1051.

Zhao, W., Y. Zhai, J. Hu, J. Wang, Z. Yang, L. Kong, and C. Chen. 2008. Economic burden of obesity-related chronic diseases in mainland China. *Obesity Reviews* 9(1):62-67.

Ziraba, A. K., J. C. Fotso, and R. Ochako. 2009. Overweight and obesity in urban Africa: A problem of the rich or the poor? *BMC Public Health* 9:465.

4

Measurement and Evaluation

The preceding chapters have outlined the scope and context of the global epidemic of cardiovascular disease (CVD), the extent of the resulting health and economic burden, and the challenge that lies ahead. This provides a compelling rationale for aggressively reducing risk factors that lead to CVD globally. Measurement is the basis for determining the scale of the global CVD epidemic and for understanding how best to intervene, and it will be critical to the success of efforts to reduce disease burden. While there is a need for CVD-specific measurement tools, existing global health efforts provide a robust foundation to draw upon and to avoid duplication as the global CVD community continues to develop and expand its evaluation of program and policy initiatives. Over the past several decades, advances in the field of global health have led to a wealth of measurement knowledge, tools, and techniques that have been developed for evaluating policy and program outcomes and impact on health status at all levels. Indeed, many of these national and global measurement initiatives are currently at risk of overlooking measurement of CVD and related chronic diseases, which will in fact be crucial in order to obtain a truly complete picture of national health needs.

This chapter[1] first describes the functions and principles of measurement, monitoring, and evaluation. The chapter then addresses several critical cross-cutting considerations that affect measurement and evaluation. This is followed by a discussion of the potential for measurement ap-

---

[1] This chapter is based in part on a paper written for the committee by Jeff Luck and Riti Shimkhada.

proaches that can provide timely feedback and guide decision making at multiple levels to achieve reductions in cardiovascular disease, including a discussion of emerging technologies to improve measurement. Finally the chapter touches on the use of measurement at the global level to inform actions to reduce the burden of CVD.

FUNCTIONS AND PRINCIPLES OF MEASUREMENT

Measurement serves a number of critical roles in the effort to address any health problem. The use of measurement to inform the cycle of decision making in addressing a public health problem is outlined in Figure 4.1. This cycle applies to decision making at any level of stakeholder, from global to local, and at any scale of intervention, from a demonstration project to a global action plan. First, it is used to assess the magnitude of the problem at the level of the population and subpopulation and informs the mitigation of risk factors. When coupled with an assessment of capacity, these can inform priorities and the setting of realistic intervention goals. This in turn guides implementation of interventions, including policies, programs, and clinical interventions at the level of the population, the provider, and the individual. Measurement then can be used to assess the processes, outcomes, and impact of the implemented interventions. This feeds back into the cycle to encourage adaptations that help ensure sustainable progress. Thus, measurement is not simply an endpoint to determine the value of an intervention; it is also the foundation for an ongoing cycle of planning, prioritizing, and operationalizing interventions.

Ultimately, measurement strategies have the potential to lead to changes in health outcomes by changing the decisions and behavior of policy makers, providers, and individuals. This derives from the fundamental purpose of measurement: to create awareness that increases understanding and motivates change. In this way, as illustrated in Figure 4.2, measurement can be viewed as a critical component of any effort to result in an impact on health outcomes, serving to guide those efforts and to accelerate the pace of change to achieve the targeted outcomes. To serve as an instrument of change, measurement needs to be ongoing and cyclical. Transparent information can increase knowledge and change intentions throughout the process of implementing an intervention approach, just as it can lead to overall changes in baseline status and new policies or programs in response to achieving a new baseline.

A number of underlying principles drive measurement as a fundamental part of efforts to decrease CVD. First, in order to be effective measurement needs to be relevant to the context in which it is implemented (Majumdar and Soumerai, 2009). Contextual elements are typically local—occurring at the level of countries, regions, cities, and villages. Context includes local

151

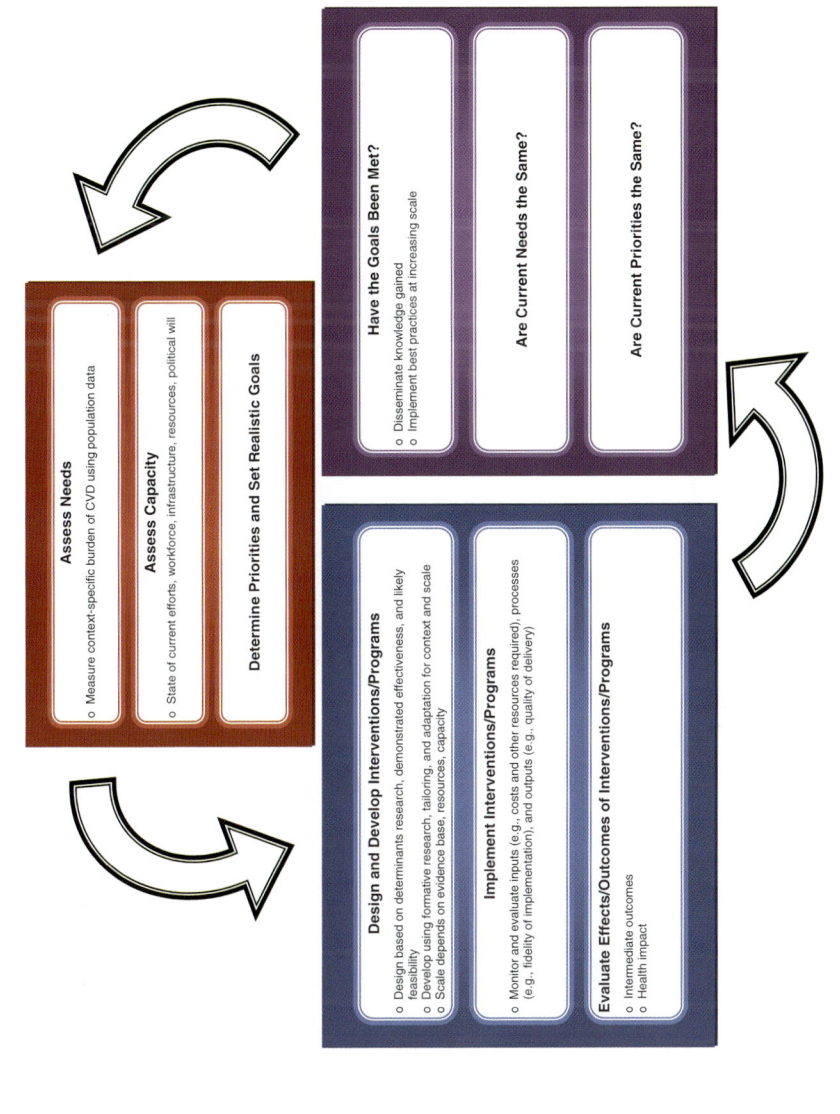

Assess Needs
o Measure context-specific burden of CVD using population data

Assess Capacity
o State of current efforts, workforce, infrastructure, resources, political will

Determine Priorities and Set Realistic Goals

Design and Develop Interventions/Programs
o Design based on determinants research, demonstrated effectiveness, and likely feasibility
o Develop using formative research, tailoring, and adaptation for context and scale
o Scale depends on evidence base, resources, capacity

Implement Interventions/Programs
o Monitor and evaluate inputs (e.g., costs and other resources required), processes (e.g., fidelity of implementation), and outputs (e.g., quality of delivery)

Evaluate Effects/Outcomes of Interventions/Programs
o Intermediate outcomes
o Health impact

Have the Goals Been Met?
o Disseminate knowledge gained
o Implement best practices at increasing scale

Are Current Needs the Same?

Are Current Priorities the Same?

FIGURE 4.1 Measurement-based decision-making cycle.

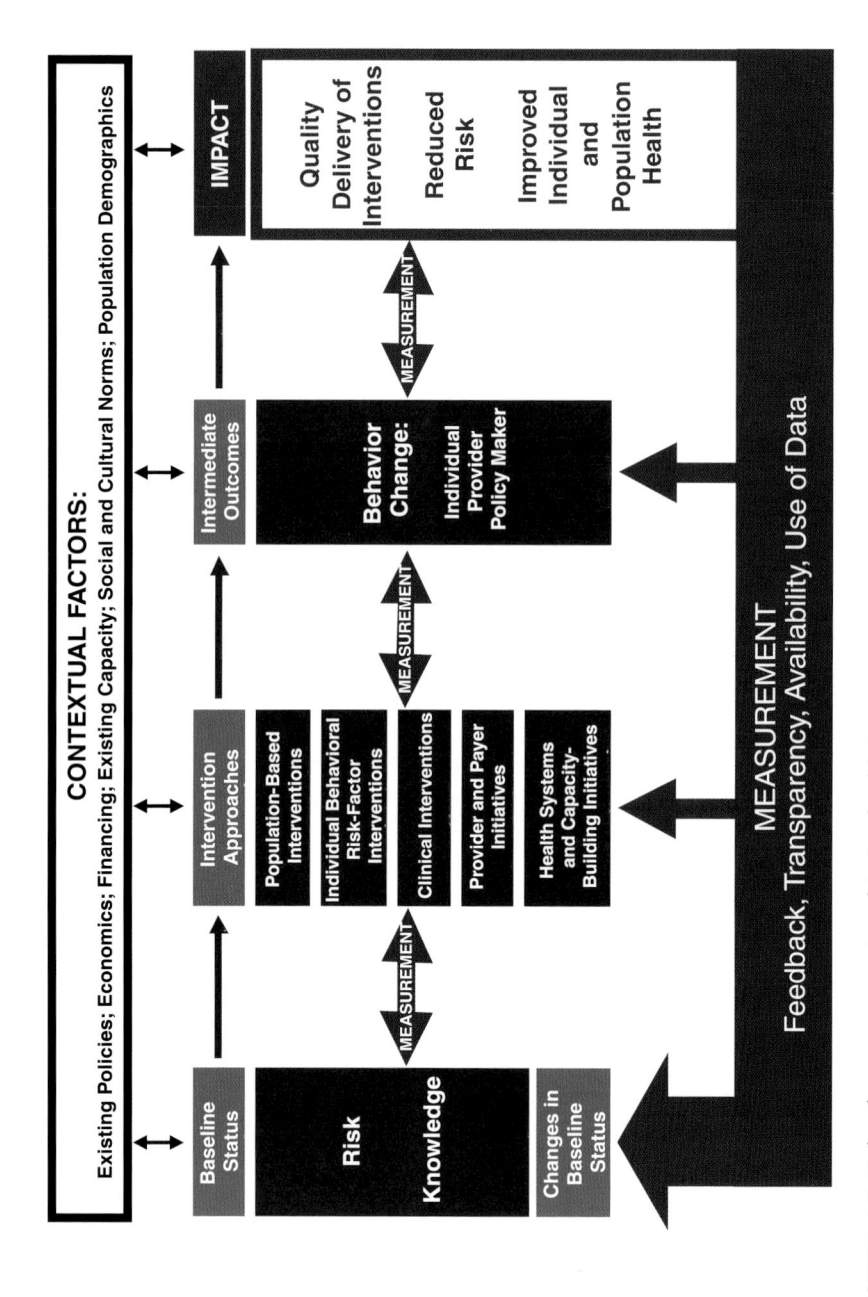

FIGURE 4.2 Role of measurement in achieving health impact.

elements of economics, financing, existing policies, existing capacity, population demographics, and social and cultural factors.

These in turn exist in a larger global context. A second principle is that measurement is most effective when it is transparent and when there are feedback mechanisms to ensure that the resulting data is widely available and widely used. Indeed, measurement alone is not sufficient—the data must actually be *used* by policy makers, providers, and individuals. Third, to truly document and maximize impact, measurement is needed at all levels, from individuals to providers to policy makers. Measurement is also needed across all kinds of interventions approaches, from clinical interventions and individual risk reduction to changes in the infrastructure to deliver interventions to policy changes and other population-based strategies. A fourth principle is that measurement needs to focus on the intermediate outcome of behavior change, for it is changes in the behavior of those at risk, of care providers, and of policy makers that will lead to lessening of the CVD burden. In order for measurement to be effective it must also be accurate, feasible, affordable, actionable, responsive, and timely (Majumdar and Soumerai, 2009). Finally, measurement outcomes should be able to be communicated clearly. Although there may be necessary complexity in the design of measurement systems, this complexity should be converted into relatively simple reporting of the data.

The number and variety of determinants that contribute to cardiovascular disease means that no single set of measures or data collection system will suffice for all goals or settings. Instead, this complexity necessitates the use of an array of measures and a variety of collection strategies, along with careful planning to set priorities for measurement and to balance feasibility with the need for comprehensive data that can be integrated and compared across countries, programs, and levels of measurement. As a final principle, it is critical in the planning and implementation of measurement strategies to make the following determinations:

- who is expected to use the data;
- what is to be measured;
- what metrics or indicators should be used;
- who will be collecting the data;
- what tools will be used to collect the data;
- who will analyze the data;
- how the data will be reported and disseminated; and
- how much it will cost to implement the measurement strategy and to analyze and disseminate the data.

CROSS-CUTTING CONSIDERATIONS IN MEASUREMENT

There are several critical cross-cutting considerations that affect measurement and evaluation that are important to discuss as the basis for interpreting the potential use of the methodologies described later in this chapter. These include standardization of indicators, data ownership and capacity for data analysis, and costs of measurement.

Standardizing Indicators for CVD Surveillance, Intervention Research, and Program Evaluation

To monitor the epidemic of CVD and ensure that there are effective intervention approaches that can be disseminated widely, it is critical to be able to gather data and make comparisons across countries, across sectors and systems, and across intervention and program evaluations. Therefore, while measurement efforts need to be tailored to the context, program, or intervention approach, some measurement strategies would benefit from standardization and global coordination of surveillance systems and evaluation systems.

The question of which indicators to use and how to prioritize them must be agreed upon by the relevant stakeholders in the international community. A number of key categories of metrics are crucial to measuring CVD and its breadth of determinants and would need to be considered. These include demographics; risk and risk mitigation including behaviors (e.g., smoking rates, physical activity, diet and nutrition) and biomedical measures (e.g., weight and height, blood pressure, cholesterol); disease outcomes (e.g., cardiovascular events); cause-specific mortality; health provider and quality improvement measures; health systems performance; economic measures; intersectoral policy measures (e.g., cigarette costs and sales data, agricultural trends, urbanization); and measures of global action. Some of these measures need to be disease specific, while others need to be harmonized and coordinated with measurement strategies for related chronic diseases and for other areas of health and development.

While there may already be consensus within a few of these indicator categories, far more are currently still being debated, and setting priorities within and across categories to balance comprehensive measurement with feasibility will not be simple. Although it was beyond the scope of this committee to do so, a minimum set of indicators with clear definitions with guidance on prioritization needs to be developed to allow for uniform and comparable data across countries and systems. Developing an indicator framework of this kind could be achieved through a consensus process involving key stakeholders such as researchers, practitioners, economists, funders, and representatives from national health and public health authorities from developing countries. This process would need to realistically consider how to balance the need for comprehensive data collection with the practicalities of timeliness and resources. In addition, a critical component for any indicator framework is what the implementation and maintenance of each measurement system would cost. The World Health Organization (WHO) has convened an epidemiology reference group, drawing on headquarters and regional offices, to develop guidance for chronic disease surveillance systems and to agree on core indicators that will be used to monitor the major chronic diseases and their risk factors (Alwan, 2009, personal communication). If this effort takes into account the considerations described here, it could be a first step in achieving an implementable indicator framework.

This need for standardization and coordination has been recognized by the global HIV/AIDS community and is addressed in large part by the United Nations' Joint Programme on HIV/AIDS (UNAIDS's) Monitoring and Evaluation Reference Group (MERG) (UNAIDS, 2009a). Created in 1998 by the UNAIDS Secretariat, the MERG provides technical guidance for HIV monitoring and evaluation and is a key driver in the harmonization of HIV indicators at the global level (Global HIV M&E Information, no date). Working through a coordinated effort with individuals at the Global Fund and the U.S. President's Emergency Plan for AIDS Relief, the MERG identified, collected, and defined high-quality indicators, making them freely accessible online (UNAIDS, 2009a, 2009b). In addition, while the indicator registry identifies which measures have been harmonized and endorsed by other stakeholders, it leaves the decision on determining the indicators that are most important to collect to the implementer, be it a national government or program manager (UNAIDS, 2009b). This use of online resources to lower the cost of use for developing countries as well as the leadership and coordination from a body with the capacity to also provide relevant technical support could provide a useful model for WHO during indicator standardization efforts for chronic diseases.

Once developed, coordinated support will be needed for the implementation of these globally comparable indicators. Technical assistance and training in surveillance, research, and evaluation will be needed to provide options for measurement tools that incorporate the uniform data from globally comparable indicators, but also to allow for national or local/program-level choices on which tools to use and which indicators to collect (beyond the minimum set) based on local and project- or program-specific priorities, resources, and needs.

Data Ownership and Capacity for Data Analysis

The collection and reporting of data, regardless of how detailed, accurate, or comprehensive, is a potential waste of time and resources unless the information is appropriately processed, analyzed, and communicated to relevant stakeholders. Currently there is a growing need to develop and maintain data analysis capacity at the local level, in an effort to help communities feel ownership of reported outcomes (Stansfield, 2009). Limits in local capacity to conduct both analysis and operations research have left some national governments hesitant to take on new measurement initiatives as they could overwhelm already fragile health information systems (Bennett et al., 2006). Thus, these absorptive capacity concerns must be kept in mind when determining how rapidly and to what degree to scale up measurement and evaluation initiatives.

Addressing these capacity needs will require a paradigm shift at the international, national, and local levels about the importance of developing locally relevant measurement solutions. Targeted funding from donors may be required not only for the development of sustainable health information systems but also to assist organizations with training of local individuals in data collection and analysis where there are shortages in this expertise, as well as with the retention of trained individuals. In order to be effective, these efforts need to be coupled with an assessment of the existing monitoring and evaluation capacity of local actors. Tools that could be used to improve measurement capacity include workshops and training sessions to instruct health authorities or program coordinators on how to set up and maintain data collection systems, implement core indicators, design evaluations, adapt preferred guidance documents to their unique situation, and analyze data. Centers of excellence in this area that are established within a developing country need not be disease specific and must have the potential to build capacity at both the national or regional level that would benefit multiple health sectors.

Expanding local analytic capacity could also potentially help to reduce the prevalence of unused data "piles" that amass in developing countries. The failure of both donors and national governments to invest in sustainable health information systems inhibits countries' abilities to routinely process these data (Stansfield, 2009). It is important to note that building the capacity to collect and analyze data is not sufficient. There is also a need to strengthen the motivation and capacity for policy makers to interpret and act on the data. To achieve this, data collection strategies could be developed in consultation with policy makers and include mechanisms for timely reporting to inform policies and programs.

In addition, the proliferation of multilateral organizations, international and local nongovernmental organizations, and the expanding private sector all place their own, often redundant measurement and evaluation demands on local actors, which adds an additional burden to local and national measurement efforts and contributes to the accumulation of unused data. Following the completion of their individual evaluation processes, the information collected is typically analyzed and disseminated within the organization itself, completely extracting it from the communities to which it refers. This practice has had two notable negative consequences: first, it limits the amount of community involvement in the measurement and evaluation process, missing an important opportunity to develop local analytic skills, and second, it propagates a culture of non-evidence-based policy making by failing to connect policy or program interventions with impact assessment results (Stansfield, 2009).

Costs of Measurement

The cost of measurement can pose an important limitation on feasibility. Along with capacity for data collection and analysis, costs must be taken into consideration when prioritizing, planning, and implementing any of the specific measurement approaches that will be described later in this chapter. Methods to collect population data, such as systematic surveillance and health information systems, can be very expensive and have required subsidization from external funders in many countries. Although there is limited publicly available information and analysis of the costs to implement population measurement strategies, some estimates for country spending on health data suggest that comprehensive measurement can be affordable for developing countries. For example, the Health Metrics Network (HMN) estimates a national health information system comprising six essential subsystems (health service statistics, public health surveillance, census, household surveys, vital events, and health resource tracking) would cost $0.53 per capita in a low income country (Stansfield et al., 2006). The health information system in Belize was implemented at an initial cost of approximately $2 per capita (Bundale, 2009). The Millennium Development Goals Africa Steering Group (2008) estimates that to support censuses, household surveys, and civil registration and vital statistics systems across Africa would cost $250 million annually (less than $1 per capita). In Tanzania, 11 information systems that generate health and poverty indicators were able to generate all but one of the indicators recommended by four major poverty reduction and reform programs, at an aggregate cost of $0.53 per capita in 2002/2003 (Rommelmann et al., 2005).

Program evaluation also requires an investment of a proportion of the project budget, but there is little publicly available information on the amount spent on measuring, monitoring, and evaluating health programs, and there is limited evidence to assess the costs, cost-effectiveness, benefit-cost ratio, or financial return on investment for different measurement strategies to evaluate these programs. Indeed, although measurement activities usually receive some funding as part of the implementation of a program, no empirical basis supports specific budget targets for measurement or monitoring and evaluation. The most explicit guidance regarding the proportion of program activities that should be devoted to monitoring and evaluation comes from the Global Fund. The Global Fund's 2009 Monitoring and Evaluation Toolkit: HIV, Tuberculosis, and Health Systems Straightening, which was co-sponsored by a number of major multilateral global health organizations, states that over the past years "global and national efforts have been made to increase financial resources for monitoring and evaluation to the widely recommended 5–10 percent of the overall program budget." It endorses this amount and offers a framework on how to allocate these funds (The Global Fund to Fight AIDS, Tuberculosis and Malaria, 2009, p. 32).

APPLYING MEASUREMENT METHODS FOR GLOBAL CVD

The following sections describe methods and tools that can serve to improve measurement for global CVD by providing information for feedback and decision making from multiple sources (such as surveillance, intervention research and program evaluation, clinical practice data, and policy analysis) and at multiple levels (including national, subnational, health systems, communities, households, and individuals). Although a distinction in levels and sources is made in the discussion that follows, it is also ideal for measurement approaches to work across different levels—for example, by using nested measures with relevance to each other. For comparable use of data across sources and levels, there also needs to be agreement on what is to be measured and how it is disseminated. To address global CVD, the methods described here draw from successful CVD measurement strategies and programs from the developed and the developing world where available, as well as from significant advances in measurement in other areas of global health, especially HIV/AIDS.

Measurement to Inform Policy

For policy makers at all levels, measurement provides information that can motivate changes in priorities and policies, influence public opinion, help select and manage intervention approaches, and set priorities for the allocation of resources. The discipline of policy analysis strives to provide objective data and analyses to support rational policy decisions (i.e., "evidence-based policy"). There is an important distinction between evidence *for* policy and evidence *on* policy. Evidence for policy supports a rationale for prioritizing and implementing policies and programs and often comes from population-level evidence as well as from system- and program-level evidence. A well-supported rationale, however, involves uncertainty as to the actual benefit or relevance, especially when being translated from other contexts.

Evidence on policy attempts to address that uncertainty by actively assessing the impact of public health and prevention policies using measurement of population endpoints, such as smoking prevalence or clinically recognized myocardial infarctions (MIs). Such research is often described as health policy and systems research in the global health literature. For example, a policy change that is phased in allows experimental data to be gathered comparing population outcomes with and without the implemented policy; this can be especially valuable in informing future policies. Policy makers also often make implementation decisions based on evaluations that assess the effectiveness and implementation of particular clinical, organizational, or public health strategies. This evaluation approach is described in more detail later in this chapter.

A recent review of the literature indicates that health policy analysis in developing countries is quite limited, especially with regard to CVD (Gilson and Raphaely, 2008). Although spending on health policy and systems research is growing, it remains low and results remain limited in rigor and generalizability compared to the needs of policy makers and providers in developing countries (Anonymous, 2008; Bennett et al., 2008). The literature on implementation science—which addresses how interventions demonstrated to be effective can be implemented in a wider range of settings—is also limited for developing countries (Madon et al., 2007). However, there is an emerging movement to use more evidence-based policy at all levels in low and middle income countries, and it is crucial to be sure that this movement does not continue to develop without being applied to policies related to chronic diseases. The strength and mix of national, regional, and local policy measurement will depend on country-specific factors, such as the governance system, the size of the relevant population, and other local attributes.

Working to fill the evidence-based policy gap in low and middle income countries, the Evidence-Informed Policy Network (EVIPNet) aims to synthesize research results into products useful to developing-country health policy makers. EVIPNet teams have now been established in Africa (van Kammen et al., 2006), Asia, and the Americas (Corkum et al., 2008). However, these efforts remain limited in scope and applicability for cardiovascular disease as none of the policy briefs currently being developed by the nine-country coalition of EVIPNet Africa relate to policy decisions on CVD risk factors (EVIPNet, 2008). The Future Health Systems: Innovations for Equity consortium is another example of an active approach to making a research–policy linkage, by working with six developing countries to develop 5-year research plans whose results will address priorities identified by policy makers (Syed et al., 2008).

While significant progress can be made by engaging national governments around measurement, the use of evidence-based policy should not be limited to national-level actors. For example, the Tanzania Essential Health Interventions Program, initiated in 1993, has attempted to identify simple tools to enable health planners at the district level to plan on the basis of evidence (IDRC, 2008). Population data and computerized decision tools were provided to two district health management teams. The goal of the program was for the data and decision support tools to assist decision makers in prioritizing their funding strategies to those diseases that cause the greatest burden. While the program focused primarily on communicable diseases, subsequent health gains were achieved in a severely low resource setting, and the potential to adapt these strategies to a chronic disease framework could be explored. To date the program has resulted in more than a 40 percent decrease in child mortality in each district (IDRC, 2008; Stansfield et al., 2006).

Cost-effectiveness analysis based on modeling is another approach that has been used to set general priorities among CVD prevention interventions in developing countries (Gaziano et al., 2007). While the broad findings on cost-effectiveness come primarily from modeling studies, countries with adequate measurement data can perform country-specific cost-effectiveness analyses of these interventions to help inform policy decisions with evidence that is more context specific. However, to date these evaluations have been limited. Cost-effectiveness analysis of CVD interventions in low and middle income countries is discussed further in Chapter 7.

A major consideration in developing better measurement for evidence on policy related to CVD is the complexity of the determinants of cardiovascular disease. Because of this complexity, policies in multiple sectors have the potential to affect CVD. Therefore, to comprehensively measure policy effects on CVD, there needs to be shared understanding of target outcomes as well as comparable indicators and integrated measurement approaches to determine the health impact on chronic diseases of policies in areas such as agriculture, urban planning, and development initiatives from donors and governments.

Population Measurement

One of the key challenges hampering many low and middle income countries is the lack of baseline and trend data on population prevalence and incidence of cardiovascular disease. Without this knowledge, ministers of health and program directors cannot know what types of interventions will be necessary, whom should be targeted to ensure these initiatives are most effective, and how long programs should remain in place. Without baseline data, resources might be misdirected to programs targeting individuals or groups who either are already managing their risk factors well or do not comprise the majority of individuals in need. Baseline data that are gathered systematically and regularly over time are also necessary in order to assess the long-term impacts and effects of policy changes across a range of sectors.

Population and subpopulation statistics on CVD and related risk factors can document outcomes that are typically easy to understand and communicate, making discussions with a wide variety of stakeholders, from policy makers to community health workers, more effective and compelling (Engelgau, 2009). Population data can also highlight opportunities to more effectively prioritize, target, or adapt CVD interventions if the data are collected in a way that allows quantification of variations in CVD outcomes, risk factors, or access to care between genders or among regions, ethnic groups, socioeconomic strata, or rural populations (Joshi et al., 2008; Kivimaki et al., 2008). In addition to informing national policies, surveys with standardized data collection methods can also be used to compare conditions and the effects of intervention approaches across countries. Showing that an intervention is effective in one country of a region, or at one level of economic development, can help convince similar countries to implement similar interventions.

There is some evidence that population-level assessments influence policy decisions in developed and developing countries, although CVD-related examples are limited. In Latin and South America, 30 countries have implemented the Pan American Health Organization's (PAHO's) Regional Core Health Data Initiative, which aims to monitor individual member states' attainment of health goals and stated obligations. The Regional Core Health Data Initiative collects information on both communicable and noncommunicable diseases, including indicators relating to cause-specific CVD mortality, overweight and smoking prevalence, and select health systems measures. However, the vast majority of indicators are related to identifying communicable disease risk (PAHO Health Analysis and Statistics Unit, 2007). This may be indicative of the current health information needs of the region, but it could also contribute to underreporting of the contribution of CVD to local disease burdens.

Of the 30 countries that have implemented the Data Initiative, 21 now report using these data to make policy decisions (Ten-year evaluation of the regional core health data initiative, 2004). For example, Mexico, following the revelation of how out-of-pocket payments led to impoverishment among low income citizens, established Seguro Popular, a new insurance program, along with other mechanisms to aid poor families (Knaul et al., 2006). As part of the Data Initiative, PAHO also produced Basic Country Health Profiles for participating countries in 2002, describing both health status and trends in each nation as well as descriptions of both policy and health systems responses (PAHO, 2007). However, follow-up surveys are needed to continue to track any progress made within countries and to identify, if possible, the level of responsiveness of national governments to changing trends in their disease burden data. Importantly, the use of standardized indicators in the Data Initiative allows comparisons of progress across countries and informs the potential transferability of effective interventions to reduce disease burden.

Over the past several decades there has been a steady growth in the number and types of methods available for collecting population data to monitor and evaluate national and global health. The following section describes methods that are currently either in use or available for population-based systematic surveillance and periodic surveys, both in developed and developing countries. These methods include vital registration systems, systematic surveillance sites and health information systems as well as periodic demographic and risk-factor surveys. Population-level methods can at minimum collect data on cause-specific mortality and cardiovascular events. To the extent feasible, these could also potentially be supplemented with more in depth analyses of demographic subpopulations and surveys of additional indicators such as behavioral and biological risk factors, disease outcome measures, biomarkers, economic measures such as national spending and household expenditures, and health-system measures such as service utilization.

Each method offers a unique opportunity for the global CVD community to draw upon existing models and lessons learned from their implementation, and in some limited cases to integrate with existing infrastructure to avoid duplication of resource expenditures. However, effective use of each of these measurement strategies is dependent on the establishment and prioritization of relevant metrics for cardiovascular disease and cardiovascular disease risk, as described earlier in this chapter.

Systematic Surveillance

Given the long time trends associated with CVD outcomes and the likelihood that funding for programmatic interventions will not include sustained, multiyear follow-up studies, the presence of active systematic surveillance mechanisms that analyze and report data is essential for identifying both program and policy impacts on CVD in developing countries. As described below, a number of surveillance systems are currently in use both in developed and developing countries that provide substantial information not only on health indicators, but also on successful methods of data collection and aggregation. However, these systems are often dominated by infectious disease data requirements, causing the unintended negative impact of constraining the amount of chronic disease-related information that can be gathered. If surveillance systems are to truly present an accurate picture of the disease and risk-factor burden in a particular country, integration with or adaptation of these systems where feasible to provide chronic disease data will be required.

Vital Registration Systems One method of collecting essential population data is through the use of vital registration systems (also called civil registration systems or sometimes death registries). These systems provide the critical information necessary to monitor a country's disease burden and associated needs through the collection of standardized cause of death statistics, including measures of CVD-related causes of mortality. The functionality and capacity of vital registration systems in developing countries varies substantially due in part to the finances and technical capacity required to initiate them (AbouZahr et al., 2007). While there has been increasing momentum recently on the international level to support the development of more comprehensive systems in low and middle income countries (Lee, 2003), there remains a lack of leadership in efforts to capitalize on this momentum because both the implementation costs and benefits are spread across a broad range of sectors at the national government level (AbouZahr et al., 2007). Given the importance of accurate cause of death reporting for understanding the impact of cardiovascular disease on population health, this presents a potential opportunity for the global CVD community to partner with existing actors to increase awareness and support for vital registration. The successful use of vital registration systems is also dependant upon regular funding, maintenance, and validation, because the most widespread data collection systems available will not be successful if the coding and recording methods used are inadequate (Joshi et al., 2009). This was seen recently in the Islamic Republic of Iran where a sampling of cases from the national vital registration system that covers 29 of the 30 Iranian provinces revealed that nearly half of the deaths that had been assigned to ill-defined causes were in fact attributable to cardiovascular disease endpoints (Khosravi et al., 2008).

In addition, more research is needed on the most effective and efficient methods for collecting vital statistics. While the majority of countries that have prioritized vital registration have attempted to establish broad, comprehensive national data collection systems, some countries, including China, India, and Tanzania have had success using sample registration and verbal autopsy to obtain an accurate picture of national trends (Mathers et al., 2005). A growing number of models have become available for this, such as the Sample Vital Registration with Verbal Autopsy (SAVVY) (MEASURE Evaluation, 2007). While implementation of SAVVY in developing countries is not well documented, the use of SAVVY to supplement current data collection methods is planned for the Central Statistics Office of Zambia (Sikanyiti and Nalishebo, 2009).

Systematic Surveillance Sites In order to collect more expansive data that can more effectively guide policy and intervention approaches, routine surveillance is needed not only on cause-specific mortality but also on CVD-related risk factors. More than 30 Health and Demographic Surveillance Sites (HDSSs) in Africa, Asia, and the Americas currently provide a basic network of routine data collection in developing countries, often through formal mechanisms such as the INDEPTH Network (Baiden et al., 2006; Krishnan et al., 2009; Ng et al., 2009). At a minimum, these sites serve to collect longitudinal data on birth rates, death rates, and population migration patterns; however, through a number of research initiatives they have been successfully supplemented with additional indicators including measures of maternal mortality, malaria prevention, and even noncommunicable diseases. This makes them an important entry point into which CVD surveillance efforts could be integrated (Baiden et al., 2006). Thus, where feasible, these systems could be augmented to include a minimum set of CVD indicators, potentially minimizing the burden associated with introducing a entirely new system and the potential future risk for creating a CVD measurement "silo." Additionally, in many developing countries the now-established HDSSs began as large program evaluation centers and were later converted for routine surveillance use, making them a potential model for ways in which program and policy interventions can contribute to the long-term sustainability of measurement capacity (Baiden et al., 2006; Ng et al., 2009).

Opportunities also exist to draw on experiences from some developed countries, where larger, routine surveillance programs that do not rely solely on sentinel sites have also been established. One example of this in the United States is the Behavioral Risk Factor Surveillance Survey (BRFSS) conducted by the Centers for Disease Control and Prevention for the past 25 years. The BRFSS is a monthly phone survey that also includes technical assistance documents, data analysis tools, and guidance on strategies to secure funding for municipalities that would like to participate. Measures of CVD risk, such as tobacco use, participation in physical activity, and previous CVD diagnoses, are included. In addition, the use of a standard set of core indicators for each survey allows for multi-site comparisons (Centers for Disease Control and Prevention, 2010). The success and relative simplicity of BRFSS suggests that this telephone survey approach may be transferable to some developing country settings, especially given the proliferation of cell phones in many regions (Tryhorn, 2009).

Health Information Systems Finally, health information systems (HISs) offer another opportunity for systematic data collection. Policies and programs that attempt to alter risk behavior among a broad cohort of individuals will often depend on these types of information systems to demonstrate the effect of their interventions. As with surveillance, efforts are currently underway to provide support to developing countries seeking to strengthen and harmonize their national HIS. Therefore, it is important for the global CVD community to ensure that metrics related to CVD and chronic diseases are integrated within these systems in developing countries, especially given the growing international focus on the integration and coordination of disparate HISs (Stansfield, 2009).

At WHO, for example, the Health Metrics Network (HMN) offers the documents a "Framework and Standards for Country Health Information Systems" and "Assessing the National Health Information System: An Assessment Tool," which are available for all nations as guidance during self-assessments of coverage and gaps in their existing HISs (WHO Health Metrics Network, 2008a, 2008b). Low and middle income countries are also eligible for additional targeted technical assistance and, in some cases, funding support (WHO Health Metrics Network, 2010). In 2006, for example, Cambodia completed the first stage of its assessment with funding from the HMN, following which they developed an HIS Strategic Plan that was disseminated at a Health Metrics Network regional workshop (Veasnakiry, 2007). Similarly, in 2007 Ethiopia completed an HIS overall assessment with the assistance of the HMN Assessment Tool as part of its Health Sector Development Plan (WHO Health Metrics Network, 2007). To date 60 developing countries have received HMN grants for a variety of HIS assessment and improvement initiatives (WHO Health Metrics Network, 2010). While the Health Metrics Network does not advise each country on the specific indicators to include in their HIS strategic plan, the inclusion of CVD measures will be important in any well-rounded health information system. Effort will be needed by the global cardiovascular disease community to ensure that other disease needs do not crowd out the inclusion and reporting of CVD metrics as efforts supported by HMN are implemented.

Population Surveys

In the past three decades, a number of major multinational surveys of patient populations in clinical settings have illuminated the growing burden of CVD worldwide and have been critical in helping to establish priorities for intervention approaches. These include the WHO Multinational Monitoring of Trends and Determinants in Cardiovascular Disease project and the European Action on Secondary Prevention by Intervention to Reduce Events (EUROASPIRE) in Europe, and the WHO PREMISE study, which included countries in the Middle East, Asia, and Latin America (EUROASPIRE Study Group, 1997; Mendis et al., 2005; Tunstall-Pedoe et al., 2003). These data collection efforts have been beneficial in three ways. First, they provide a cross-sectional view of the epidemic. Second, they provide a richer estimation of what measurement can tell us about the epidemic through the inclusion of more detailed indicators and analysis, which, if particularly useful, would expand and guide future measurement efforts. Third, they set standards for more rigorous collection and validation processes. However, due to the lack of repetition for most of these collection efforts, limited analysis can be done regarding temporal trends. In addition, implementing, coordinating, and funding a multinational survey of such detail is less likely to be feasible in a developing-country setting.

By contrast, routine surveys done at the national or cross-national level, supported by national governments and/or multinational organizations and implemented every 1, 2, or 5 years, can provide ongoing data collection that is critical to measure the scale and scope of CVD as well as trends in disease burden over time. While the cost of these surveys, both to the national government and implementing partners, limits the frequency with which they can be conducted, strong models, such as the Demographic and Health Surveys (DHS), do exist and have been successfully conducted in a wide variety of developing countries. DHS survey templates have been developed for a range of topics; however one is not yet publicly available for CVD or CVD risk-factor prevalence (MEASURE DHS, 2010). Other tools for population-level data collection in developing countries are being developed at the Institute for Health Metrics and Evaluation (IHME), most notably in the area of modeling for disease prevalence, health outcomes, and coverage of health interventions. In addition, IHME has the capacity to develop needs-specific survey instruments for data collection (University of Washington, 2010). Organizations such as MEASURED HS and IHME represent key actors with extensive knowledge of successful developing country survey strategies and, in some cases, established infrastructure. Therefore, they have the potential to be future partners in CVD burden data collection efforts.

One major effort to develop chronic disease-specific survey tools is WHO's STEPwise Approach to Chronic Disease Risk Factor Surveillance (STEPS). STEPS has been piloted and implemented in a demonstration capacity in 41 different countries spanning all income categories (WHO, 2010a). The goal of the STEPS program is to provide flexible options for countries seeking to assess their chronic disease and risk-factor burden in the form of core, expanded, or optimal sets of indicators depending on the technical and financial capacity of the individual government (WHO Noncommunicable Diseases and Mental Health Cluster Surveillance Team, 2001). In addition to the basic implementation tool with a spectrum of measurements, WHO also provides a variety of blank templates, implementation guidance, and analytical software (WHO, 2010b).

The STEPS program advances the possibility of implementing routine population surveys in multiple countries using comparable indicators and survey methodologies. For example, PAHO has worked with countries to adapt STEPS for local context in Latin American countries. Their version, called PanAm STEPS, contains many of the same core questions, but has alternative indicators in the area of food and cigarette consumption that take into account regional and contextual issues (PAHO, 2008). The next steps are to evaluate the feasibility of implementing STEPS on a larger scale as a population-level surveillance tool in developing-country settings. This will require evaluation of costs of implementation and the sustainability of these methodologies for serial surveillance, for example, by evaluating the potential burden associated with different numbers and types of indicators.

As with the expansions of surveillance and health information systems, future assessments of STEPS and other population surveys should also consider the opportunity costs of committing local capacity to assessing CVD and behavioral risk factors compared to other priorities. In some cases, surveys to collect new information on cardiovascular disease can make use of existing resources and capacity by being integrated into existing data collection efforts. For example, STEPS was recently successfully integrated into nine sites in five Asian nations that are part of the INDEPTH Network in order to establish baseline CVD risk-factor data that could inform policy makers (Ng et al., 2009). It will also be important to consider questions of local data ownership and empowerment to adapt survey design, implementation, and analysis. These questions speak to the need to avoid costs without benefit and data without utility (Stansfield, 2009).

In a more narrowly targeted risk-factor survey, the Global Youth Tobacco Survey (GYTS), and the subsequent Global Adult Tobacco Survey, are additional sources that already provide critical information on smoking and tobacco use prevalence internationally within predefined geographic regions (Warren et al., 2008). The standardized methodology employed by the GYTS sites allows for cross-national comparisons of results and analyses to identify where or if progress occurs. Present in 142 nations and recording indicators that cover tobacco use, knowledge and attitudes, advertising levels, and school-based curricula (Asma, 2009), the GYTS may provide either sufficient information on youth tobacco use that does not need to be replicated, or an opportunity to partner with a broad, well-established systematic data collection effort in order to address other risk factor topics. In addition, the indicators in successful surveys of this kind that are currently validated and in use should also be considered during efforts to establish internationally agreed upon measures, as discussed earlier in this chapter.

Conclusion 4.1: *Gaining knowledge about the specific nature of the CVD epidemic in individual countries and about what will work in developing-country settings is a high priority. Improved country-level population data would serve to inform policies and programs.*

Recommendation: Improve Local Data

National and subnational governments should create and maintain health surveillance systems to monitor and more effectively control chronic diseases. Ideally, these systems should report on cause-specific mortality and the primary determinants of CVD. To strengthen existing initiatives, multilateral development agencies and WHO (through, for example, the Health Metrics Network and regional chronic disease network, NCDnet) as well as bilateral public health agencies (such as the Centers for Disease Control and Prevention [CDC] in the United States) and bilateral development agencies (such as United States Agency for International Development [USAID]) should support chronic disease surveillance as part of financial and technical assistance for developing and implementing health information systems. Governments should allocate funds and build capacity for long-term sustainability of disease surveillance that includes chronic diseases.

Efforts to scale up, expand, or adapt any of the existing routine data collection methods described above to develop better chronic disease measurement in low and middle income countries need to take into account potential areas of duplication of efforts and resources and to carefully consider how best to incorporate or take advantage of existing international initiatives. It will be a major challenge for developing countries to invest in chronic disease measurement capacity while the burden of infectious and perinatal disease still remains high (Boutayeb, 2006; Ezzati et al., 2005). Policy makers should strive to identify the minimum scope of data that must be collected to support CVD control programs in their country. Program- or funder-specific data collection may help developing countries meet some of these needs but may also perpetuate information "silos" (Stansfield et al., 2006) that can hinder the efficiency of managing chronic disease programs that simultaneously address multiple risk factors. This leads to a compelling rationale for leveraging resources and capacity by building the collection of new CVD information into integrated data collection efforts with existing surveillance mechanisms, which in many countries focus on infectious diseases and maternal and child health. New efforts to expand population measurement to include chronic disease should be conceptualized in the context of building and strengthening national systems for data collection rather than competing for limited resources. Although challenging, opportunities exist to promote collaboration rather than rivalry by using new technologies, disseminating findings, working with civil society, and training transferrable skilled analysts.

However, it is also important to note that there are inherent differences between chronic and infectious diseases that may limit the direct overlap of infectious disease surveillance methods with CVD and other chronic diseases (Nsubuga et al., 2006). For example, unlike the long-term, sustained services needed to address chronic diseases, many infectious diseases have a narrow range of treatment or vaccine options (which in some cases confer lifetime protection), and a response time frame for intervention outcomes of weeks, compared to decades for chronic diseases. The contributing factors to disease incidence can also be much less complex when there is a single infectious agent and a defined path or vector for transmission. HIV and tuberculosis (TB), the so-called chronic infectious diseases, are probably most analogous to CVD due to their need for chronic care, the role of lifestyle risk factors, and the need for extensive prevention efforts. Elements from HIV and TB surveillance that can most directly inform CVD surveillance include risk-factor measurement, maintenance of disease registries for managing treatment and secondary prevention, and techniques for monitoring service management effectiveness (Diaz et al., 2009).

Measurement of Health Systems

Over the past decade, there has been growing recognition that achieving many of the current global health priorities will require strengthening of health systems rather than simply concentrating efforts on disease-specific programs. Measurement of health systems performance is a critical component for national governments and donors to use in evaluating the capacity of countries to promote the health of their citizens, the effectiveness of health programs, and the transferability of successful health systems reforms from one country to another.

There is ongoing debate within the policy and global health communities over how to define health systems and their impact (IOM, 2009a; Kruk and Freedman, 2008; Murray and Frenk, 2000; Shengelia et al., 2003). A number of different frameworks for measuring health systems performance have been proposed. These vary in the definition of the scope and primary objectives of health systems and therefore what aspects should be evaluated to assess their performance, ranging from a narrow focus on health services to a broader inclusion of public health efforts (Arah et al., 2003; Kruk and Freedman, 2008). In any of these frameworks, a clear definition of the goals of a health system is the essential first step to performance evaluation (Kruk and Freedman, 2008; Murray and Frenk, 2000).

The variability in existing efforts to assess health systems performance highlights two of the biggest current challenges: the lack of available data and the lack of an internationally standardized framework or set of indicators. Determining how to measure health systems in a standardized way that is valid, reliable, and locally relevant, with feasible and implementable data collection, is an important item on the global health research agenda (Kruk and Freedman, 2008). A number of major initiatives are currently being used to standardize health systems metrics to be used globally, including the United Nations' Interagency and Expert Group on Millennium Development Goal Indicators, the WHO-based HMN, and the IHME at the University of Washington (Kruk and Freedman, 2008). Coordination among these initiatives will be essential to avoid duplicate systems of measurement and to maximize the limited resources for evaluation and measurement.

Thus, measurement and evaluation of health systems is another area in which it is important for the global CVD community to engage in these emerging initiatives and ensure that metrics that are relevant to the quality, costs, and financing of chronic care are integrated as health systems indicators are developed. This will help ensure that measurement of health systems going forward will be informative in terms of the capacity of these systems to address CVD and related chronic diseases.

Measurement of Quality of Care

The quality of clinical practice, which relies on measurement and feedback, is critical to translating evidence based-practices into effectiveness. The fundamental importance of evaluations of the quality of clinical care is that they relate risk factors to the successful application of interventions such as treatment of hypertension and hypercholesterolemia and other areas where clinical interventions mitigate risk, including counseling about diet indiscretions, tobacco use, and exercise. Improving the quality and effectiveness of patient care can also reduce waste and inefficiencies, which is especially important for CVD treatment within health systems and clinics in low-resource settings. These measures also have the advantage of being more readily obtained than an outcome event (e.g., an MI) and are by definition aimed at the provider behavior that needs to change to improve health.

A number of methods are available for measuring practitioner performance: provider self-report, patient vignettes, patient self-report, and record reviews. The Institute of Medicine (IOM, 2001) recommends that quality be defined along six dimensions, as timely, effective, safe, equitable, cost-effective, and patient centered. Measures of quality ideally reflect these dimensions in addition to being amenable to improvement, able to account for differences in the type of patients treated by different providers, and economically feasible to use over time and across systems (Epstein, 2006;

Spertus et al., 2003). Measures should also be reliable and valid, and not be able to be "gamed" (Petersen et al., 2006).

Currently, a variety of studies have been published that identify indicators for use in high income countries, which cover a broad range of illnesses and areas. However, the current challenge with many of these indicators is that they may not always be suitable in all contexts, meaning they will need to be developed and adapted to be locally relevant (Engelgau, 2009). However, with feedback mechanisms established, these measurements could be used to more effectively target problem areas of service provision in low-resource settings.

A set of evidence-based measures specific to quality of CVD care have been developed by the American College of Cardiology (ACC) and the American Heart Association (AHA). These include performance measures that can be used for reporting and evaluation (Bonow et al., 2008). As defined by ACC and AHA, quality measures largely reflect the "processes of care for which recommendations in practice guidelines are of adequate strength that the failure to follow the recommendations is likely to result in suboptimal patient outcomes." Examples of such measures include prescribing warfarin for patients with nonvalvular atrial fibrillation, beta blockers after MI, and angiotensin-converting enzyme inhibitors or angiotensin receptor antagonists for heart failure with left ventricular systolic dysfunction. Quality metrics recommended by ACC and AHA also include structural measures, such as staffing ratios, and patient outcomes, such as post-MI mortality. Performance measures—a subset of quality indicators used for public reporting, incentive-based programs, and comparisons across providers—have also been developed by ACC and AHA for heart failure, acute MI, cardiac rehabilitation, and atrial fibrillation.

Intervention Research and Program Evaluation

Measurement can be used to determine the effectiveness of an intervention in an experimental trial, but it is also the foundation for planning, prioritizing, and operationalizing interventions and programs When interventions that have been demonstrated to be effective are implemented on a larger scale as part of programs at scale, whether or not they are part of a trial, program evaluation can be used to monitor their outcomes. In addition, a cycle of ongoing evaluation can be used formatively by program implementers to assess and improve their programs and make adaptations that encourage sustainability.

An extensive review of methodologies for intervention research and program evaluation is beyond the scope of this report and is information that can be found elsewhere in the literature for evaluations not only of programs for CVD and related chronic disease but also for HIV/AIDS, mental illness and substance abuse, and other areas of health that warrant a similar range of intervention approaches from health promotion and prevention to treatment and disease management. Therefore, only a brief overview of some key points is presented here. Although intervention research and program evaluation are described separately in this section, in reality they overlap significantly. A program can also be implemented at scale as part of an experimental trial, such that evaluation data also serve as outcome data for the intervention trial. In addition, elements of program design such as formative research and tailoring of intervention components are applicable to both experimental intervention trials and programs. In addition, given limited financial resources, careful advance planning is necessary in prioritizing intervention research and program evaluation design and methods.

Although there are an increasing number of CVD risk-reduction and treatment programs currently underway in developing countries addressing an array of local needs, information regarding their effectiveness and impact on health status is very limited and, even when available, not readily conveyed to other locations struggling with similar disease burdens. For some of these programs, improved program evaluation strategies and more reliable and rigorous measurement are needed to document and assess their progress. In other cases, accurate data collection may be occurring, but the transfer of this information is hampered by limited mechanisms available to facilitate dissemination of the results. The available evidence base for intervention research and program evaluation for CVD and related chronic diseases in low and middle income countries will be discussed in more detail in Chapters 5, 6, and 7.

Intervention Research

The goal of intervention research is to examine a program's effects and whether a program can be implemented with sufficient effectiveness and fidelity in different communities and at scale. Intervention research can be used to assess efficacy (impact under ideal conditions) or effectiveness (impact under conditions that are likely to occur in a real-world implementation). This assessment can be made through comparison to a control condition or as a comparison between two types of intervention. Intervention research can also be used to experimentally evaluate approaches to implement, adapt, scale up, and sustain an intervention over time (Flay et al., 2005; IOM, 2009b; Kellam and Langevin, 2003; Pangea Global AIDS Foundation, 2009).

Randomized trials are often seen as the highest standard for intervention research, and they do allow for rigorous conclusions about intervention effects and causal inferences. However, a randomized trial is often not a feasible approach to evaluate interventions in real-world settings. Other methodologies for the experimental design, measurement, and analysis of the effects of preventive interventions include waitlist comparisons, interrupted time series, and pre-post comparisons. Interventions can also be assessed when natural experiments occur as well as through modeling approaches (Flay et al., 2005; IOM, 2009b; Kellam and Langevin, 2003).

CVD prevention research often focuses on intermediate outcomes such as behavioral measures, which can be a reasonable endpoint if causal links have been well established, for example, between behaviors and improved outcomes. When feasible, more direct measures of effect can include measure of biological risk factors or disease outcome measures, such as cardiac events. To truly assess the feasibility of interventions, economic measures such as cost-effectiveness or benefit-cost analysis are critical as well as measures of implementation processes.

Program Evaluation

When intervention programs are implemented, measurement is a critical tool both to assess whether the program is having the intended effect and to provide feedback to program managers and providers to help them assess and improve the program and their own performance. Data collection and reporting for programs are typically left to the program implementers depending on their evaluation needs and on the reporting needs of the organization under which they operate or from whom they receive their funding. Although universal program evaluation guidance may not be warranted, organized national, regional, or international reporting mechanisms can maximize the potential for sharing results or best practices. With the growing international emphasis on impact evaluations at the programmatic, community, and national levels, the importance of preplanned and rigorous program evaluations that include data that can be integrated with other measurement systems has never been more important.

Along with this growing emphasis on evaluation in global health efforts, many tools have been developed that provide models and support for program evaluation in low and middle income countries. The majority of these have been either developed or initiated by the infectious disease community, but the principles and approaches have the potential to be adapted for CVD and related chronic diseases. There are more than 200 program evaluation tools currently in use in the HIV/AIDS community (Family Health International, 2010). These have varying degrees of disease specificity. While some are directed at unique components of the HIV/AIDS epidemic or infectious diseases more broadly, there are also frameworks outlining the principles of measurement as well as guidance documents for developing evaluation and analysis plans ready for adaptation by the CVD community (Family Health International, 2010). For example, MEASURE

Evaluation provides an online basic measurement and evaluation Fundamentals Self-Guided Mini Course, originally developed for USAID, which includes discussions on how to identify indicators, plan and conduct intervention evaluations, and analyze the results (Frankel and Gage, 2007). The Global Fund to Fight HIV/AIDS, Tuberculosis and Malaria has also developed a Monitoring and Evaluation Toolkit that addresses not only HIV and TB but also efforts to strengthen health systems (The Global Fund to Fight AIDS, Tuberculosis and Malaria, 2009). Given the potential role of health systems strengthening programs in addressing the global burden of CVD, adaptation of this toolkit could provide an opportunity to harmonize relevant chronic and infectious disease health systems indicators. The Global Fund Guide for Operational Research offers the addition of process measures for long-term adaptation and sustainability of ongoing programs. This kind of operational research is particularly critical for programs to address CVD, which requires ongoing intervention. Indeed, new research may also be needed to develop program evaluation strategies that can address the long-term needs of measurement follow-up and impact evaluation, as the reality is that many of the benefits of CVD risk-factor interventions will not accrue until years or decades after individual programs have been completed.

Impact measures for programs to prevent and manage CVD would follow principles similar to those for intervention research, including both CVD-related outcomes and economic measures, as well as process measures to monitor program implementation. Although measurement strategies need to be tailored to specific interventions or programs, some standardization would provide an opportunity for a better continuum from intervention trials through implementations of interventions at scale, with a set of streamlined indicators that would be useful to assess whether the original effectiveness is being maintained. The incorporation of some agreed-upon standardized metrics would also allow for comparisons across programs and over time and greater long-term feasibility of program evaluation.

As intervention programs increase in scale, so do their data collection and reporting needs, and their risk of developing duplicate systems that operate alongside national health information systems. A review of how reporting mechanisms for major global HIV/AIDS programs interact with national data collection efforts showed that this can lead to inefficient use of resources on parallel reporting structures, a failure to develop one coherent national picture of impact, and an increased burden on program implementers (Oomman et al., 2008). Avoiding this duplication by identifying CVD indicators that can meet the needs of both the program and the health information system as well as encouraging the integration of reporting with the national systems where appropriate will be important considerations as global CVD programs expand in developing countries.

Measurement of Individual Health Status

Measurement of individual behavioral or biological risk factors can be useful to motivate changes in a person's behavior if the data are meaningful enough for the individual to be able to act upon the results. This requires that the data be presented in clear terms alongside health counseling or education initiatives to establish clinically relevant behavior-change goals for individuals.

Several decades of behavioral research in developed-country settings indicate that an individual's knowledge of his or her health status and/or risk for disease is a necessary (albeit insufficient) precursor to behavior change. This theoretical principle is supported by research of several cardiovascular risk behaviors. For example, regular self-weighing has been associated in several studies with weight loss and weight maintenance (Butryn et al., 2007; Linde et al., 2005; VanWormer et al., 2009). Also, a recent review found that the use of pedometers to track the number of steps a person takes, particularly if a goal for steps was set, was consistently associated with increased physical activity (Bravata et al., 2007). In addition, limited data indicate that simply the knowledge of cholesterol levels can influence fat intake (Aubin et al., 1998).

In addition to providing feedback to individuals and providers to motivate and guide individual behavior change, individual measures can also be aggregated to improve provider performance, to inform measurement of health systems, or to reflect populations at a broader level when it is statistically appropriate to do so and appropriate methods are used. However, an important consideration in individual-level measurement is whether standards and norms are replicable in different populations. This is true for single measures, such as body mass index, and especially for methods used to score aggregate risk.

Emerging Technologies to Support Measurement Methods

The emergence of electronic health (e-health) and mobile health (m-health) initiatives in both developed and developing countries have opened the door to an enormous new set of potential efforts to help make both health care delivery and measurement more effective and efficient. These technologies cut across all levels of measurement and interact with each to varying degrees. While there is a need for much more research on the training, infrastructure, and cost barriers to introducing new technology and mobile data collection devices, they present a rapidly growing field of research and investment on which global health initiatives have already begun to capitalize (United Nations Foundation, 2010). Thus, it is in the interests of the global CVD community to actively pursue involvement in ongoing efforts to improve these nascent systems.

A recent review of e-health initiatives in developing countries showed that technology is already being used in resource-poor settings with some success for a wide variety of projects, ranging from electronic health records to laboratory and pharmacy management systems to data collection and evaluation tools (Blaya et al., 2010). E-health and m-health technology are also emerging to support measurement through new tools to conduct population-based surveys and surveillance, to link data to geographic information, and to present that data to policy makers in more coherent and compelling manners (Gapminder Foundation, 2010; IDRC, 2009; Tegang et al., 2009).

In particular, the potential application of new tools to track patient status over the long term and to integrate information with health systems is uniquely suited to chronic disease management. For example, the use of electronic medical records systems in health care settings is one potential mechanism for improved data collection and analysis. These systems are already in use in a number of developing countries for monitoring patients on antiretroviral therapy (Braitstein et al., 2009; Forster et al., 2008; Kalogriopoulos et al., 2009), and a variety of both proprietary and open source software tools are available. However, it is important that these be adapted to local needs in order to prevent inefficiencies caused by a failure to ensure the collection of all necessary data or by the use of multiple systems to cover duplicate reporting needs (Forster et al., 2008; Kalogriopoulos et al., 2009; OpenMRS, 2010). Some organizations, such as AMPATH in Kenya, have already begun to adapt their antiretroviral therapy focused electronic medical records systems to include measures for diabetes and cardiovascular disease (Braitstein et al., 2009). In addition to assisting with the management of patient-level data, electronic medical records systems, if designed appropriately, also have the potential to incorporate measures that can be aggregated to inform health systems priorities. The use of mobile health approaches to improve patient outcomes is discussed further in Chapter 5.

GLOBAL USES OF MEASUREMENT

The use of measurement data compiled and analyzed at the global level is crucial to the success of current and future initiatives as it can serve to raise awareness and to prioritize and coordinate efforts among global stakeholders. As described in Chapters 1 and 2, analyses of the global burden of CVD have been critical in illuminating the scope and magnitude of the CVD epidemic and advancing the advocacy message of the CVD community.

Burden-of-disease analyses are an important method of data aggregation and modeling, which can lay out mortality and morbidity estimates, showing changes in the epidemic across countries and linking this information to economic data (Abegunde et al., 2007; Lopez et al., 2006). In addition to these aggregated analyses, individual country efforts need to be tracked in a coordinated manner in order to inform global efforts, learn from emerging best practices, prevent duplication, and identify where additional resources and focus should be directed.

A number of broad measures of progress would benefit from leadership at the global level, including the evaluation and dissemination of the impact and implementation of global efforts, behavioral and biomedical surveillance and its integration into national surveillance systems at the population level, infrastructure, training, health education, and tracking and evaluating the effectiveness of funding and expenditures. In addition, all new policies by major global players should be backed by a financial assessment of the implementation cost and should describe means by which pledges and commitments will be reported.

A variety of stakeholders are currently responsible for either coordination or measurement at the international level. First and foremost an extensive list of measures was proposed in the 2008 WHO Noncommunicable Disease Action Plan to track global progress and characterize the different actions underway in member states. WHO is scheduled to release a preliminary progress report on a select number of these metrics (WHO, 2008). In addition, globally coordinated research efforts, such as the newly created Global Alliance for Chronic Disease (Daar et al., 2009), will need to establish indicators for tracking the distribution of funds, demonstrating the impact of their efforts, and identifying successful coordination strategies. Given the overlapping interest of many of these multilateral organizations, the development of harmonized indicators is an essential next step, as described previously in this chapter. An epidemiology reference group has also been working with WHO staff from headquarters and regional offices to develop guidance for chronic disease surveillance systems and to agree on core indicators that will be used to monitor the major chronic diseases and their risk factors (Ala Alwan, World Health Organization, 2009, personal communication). Finally, the creation of a routine global reporting mechanism that convenes to compare and disseminate results is also needed. Mechanisms for developing this are discussed further in Chapter 8.

CONCLUSION

Measurement is crucial to the success of efforts at every stage of the process to avert the rise of CVD in developing countries. Stakeholders of all kinds, from national governments to development agencies and other donors, who have committed to taking action to address the burden of chronic diseases will need to carefully assess the needs of the population they are targeting, the state of current efforts, the available capacity and infrastructure, and the political will to support the available opportunities for action. This assessment will inform priorities and should lead to specific and realistic goals for intervention strategies that are adapted to local baseline capacity and burden of disease and designed to improve that baseline over time. These goals will determine choices about the implementation of both evidence-based policies and programs and also capacity-building efforts. Ongoing evaluation of implemented strategies will allow policy makers and other stakeholders to determine if implemented actions are having the intended effect and meeting the defined goals, and to reassess needs, capacity, and priorities over time.

Over the past two decades great progress has been made toward identifying risk-factor prevalence and CVD incidence, prevalence, severity, and mortality, as described in Chapter 3. At the global level, this has fulfilled the first step in the cycle of measurement for CVD. However, many low and middle income countries still lack sufficient local data to inform their decisions about how to prioritize actions to target CVD. In addition, while basic epidemiologic knowledge has been expanding, other core functions of measurement, such as policy analysis, health services research, intervention research, and program impact evaluation, have not been keeping pace. As a result, although there exists greater awareness about which risk factors require the most attention, less is known about what intervention approaches will be most effective and feasible in the resource-constrained settings of low and middle income countries. This lack of knowledge about program and policy effectiveness within local realities not only constrains program implementers, but also prevents national governments, nongovernmental organizations, and multilateral organizations from effectively making and implementing decisions to address the cardiovascular disease epidemic.

For some CVD measurement needs, there are well-established models for evaluation and data collection in developing countries, such as models for national surveillance, behavioral surveys, electronic medical records, and tools for program evaluation. For other purposes, new tools need to be developed. In either case, it is important, when feasible, to build upon current approaches used in monitoring and evaluation both locally and globally in order to take advantage of existing infrastructure, to build capacity in measurement and monitoring, and to avoid the inefficiencies of duplicate systems. Finally, for comparable use of data across programs and countries, there also needs to be international agreement on what is to be measured and how the information is disseminated.

REFERENCES

Abegunde, D. O., C. D. Mathers, T. Adam, M. Ortegon, and K. Strong. 2007. The burden and costs of chronic diseases in low-income and middle-income countries. *Lancet* 370(9603):1929-1938.
AbouZahr, C., J. Cleland, F. Coullare, S. B. Macfarlane, F. C. Notzon, P. Setel, S. Szreter, R. N. Anderson, A. A. Bawah, A. P. Betran, F. Binka, K. Bundhamcharoen, R. Castro, T. Evans, X. C. Figueroa, C. K. George, L. Gollogly, R. Gonzalez, D. R. Grzebien, K. Hill, Z. Huang, T. H. Hull, M. Inoue, R. Jakob, P. Jha, Y. Jiang, R. Laurenti, X. Li, D. Lievesley, A. D. Lopez, D. M. Fat, M. Merialdi, L. Mikkelsen, J. K. Nien, C. Rao, K. Rao, O. Sankoh, K. Shibuya, N. Soleman, S. Stout, V. Tangcharoensathien, P. J. van der Maas, F. Wu, G. Yang, S. Zhang. 2007. The way forward. *Lancet* 370(9601):1791-1799.
Anonymous. 2008. The state of health research worldwide. *Lancet* 372(9649):1519.
Arah, O. A., N. S. Klazinga, D. M. J. Delnoij, A. H. A. Ten Asbroek, and T. Custers. 2003. Conceptual frameworks for health systems performance: A quest for effectiveness, quality, and improvement. *International Journal for Quality in Health Care* 15(5):377-398.
Asma, S. 2009. Global tobacco surveillance system. Presentation at the Public Information Gathering Session for the Institute of Medicine Committee on Preventing the Global Epidemic of Cardiovascular Disease, Washington, DC.
Aubin, M., G. Godin, L. Vezina, J. Maziade, and R. Desharnais. 1998. Hypercholesterolemia screening. Does knowledge of blood cholesterol level affect dietary fat intake? *Canadian Family Physician* 44:1289-1297.
Baiden, F., A. Hodgson, and F. N. Binka. 2006. Demographic surveillance sites and emerging challenges in international health. *Bulletin of the World Health Organization* 84(3):163.
Bennett, S., J. T. Boerma, and R. Brugha. 2006. Scaling up HIV/AIDS evaluation. *Lancet* 367(9504):79-82.
Bennett, S., T. Adam, C. Zarowsky, V. Tangcharoensathien, K. Ranson, T. Evans, and A. Mills. 2008. From Mexico to Mali: Progress in health policy and systems research. *Lancet* 372(9649):1571-1578.
Blaya, J., H. S. Fraser, and S. Holt. 2010. E-health technologies show promise in developing countries. *Health Affairs* 29(2):245-251.
Bonow, R. O., F. A. Masoudi, J. S. Rumsfeld, E. Delong, N. A. Estes, 3rd, D. C. Goff, Jr., K. Grady, L. A. Green, A. R. Loth, E. D. Peterson, I. L. Pina, M. J. Radford, and D. M. Shahian. 2008. ACC/AHA classification of care metrics: Performance measures and quality metrics: A report of the American College of Cardiology/American Heart Association Task Force on Performance Measures. *Journal of the American College of Cardiology* 52(24):2113-2117.
Boutayeb, A. 2006. The double burden of communicable and non-communicable diseases in developing countries. *Transactions of the Royal Society of Tropical Medicine and Hygiene* 100(3):191-199.
Braitstein, P., R. M. Einterz, J. E. Sidle, S. Kimaiyo, W. Tierney, P. Braitstein, R. M. Einterz, J. E. Sidle, S. Kimaiyo, and W. Tierney. 2009. "Talkin' about a revolution": How electronic health records can facilitate the scale-up of HIV care and treatment and catalyze primary care in resource-constrained settings. *Journal of Acquired Immune Deficiency Syndromes: JAIDS* 52(Suppl 1):S54-S57.
Bundale, B. 2009. Company's software benefits Belize. *New Brunswick Business Journal*, 8 June.
Butryn, M. L., S. Phelan, J. O. Hill, and R. R. Wing. 2007. Consistent self-monitoring of weight: A key component of successful weight loss maintenance. *Obesity (Silver Spring)* 15(12):3091-3096.

Centers for Disease Control and Prevention. 2010. *CDC's behavioral risk factor surveillance system.* http://www.cdc.gov/brfss/ (accessed October 8, 2009).

Corkum, S., L. G. Cuervo, and A. Porras. 2008. EVIPNet Americas: Informing policies with evidence. *Lancet* 372(9644):1130-1131.

Daar, A. S., E. G. Nabel, S. K. Pramming, W. Anderson, A. Beaudet, D. Liu, V. M. Katoch, L. K. Borysiewicz, R. I. Glass, J. Bell. 2009. The global alliance for chronic diseases. *Science* 324(5935):1642.

Diaz, T., J. M. Garcia-Calleja, P. D. Ghys, and K. Sabin. 2009. Advances and future directions in HIV surveillance in low- and middle-income countries. *Current Opinion in HIV AIDS* 4(4):253-259.

Engelgau, M. M. 2009. Measuring success: Using tools we already have. Presentation at the Public Information Gathering Session of the Committee on Preventing the Global Epidemic of Cardiovascular Disease, Washington, DC.

Epstein, A. J. 2006. Do cardiac surgery report cards reduce mortality? Assessing the evidence. *Medical Care Research and Review* 63(4):403-426.

EUROASPIRE Study Group. 1997. EUROASPIRE: A European Society of Cardiology survey of secondary prevention of coronary heart disease: Principal results. *European Heart Journal* 18(10):1569-1582.

EVIPNet. 2008. *Evidence informed policy network: For better decision making.* Geneva: World Health Organization.

Ezzati, M., S. Vander Hoorn, C. M. Lawes, R. Leach, W. P. James, A. D. Lopez, A. Rodgers, and C. J. Murray. 2005. Rethinking the "Diseases of affluence" paradigm: Global patterns of nutritional risks in relation to economic development. *PLoS Med* 2(5):e133.

Family Health International. 2010. *An inventory of program evaluation tools and guidelines.* Arlington, VA: Family Health International.

Flay, B. R., A. Biglan, R. F. Boruch, F. G. Castro, D. Gottfredson, S. Kellam, E. K. Moscicki, S. Schinke, J. C. Valentine, and P. Ji. 2005. Standards of evidence: Criteria for efficacy, effectiveness and dissemination. *Prevention Science* 6(3):151-175.

Forster, M., C. Bailey, M. W. Brinkhof, C. Graber, A. Boulle, M. Spohr, E. Balestre, M. May, O. Keiser, A. Jahn, and M. Egger. 2008. Electronic medical record systems, data quality and loss to follow-up: Survey of antiretroviral therapy programmes in resource-limited settings. *Bulletin of the World Health Organization* 86(12):939-947.

Frankel, N., and A. Gage. 2007. *M&E fundamentals: A self-guided mini course.* Chapel Hill, NC: MEASURE Evaluation.

Gapminder Foundation. 2010. *For a fact-based world view.* http://www.gapminder.org/ (accessed March 9, 2010).

Gaziano, T. A., G. Galea, and K. S. Reddy. 2007. Scaling up interventions for chronic disease prevention: The evidence. *Lancet* 370(9603):1939-1946.

Gilson, L., and N. Raphaely. 2008. The terrain of health policy analysis in low and middle income countries: A review of published literature 1994-2007. *Health Policy Plan* 23(5):294-307.

The Global Fund to Fight AIDS, Tuberculosis and Malaria. 2009. *Monitoring and evaluation toolkit: HIV, tuberculosis, and malaria and health systems strengthening.* Geneva: The Global Fund.

Global HIV M&E Information. *MERG background.* http://www.globalhivmeinfo.org/AgencySites/Pages/MERG%20Background.aspx (accessed February 2, 2010).

IDRC (International Development Research Centre). 2008. *Fixing health systems, 2nd edition—executive summary.* Ottawa, Canada: International Development Research Centre.

IDRC. 2009. *Assessing the use of PDAs for household surveys in Tanzania.* http://www.idrc.ca/en/ev-88026-201-1-DO_TOPIC.html (accessed March 9, 2010).

IOM (Institute of Medicine). 2001. *Crossing the quality chasm: A new health system for the 21st century.* Washington, DC: National Academy Press.
IOM. 2009a. *State of the USA health indicators: Letter report.* Washington, DC: The National Academies Press.
IOM. 2009b. *Preventing mental, emotional, and behavioral disorders among young people: Progress and possibilities.* Washington, DC: The National Academies Press.
Joshi, R., S. Jan, Y. Wu, and S. MacMahon. 2008. Global inequalities in access to cardiovascular health care: Our greatest challenge. *Journal of the American College of Cardiology* 52(23):1817-1825.
Joshi, R., A. P. Kengne, and B. Neal. 2009. Methodological trends in studies based on verbal autopsies before and after published guidelines. *Bulletin of the World Health Organization* 87(9):678-682.
Kalogriopoulos, N. A., J. Baran, A. J. Nimunkar, and J. G. Webster. 2009. Electronic medical record systems for developing countries: Review. *Conference Proceedings Engineering in Medicine and Biology Society* 1:1730-1733.
Kellam, S. G., and D. J. Langevin. 2003. A framework for understanding "evidence" in prevention research and programs. *Prevention Science* 4(3):137-153.
Khosravi, A., C. Rao, M. Naghavi, R. Taylor, N. Jafari, and A. D. Lopez. 2008. Impact of misclassification on measures of cardiovascular disease mortality in the Islamic Republic of Iran: A cross-sectional study. *Bulletin of the World Health Organization* 86(9):688-696.
Kivimaki, M., M. J. Shipley, J. E. Ferrie, A. Singh-Manoux, G. D. Batty, T. Chandola, M. G. Marmot, and G. D. Smith. 2008. Best-practice interventions to reduce socioeconomic inequalities of coronary heart disease mortality in UK: A prospective occupational cohort study. *Lancet* 372(9650):1648-1654.
Knaul, F. M., H. Arreola-Ornelas, O. Mendez-Carniado, C. Bryson-Cahn, J. Barofsky, R. Maguire, M. Miranda, and S. Sesma. 2006. Evidence is good for your health system: Policy reform to remedy catastrophic and impoverishing health spending in Mexico. *Lancet* 368(9549):1828-1841.
Krishnan, A., B. Nongkynrih, S. K. Kapoor, and C. Pandav. 2009. A role for INDEPTH Asian sites in translating research to action for non-communicable disease prevention and control: A case study from Ballabgarh, India. *Global Health Action* 2.
Kruk, M. E., and L. P. Freedman. 2008. Assessing health system performance in developing countries: A review of the literature. *Health Policy* 85(3):263-276.
Lee, J. 2003. Global health improvement and WHO: Shaping the future. *Lancet* 362(9401): 2083-2088.
Linde, J. A., R. W. Jeffery, S. A. French, N. P. Pronk, and R. G. Boyle. 2005. Self-weighing in weight gain prevention and weight loss trials. *Annals of Behavioral Medicine* 30(3): 210-216.
Lopez, A. D., C. D. Mathers, M. Eszati, D. T. Jamison, and C. J. L. Murray. 2006. *Global burden of disease and risk factors.* Washington, DC: World Bank.
Madon, T., K. J. Hofman, L. Kupfer, and R. I. Glass. 2007. Public health. Implementation science. *Science* 318(5857):1728-1729.
Majumdar, S. R., and S. B. Soumerai. 2009. The unhealthy state of health policy research. *Health Affairs (Millwood).*
Mathers, C. D., D. Ma Fat, M. Inoue, C. Rao, and A. D. Lopez. 2005. Counting the dead and what they died from: An assessment of the global status of cause of death data. *Bulletin of the World Health Organization* 83:171-177c.
MEASURE DHS. 2010. *Demographic and health surveys: Measure DHS: Surveys and methodology.* http://www.who.int/healthmetrics/library/countries/HMN_8Board_4hi_khm.pdf (accessed March 9, 2010).

MEASURE Evaluation. 2007. *Sample vital registration with verbal autopsy: An overview.* Chapel Hill, NC: Carolina Population Center. http://www.cpc.unc.edu/measure/tools/monitoring-evaluation-systems/savvy (accessed March 8, 2010).

Mendis, S., D. Abegunde, S. Yusuf, S. Ebrahim, G. Shaper, H. Ghannem, and B. Shengelia. 2005. WHO study on prevention of recurrences of myocardial infarction and stroke (WHO-premise). *Bulletin of the World Health Organization* 83(11):820-828.

Millennium Development Goals Africa Steering Group. 2008. *Achieving the millennium development goals in Africa.* New York: United Nations.

Murray, C. J., and J. Frenk. 2000. A framework for assessing the performance of health systems. *Bulletin of the World Health Organization* 78(6):717-731.

Ng, N., H. Van Minh, S. Juvekar, A. Razzaque, T. Huu Bich, U. Kanungsukkasem, A. Ashraf, S. Masud Ahmed, and K. Soonthorntada. 2009. Using the INDEPTH HDSS to build capacity for chronic non-communicable disease risk factor surveillance in low and middle-income countries. *Global Health Action* 2.

Nsubuga, P., M. E. White, S. B. Thacker, M. A. Anderson, S. B. Blount, C. V. Broome, T. M. Chiller, V. Espitia, R. Imtiaz, D. Sosin, D. F. Stroup, R. V. Tauxe, M. Vijayaraghavan, and M. Trostle. 2006. Public health surveillance: A tool for targeting and monitoring intervention. In *Disease control priorities in developing countries.* 2nd ed. New York: Oxford University Press. Pp. 997-1018.

Oomman, N., M. Bernstein, and S. Rosenzweig. 2008. *Seizing the opportunity on AIDS and health systems.* Washington, DC: Center for Global Development.

OpenMRS. 2010. *OpenMRS.* http://openmrs.org/ (accessed February 1, 2010).

PAHO (Pan American Health Organization). 2007. *Basic country health profiles for the Americas: Summaries.* http://www.paho.org/English/DD/AIS/cp_index.htm (accessed October 20, 2009).

PAHO. 2008. *Pan American version of STEPS.* Washington, DC: Pan American Health Organization.

PAHO Health Analysis and Statistics Unit. 2007. *Regional core health data initiative: Indicators glossary.* Washington, DC: Pan American Health Organization.

Pangea Global AIDS Foundation. 2009. *Report from the Expert Consultation on Implementation Science Research: A requirement for effective HIV/AIDS prevention treatment and scale-up.* Cape Town, South Africa: Pangea Global AIDS Foundation.

Petersen, L. A., L. D. Woodard, T. Urech, C. Daw, and S. Sookanan. 2006. Does pay-for-performance improve the quality of health care? *Annals of Internal Medicine* 145(4):265-272.

Rommelmann, V., P. W. Setel, Y. Hemed, G. Angeles, H. Mponezya, D. Whiting, and T. Boerma. 2005. Cost and results of information systems for health and poverty indicators in the United Republic of Tanzania. *Bulletin of the World Health Organization* 83(8):569-577.

Shengelia, B., C. Murray, and O. Adams. 2003. Beyond access and utilization: Defining and measuring health system coverage. In *Health systems performance assessment: Debates, methods and empiricism.* Edited by C. Murray and D. Evans. Geneva: World Health Organization. Pp. 221-234.

Sikanyiti, P., and S. Nalishebo. 2009. Sample vital registration with verbal autopsy: Background, scope, and methodology. Presentation at the 2nd Global HIV/AIDS Surveillance Meeting, Bangkok, Thailand.

Spertus, J. A., M. J. Radford, N. R. Every, E. F. Ellerbeck, E. D. Peterson, and H. M. Krumholz. 2003. Challenges and opportunities in quantifying the quality of care for acute myocardial infarction: Summary from the Acute Myocardial Infarction Working Group of the American Heart Association/American College of Cardiology First Scientific Forum on Quality of Care and Outcomes Research in Cardiovascular Disease and Stroke. *Circulation* 107(12):1681-1691.

Stansfield, S. K. 2009. Cardiovascular disease in developing countries: Meeting the challenge. Presentation at the Public Information Gathering Session for the Institute of Medicine Committee on Preventing the Global Epidemic of Cardiovascular Disease, Washington, DC.

Stansfield, S. K., J. Walsh, N. Prata, and T. Evans. 2006. Information to improve decision making for health. In *Disease control priorities in developing countries*. 2nd ed. New York: Oxford University Press. Pp. 1017-1030.

Syed, S. B., A. A. Hyder, G. Bloom, S. Sundaram, A. Bhuiya, Z. Zhenzhong, B. Kanjilal, O. Oladepo, G. Pariyo, and D. H. Peters. 2008. Exploring evidence-policy linkages in health research plans: A case study from six countries. *Health Research Policy and Systems* 6:4.

Tegang, S., G. Emukule, S. Wambugu, I. Kabore, and P. Mwarogo. 2009. A comparison of paper-based questionnaires with PDA for behavioral surveys in Africa: Findings from a behavioral monitoring survey in Kenya. *Health Informatics in Developing Countries* 3(1):22-25.

Ten-year evaluation of the regional core health data initiative. 2004. *Epidemiological Bulletin* 25(3):1-7.

Tryhorn, C. 2009. Developing countries drive explosion in mobile phone use. *The Guardian*, March 2, 2009.

Tunstall-Pedoe, H., K. Kuulasmaa, H. Tolonen, M. Davidson, S. Mendis, and WHO MONICA Project. 2003. *MONICA monograph and multimedia sourcebook: World's largest study of heart disease, stroke, risk factors, and population trends 1979-2002*. Geneva: World Health Organization.

UNAIDS (United Nations Joint Programme on HIV/AIDS). 2009a. *New HIV indicator registry improves access to high-quality indicators*. http://www.unaids.org/en/KnowledgeCentre/Resources/FeatureStories/archive/2009/20090313_Propertyright_UNDP.asp (accessed February 2, 2010).

UNAIDS. 2009b. *UNAIDS: Indicator registry*. http://www.indicatorregistry.org (accessed February 2, 2010).

United Nations Foundation. 2010. *United Nations foundation: Mhealth alliance*. http://www.unfoundation.org/global-issues/technology/mhealth-alliance.html (accessed March 9, 2010).

University of Washington. 2010. *Institute for Health Metrics and Evaluation (IHME)*. http://www.healthmetricsandevaluation.org/ (accessed March 9, 2010).

van Kammen, J., D. de Savigny, and N. Sewankambo. 2006. Using knowledge brokering to promote evidence-based policy-making: The need for support structures. *Bulletin of the World Health Organization* 84(8):608-612.

VanWormer, J. J., A. M. Martinez, B. C. Martinson, A. L. Crain, G. A. Benson, D. L. Cosentino, and N. P. Pronk. 2009. Self-weighing promotes weight loss for obese adults. *American Journal of Preventive Medicine* 36(1):70-73.

Veasnakiry, L. 2007. *Cambodia briefing note*. Geneva: WHO Health Metrics Network, World Health Organization.

Warren, C. W., N. R. Jones, A. Peruga, J. Chauvin, J. P. Baptiste, V. Costa de Silva, F. el Awa, A. Tsouros, K. Rahman, B. Fishburn, D. W. Bettcher, and S. Asma. 2008. Global youth tobacco surveillance, 2000-2007. *MMWR Surveillance Summaries* 57(1):1-28.

WHO (World Health Organization). 2008. *2008-2013 action plan for the global strategy for the prevention and control of noncommunicable disease*s. Geneva: World Health Organization.

WHO. 2010a. *STEPS country reports*. http://www.who.int/chp/steps/reports/en/index.html (accessed October 8, 2009).

WHO. 2010b. *STEPS resources*. http://www.who.int/chp/steps/resources/en/index.html (accessed October 8, 2009).

WHO Health Metrics Network. 2007. *Assessment of the Ethiopian national health information system: Final report.* Geneva: World Health Organization.

WHO Health Metrics Network. 2008a. *Assessing the national health information system: An assessment tool.* Geneva: World Health Organization.

WHO Health Metrics Network. 2008b. *Framework and standards for country health information systems.* Geneva: World Health Organization.

WHO Health Metrics Network. 2010. *How can countries benefit from HMN?* http://www.who.int/healthmetrics/about/howcancountriesbenefitfromhmn/en/index.html (accessed March 9, 2010).

WHO Noncommunicable Diseases and Mental Health Cluster Surveillance Team. 2001. *STEPS instruments for NCD risk factors (core and expanded version 1.4): The WHO STEPwise approach to surveillance of noncommunicable diseases (STEPS).* Geneva: World Health Organization.

5

Reducing the Burden of Cardiovascular Disease: Intervention Approaches

The preceding chapters have described the many interrelated risk factors that influence cardiovascular health, which involve aspects of economies and societies that extend far beyond public health and health systems. This underscores the complexity of any undertaking to promote cardiovascular health and to prevent and manage cardiovascular disease (CVD). In addition to being complex, CVD is also a long-term problem. It cannot be addressed through a singular, time-limited commitment but rather requires long-term interventions and sustainable solutions.

This chapter first outlines the ideal vision of a comprehensive approach to promote cardiovascular health and reduce the burden of cardiovascular disease. The chapter then turns to a more pragmatic and focused discussion, starting first with a description of the committee's approach to the evidence. This is followed by a more thorough consideration of the rationale and evidence for components of the ideal approach, which include population-based approaches such as policies and communications campaigns; delivery of health care; and community-based programs. Recognizing the complexity of the disease and the local realities and practical constraints that exist in developing countries, the goal of this final section of the chapter is to identify, based on the totality of the available evidence, what is most advisable and feasible in the short term and what might hold promise as part of longer-term strategies.

IDEAL STRATEGY TO ADDRESS GLOBAL CVD IN THE DEVELOPING WORLD

The factors described in Chapters 2 and 3 that contribute to the burden of CVD and related chronic diseases are the targets for change in the quest to promote global cardiovascular health. These can be divided into behavioral factors (such as tobacco use, diet, and physical activity); biological factors (such as blood pressure, cholesterol, and blood glucose); psychosocial factors (such as depression, anxiety, acute and chronic life stressors, and lack of social support); health systems factors (such as access to care, screening, diagnosis, and quality of care); and intersectoral factors (such as tobacco control policies and agricultural policies). The evidence describing the interrelated determinants of CVD provides a strong conceptual basis for a strategy that coordinates across multiple sectors and integrates health promotion, prevention, and disease management as part of a long-term, comprehensive approach. This approach would employ multiple intervention strategies in a mix of programs and policies that accomodate variations in need according to context and locale.

The ideal approach would take advantage of opportunities for intervention at all stages of the life course in order to promote cardiovascular health by preventing acquisition and augmentation of risk, detecting and reducing risk, managing CVD events, and preventing the progression of disease and recurrence of CVD events. Policies and programs to change the factors that contribute to CVD would be designed to work through population-wide approaches; through interventions within health systems; and through community-based programs with components in schools, worksites, and other community settings. A comprehensive strategy of this kind that takes into account the full range of complex determinants of CVD, illustrated in Figure 5.1, would have the theoretical potential to produce a synergistic interaction among approaches at individual and population levels. Concurrent modalities could include policy and regulatory changes, health promotion campaigns, innovative applications of communications technologies, efficient use of medical therapies and technologies, and integrated clinical programs. For individuals already at high risk or with existing disease, this approach would combine education, support, and incentives to both address behavioral risk factors and improve adherence to clinical interventions. Participation in this approach extends beyond clinical providers and public health approaches to also include public media outlets, community leaders, and related sectors, especially food and agriculture policy, transportation and urban planning, and private-sector entities such as the food and pharmaceutical industries. All these players are potential partners both in assessing needs and capacity and in developing and implementing solutions.

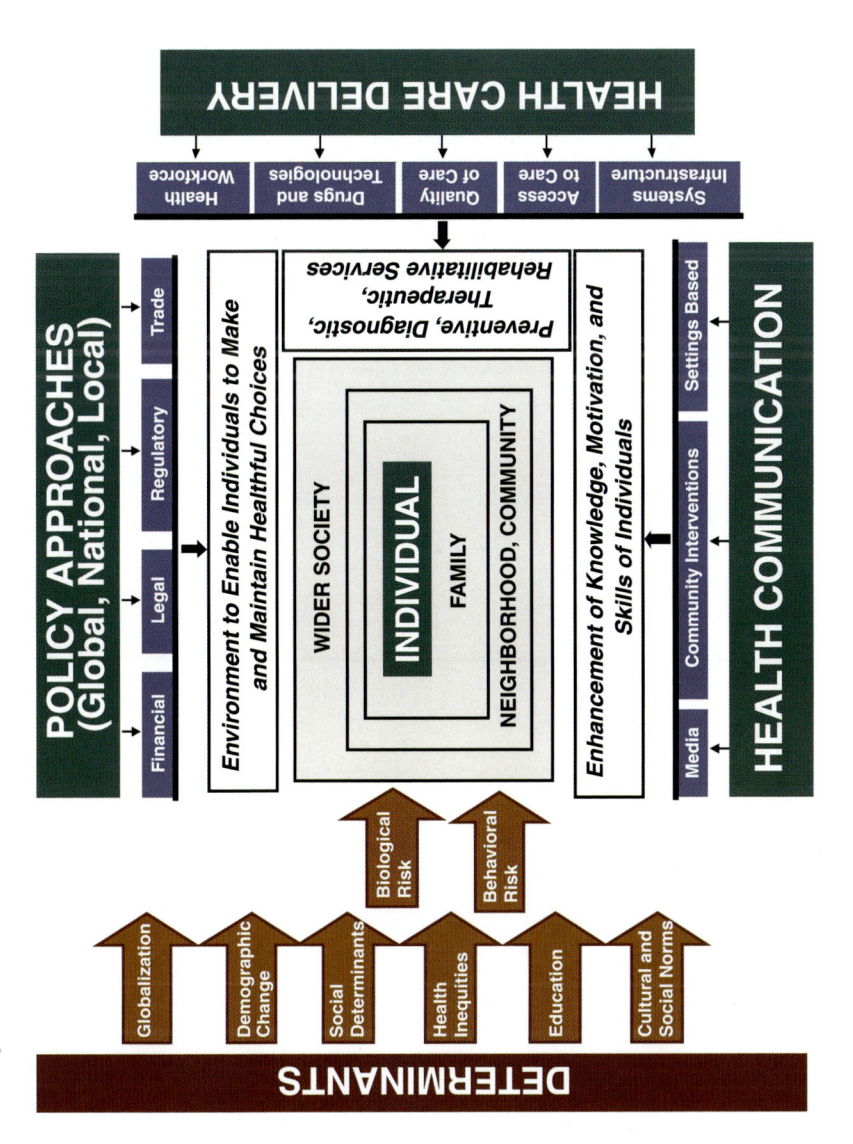

FIGURE 5.1 Comprehensive strategy to address cardiovascular disease.

Such a comprehensive approach stands as an ideal for countries facing the burden of CVD and for global stakeholders in the fight against CVD and related chronic diseases. Reality, of course, complicates this ideal considerably. A comprehensive integrated approach of this kind has not been successfully implemented in a model that can be readily replicated in low and middle income country settings. Progress in high income countries points to models for many of the components that could make up such an ideal approach to CVD, but interventions that may be efficacious in certain settings cannot be assumed to be effective if they are implemented in settings that have significantly different available resources and differ significantly at the level of policy or population characteristics. Most of the intervention components described as part of the ideal approach do not have sufficient evidence to support scale-up for widespread implementation in low and middle income countries in the immediate term. Even with sufficient evidence to support implementation, many low and middle income country governments might not have adequate resources in place to undertake ambitious, comprehensive, full-scale approaches.

Nevertheless, although the components are likely to work best in synergy with each other, the lack of readiness and capacity to accomplish the comprehensive ideal is not reason to do nothing. An impact on the very high burden of CVD is possible even without doing everything that makes up the ideal. Indeed, developing countries will want to focus more pragmatically on efforts that promise to be economically feasible, have the highest likelihood of intervention success, and have the largest morbidity impact. The goal of this chapter is to provide an analysis to help determine (1) what policies, programs, and clinical interventions have sufficient evidence for priority implementation in developing countries in the near term and (2) what approaches have a solid conceptual basis but require greater knowledge based on specific policies and programs with demonstrated effectiveness and implementability in developing-country settings in order to make progress toward implementation in the medium and long term. Chapter 7 will continue the discussion of feasibility and prioritizing the use of limited resources in low and middle income countries with a synthesis of the available economic evidence and future economic research needs for the intervention approaches described in this chapter.

Building a Strategy to Address CVD

The following briefly outlines the series of components needed for countries and supporting global stakeholders to build a strategy to promote cardiovascular health. As described above, these components would ideally be integrated to work toward a comprehensive intervention strategy. The intent is to develop a supportive policy environment and build the capacity to develop, implement, and evaluate intervention programs, with the ultimate goal of reducing the burden of CVD through reduction of risk factors and management of disease. This includes "top-down" policies and complementary "bottom-up" approaches in health care delivery systems and in community-based education and health promotion programs. The specific components within each of these steps and examples of the available evidence to support their implementation are described later in the chapter, along with more discussion of the limitations, taking into account gaps in the evidence and variations among countries in baseline capacity, economic status, and level of infrastructure.

Needs and Capacity Assessment

A crucial basis for developing policies and programs is for governments and communities to estimate and, where possible, measure the nature of the problem as it occurs in the local context where approaches will be implemented; to assess the needs of the population; to catalog current efforts; to assess the available capacity and infrastructure to address CVD and related chronic diseases; and to gauge the political will to support the available opportunities for action. This assessment will inform priorities and determine choices about the implementation of evidence-based policies and programs as well as capacity-building efforts. This should lead to specific and realistic goals for intervention strategies that are adapted to local baseline capacity and burden of disease and that also aim to improve that baseline capacity. This critical underlying step was discussed in full in Chapter 4.

Country-level measurement, assessment, and prioritization of this kind can occur at the level of national or local governments, such as provincial or city-level health authorities. In many low and middle income countries, this will require the development of sufficient capacity and infrastructure to carry out population-based approaches for measuring cause-specific mortality and behavioral and biological risk factors. In countries with very limited capacity at baseline, at first it may be nongovernmental organizations, foreign assistance agencies, and other donors who need to carry out a needs assessment and prioritization before implementing programmatic efforts. Regardless of the driving force behind the initiated action, this strategic planning can, to the extent possible, involve local authorities, be harmonized with local efforts, and be designed as an opportunity to improve local baseline capacity over time.

Policy Strategies

When a baseline is established and priorities are determined based on country-level data, the starting place for developing intervention approaches is policy strategies for population-based prevention. The primary population approach can be based on setting or changing policies, incentives, and regulations, especially those related to food, agriculture, and tobacco. There is evidence to support the implementation of some of these policies in the immediate term. For those developing countries where there exist democratic means to develop policies, where regulatory and enforcement capacity is sufficient, these policy changes may include, for example, taxation and regulations on tobacco production and sales; regulations on tobacco and food marketing and labeling; alterations in subsidies for foods and other food and agricultural policies; and strategies to make rapid urbanization more conducive to health. Regulatory change usually needs to be incremental and should be proportional to the possible impact and cost.

Health Communications

Both in coordination with policy changes and as a separate strategy for affecting crucial CVD-related behaviors, there is substantial promise in implementing health communications and education efforts. Public communication interventions that are coordinated with select policy changes can enhance the effectiveness of both approaches, which together can help create an environment in which more targeted programs in health systems and communities can succeed. Even in the absence of an ideal policy environment, well-constructed stand-alone population-level health communication efforts have the potential to be effective in encouraging population behavior change, for example, in areas such as smoking initiation and salt and fat consumption. Depending on the governmental infrastructure within a country, policies with coordinated communication and health education efforts can occur at the level of national or local authorities.

Delivery of Quality Health Care

Along with select population-based approaches, a key step in addressing CVD is to strengthen health systems to deliver high-quality, responsive care for the prevention and management of CVD. Improving health care delivery includes, for example, provider-level strategies, financing, integration of care, workforce development, and access to essential medical products. The need to strengthen health systems in low and middle income countries is not specific to CVD, and it is important that ongoing efforts in this area take into account not only traditional focus areas such as infectious disease and maternal and child health but also CVD and related chronic diseases as well as chronic care needs that are shared among chronic non-infectious diseases and chronic infections such as HIV/AIDS and tuberculosis (TB).

Community-Based Programs

Along with efforts to implement population-based approaches and to strengthen health systems, an ideal comprehensive integrated approach would also include community-based programs that offer opportunities to access individuals where they already gather, such as schools, worksites, and other community organizations. Depending on local priorities, there is potential for synergism in both effectiveness and economic feasibility through coordinated interventions that target multiple risk factors, are conducted in multiple settings in communities, and coordinate the health systems and population-based strategies described above with related, community-specific strategies. Because of the lack of community-based models that have been successfully implemented, evaluated, and sustained in low and middle income country settings, the critical next step in these settings is to support research to develop and evaluate demonstration projects through implementation trials. In many cases, the focus can be on adapting and evaluating programs with demonstrated success in developed countries. The design of demonstration programs will need to take into account local infrastructure and capacity to develop and maintain such programs over time, particularly if they are ultimately intended to affect a large portion of the population and operate on a large scale.

Scale-Up and Dissemination

The ultimate goal when intervention approaches in all these domains are demonstrated to be effective and feasible is scale-up, maintenance, and dissemination. In addition to implementing best practices and evidence-based policies and programs on a larger scale, this includes disseminating in a broader global context, by sharing knowledge among similar countries with analogous epidemiological characteristics, capacity, and cultural norms and expectations.

Ongoing Monitoring, Evaluation, and Assessment

As described in Chapter 4, ongoing surveillance and evaluation of implemented strategies will allow policy makers and other stakeholders to determine if implemented actions are having the intended effect and meeting the defined goals, and to reassess needs, capacity, and priorities over time. This will be critical to alter policies and programs as priorities change, as new lessons are learned, and as a country goes through inevitable transitions in its economy and its health or social environments.

Global Support

As described in more detail in Chapter 8, international agencies can play an important role in working toward comprehensive country-level approaches. These agencies can help initiate and enrich any country's CVD prevention and management process through direct financial and technical assistance. In addition, external aid and coordination can facilitate the transfer of lessons learned among countries, allowing each country to actively contribute to the international repertoire of prevention strategies.

APPROACH TO THE EVIDENCE

This chapter is concerned with what works. The challenge is to define what qualifies as an intervention that works, to martial these findings together to establish a coherent evidence base, and then to use this as the basis to necessarily prioritize approaches. This section of the chapter briefly discusses the committee's approach to considering evidence for evaluating intervention approaches for CVD at all levels. This includes how the methodology for evaluating large-scale programs and population-based and policy interventions differs from clinical interventions and small-scale projects as well as a special emphasis on the importance of effectiveness and implementation evidence in relevant contexts.

The attempt to define a broad-based set of effective approaches available for CVD promotion and prevention rests on data standards—notably data standards that continue to evolve. The aspirational standard is evidence that describes causal linkages between intervention and better health status (i.e., outcomes). These data should meet the additional standards of contextual generalizability so that the reported findings are feasible based on implementation evidence and economic evaluation and adaptable in a variety of settings.

The intent is that good epidemiologic observational data on the role of risk factors and the preventive effects of reductions in those risk factors will lead to hypotheses about causal pathways that interventions are designed to influence. Ideally, these hypotheses will be confirmed by prospective interventional studies that are repeated and reaffirmed in a variety of settings. Evidence from randomized trials can be highly valuable to infer causality. As a rigid evidence standard, however, this is not always available, feasible, necessary, or even optimal. For many intervention approaches, the best available evidence can also come from, for example, cohort evaluations and qualitative assessments as well as other research methodologies that support plausible causal linkages. For policy and public health approaches in particular, traditionally defined rigorous evaluation standards are often unrealistic, and it is instead a comprehensive perspective on the totality of the available evidence that is weighed alongside other policy pressures to drive implementation decisions. Therefore, the committee did not apply randomization as a standard of evidence for consideration of the illustrative examples included in this chapter. However, the committee did restrict its review of the evidence to published studies that included some comparison condition, either through a control group or a comparison to before and after an intervention was implemented.

The second standard for evidence set out by the committee is one of relevancy, an issue of particular importance here, although it is by no means exclusive to low and middle income countries. Conceptually, the ideal is not narrowly defined evaluations focused on internal validity but instead evaluations that look beyond efficacy—the estimation of what is possible—to effectiveness—the determination of what actually was accomplished by an intervention in a real-world setting. This refers to what is often a tension between confident findings of causal influence and confident findings of the relevance of evidence. Studies imposing enough controls on the context to support strong causal statements often in the process have to create a context that is distant from the messy environment and constraints in which programs at scale will be implemented, particularly in low and middle income countries. This review of evidence by the committee respects that tension, and then puts substantial emphasis on relevance.

Beyond effectiveness and relevance, the ultimate ideal standard to inform large investments in programs and intervention approaches is evidence from implementation research, operations research, and health services research. In addition, evidence on economic feasibility is a critical factor in determining implementation readiness and prioritizing intervention approaches. The available evidence from economic evaluations of intervention approaches is the subject of Chapter 7.

Applying the standards described here to the available evidence for CVD in developing countries revealed significant gaps in the evidence base, especially given the desire to have a concrete basis for advocating policy change, system change, or program implementation. The committee, however, does not intend that the message about higher data mandates with a responsible exposure of these data gaps be equated with a suggestion of inaction. A principle throughout the report is one of being action-oriented based on available findings. The committee's review of the available evidence according to these standards informed an analysis of which potential components of the ideal comprehensive approach warrant priority for implementation or, if near-term implementation is not supported, which components warrant other intermediate steps to develop the evidence base in support of implementation in the longer-term.

Given the broad and global scope of this study, a comprehensive systematic review of all available evidence related to every aspect of CVD and related chronic diseases was not within the scope of this project. Nor was it feasible for this report to catalog every intervention approach that has been attempted and documented across all countries. Instead, to present the rationale put forth by the committee, the following sections include illustrative examples that represent the best available evidence to support the committee's findings on the implementation potential for component strategies. In order to limit the length of this document and to avoid replication of existing work, the committee sought existing relevant, high-quality, systematic and narrative reviews. In content areas where these were available, this chapter includes summaries of key findings, but otherwise refers the reader to the available resources for more detailed information.

The focus is on intervention approaches for CVD with evidence for effectiveness and implementation in developing countries. Where this evidence is limited, generalizable examples are offered with evidence for effectiveness and implementation from both CVD-specific approaches in developed countries and developing-country evidence for non-CVD health outcomes. An assessment of the transferability of the evidence for these approaches is included. For components where there is limited or no effectiveness or implementation data, the logical basis for intervention approaches is discussed as being derived from knowledge about the determinants of CVD, modifiable risk factors, and characteristics of ideal intervention design and implementation.

Conclusion 5.1: *Context matters for the planning and implementation of approaches to prevent and manage CVD, and it also influences the effectiveness of these approaches. While there are common needs and priorities across various settings, each site has its own specific needs that require evaluation. Additional knowledge needs to be generated not only about effective interventions but also about how to implement these interventions in settings where resources of all types are scarce; where priorities remain fixed on other health and development agendas; and where there might be cultural and other variations that affect the effectiveness of intervention approaches. Translational and implementation research will be particularly critical to develop and evaluate interventions in the settings in which they are intended to be implemented.*

COMPONENTS OF A STRATEGY TO REDUCE THE BURDEN OF CVD

This section presents in more detail the rationale for the ideal approach described previously and the evidence for the main components, which include population-based approaches such as policies and health communications campaigns; delivery of health care; and community-based programs. Recognizing the complexity of the disease and the local realities and practical constraints that exist in developing countries, the goal of this final section of the chapter is to identify, based on the totality of the available evidence, policies, programs, and strategies to improve clinical care that have sufficient evidence for advisable and feasible implementation in developing countries in the near term as well as approaches that have a solid conceptual basis but need more evidence for specific policies and programs with demonstrated effectiveness and implementability in developing country settings to progress toward implementation in the medium and long term.

Intersectoral Policy Approaches[1]

Chapter 2 described the complexity of the determinants of CVD, which are drawn from a range of broad social and environmental influences. As a result, many of the crucial actions that are needed to support the reduction of CVD burden are not under the direct control of health ministries, but rather include other governmental agencies as well as private-sector entities. For example, they rely on tax rates on tobacco set by economic agencies, food subsidy policies set at agricultural agencies, access rules for public service advertising set by communication agencies, curricular choices by education agencies, and commitments to product reformulation by multinational corporations. Thus, success in achieving the specific priority goals for CVD programs will rely heavily on decisions made outside of health agencies, and that success will only come if there is substantial intersectoral collaboration.

The specifics of how that collaboration will come about will vary with the particular political arrangements in a country, but there will be a common theme: success will depend on building a shared commitment across sectors in the whole of government. This will require engaging not only those already motivated by health-related goals but also those who have very different pressures and considerations driving their decision making. Therefore, it is important to acknowledge the different forces that drive policy decisions in different sectors in order to seek out shared objectives, including economic objectives. To this end, there will be a need not only to make a case that the population as a whole will benefit from addressing CVD, but also to make the specific case that work to target CVD-related behaviors and outcomes will be in the interest of each collaborating agency or stakeholder in the private sector. For example, it may not be enough to

---

[1] This section is based in part on a paper written for the committee by Marie-Claude Jean and Louise St-Pierre.

talk up health benefits to encourage increased taxation on tobacco; evidence bearing on the likely gains and losses in revenues associated with such increased taxation and reduced tobacco consumption may have higher priority. To this end, a pragmatic approach will require a realistic assessment of what the fundamental requirements are for CVD-related needs, and what aspects of a proposed policy might be negotiable.

Intersectoral policy approaches for CVD will not be simple to implement, and a central part of intervention will be to form a strategy to stimulate such actions. In addition, just as with all interventions, policies need to be context specific and culturally relevant, and need to take into account infrastructure capacity and economic realities. A review commissioned for this committee identified the key success factors for implementing intersectoral approaches (Jean and St-Pierre, 2009). These include elements related to context, including political will and support; a favorable legislative, economic and organizational environment; and community support. There also needs to be a well-defined problem targeting an issue that is widely significant with a clear rationale for intersectoral action. Planning is also an important aspect of intersectoral approaches and requires credible organizers, as well as carefully chosen partners with a shared vision, clearly defined roles and responsibilities, and sufficient authority. It is also crucial to have evaluation based on concrete and measurable objectives. The final key success factor is a system for adequate communication, flexible and adaptable decision making, and conflict resolution.

The following sections present a more detailed discussion of the policy levers that have the most potential to affect the future course of CVD within an intersectoral approach by addressing specific goals, including tobacco control, reduced consumption of salt and unhealthful food, and increased physical activity. The rationale for these policy approaches are described, along with precedent for implementation. The focus is on examples from low and middle income countries when possible. Evaluations of policy interventions are not common, especially in low and middle income country settings, but where an evaluation has generated evidence on policy this is presented as well.

Tobacco Control Policies

Tobacco control, including efforts to reduce both tobacco use and exposure to secondhand smoke, is one of the most well-developed areas of CVD-related policy. Strategies for tobacco control in high income countries have been reviewed extensively elsewhere and will not be repeated here (Breslow and Johnson, 1993; Frieden and Bloomberg, 2007; IOM, 2010; Jha et al., 2006). This precedent in high income countries provides a strong rationale for policy measures of this type in low and middle countries with adequate regulatory and enforcement capacity.

Indeed, strategies for tobacco control worldwide were laid out exhaustively as part of the World Health Organization (WHO) Framework Convention on Tobacco Control (FCTC) (WHO, 2008b). The FCTC emphasizes the importance of both demand reduction and supply control strategies, including taxation measures on tobacco products, protection from exposure to tobacco smoke, packaging and labeling of tobacco products to include health warnings and to ban misleading terms like "light" and "mild," education and public awareness campaigns, controls on tobacco advertising, tobacco cessation services, control of illicit trade in tobacco products, control of sales to minors, and provision of support for economically viable alternative economic activities. WHO has also presented a policy package for tobacco control to support implementation of the FCTC (WHO, 2008b). Known as the MPOWER package, the focus is on six key policy areas: monitor tobacco use, protect people from tobacco smoke, offer help to quit tobacco use, warn about the dangers of tobacco, enforce bans on tobacco advertising and promotion, and raise taxes on tobacco products.

However, although many low and middle income countries have signed the FCTC treaty, implementation has been achieved in only a limited number (Bump et al., 2009). Indeed, there are only a few well-documented examples of implementation of tobacco control policies in low and middle income countries to serve as models, including Bangladesh, Brazil, Poland, Thailand, and South Africa (de Beyer and Brigden, 2003). Therefore, evaluation strategies are needed to examine the effects of tobacco control policies in low and middle income settings, and there is a need for more knowledge and analysis of the barriers to successful implementation and how to overcome them (Bump et al., 2009).

In Bangladesh, systematic and concerted efforts by nongovernmental organizations (NGOs) provide a model of very low-budget advocacy (Efroymson and Ahmed, 2003). Similarly, in Thailand tobacco control policy has been significantly influenced by NGOs in the health sector with direct access to government officials (Vateesatokit, 2003). In Brazil, by contrast, persistent action led from within the government resulted in strong legislation and a nationwide, decentralized program, with training and support cascading down the levels of government (da Costa and Goldfarb, 2003). In South Africa, political and social change created new environments and policy windows that public health advocates were able to turn to their advantage. Comprehensive legislation was enacted in two steps, with a second law strengthening the first. Legislative efforts began with policies to inform consumers and to restrict smoking and advertising. Later, tax increases were put in place and helped reduce consumption. The availability of strong local evidence, especially on the economic implications of tax increases, was very important in this case (Malan and Leaver, 2003).

Food and Agriculture Policies

Policies related to dietary changes can be thought of in terms of an integrated food system that goes from "farm to fork." This system includes food production, food processing, supply chain including food delivery and food availability, food marketing, and food choices both at point of purchase and in individual dietary choices. This system can be influenced by a variety of policies and initiatives in the agriculture sector, the public health sector, and the private sector. By facilitating greater consumption of specific foods, which often replace more healthful traditional foods, changes in agricultural production and policy can be linked with the "nutrition transition," much of which contributes to rising levels of CVD (Hawkes, 2006). Therefore, it is reasonable to conclude that there is potential for cardiovascular health to be promoted by finding economically feasible ways to globalize agricultural and food policies that promote more healthful food production and make more healthful foods affordable to developing country populations, including the poor.

In the past 25 years, agricultural production has increased for all major food groups around the world; however, the rate of increase has been markedly steeper for some foods associated with CVD and other diet-related chronic diseases. One example is Latin America—a major producer of vegetable oils, meat, fish, sugar, and fruit. As part of globalization, agricultural policy in the region shifted in the early 1990s from production to market-led policies. The food-consuming industries (distributors, manufacturers, processors, and retailers) played a key role in this shift. Case studies from Brazil, Colombia, and Chile show that these changes in agricultural policy are linked to changing consumption patterns. In Brazil the government instituted a series of market-led reforms in the early 1990s, which opened up the soybean oil market and encouraged production and enabled greater consumption in export markets (Hawkes, 2006). After investments in technology and infrastructure and trade liberalization during the 1980s in Colombia, the government implemented a market liberalization program, called "Apertura," which eased imports on feed ingredients and reduced import duties in the early 1990s (Hawkes, 2006). In line with the market-led paradigm, the government in Chile deregulated agricultural policy, privatized land ownership, cut labor costs by dismantling organized activity, provided more favorable conditions for foreign investment, and liberalized trade. These actions increased foreign investment in the fruit industry and were strengthened in the mid-1980s, with the provision of tax incentives to boost exports, increased investment in export-oriented agriculture, and more provisions to further increase foreign investment (Hawkes, 2006).

Agriculture is also a heavily traded sector, and trade policies affect what food is available within a country and its trading partners. The United States and Europe are major food exporters, and the composition of food available in their developing-country trading partners shows the influence of agricultural subsidies for animal-based products and coarse grains that provide animal feed. A recent study illustrates this by examining the increase in agricultural trade between the United States and Central America, following a new trade pact in 2004. The analysis suggests that "food availability change associated with trade liberalization, in conjunction with social and demographic changes, has helped to facilitate dietary change in Central American countries towards increased consumption of meat, dairy products, processed foods and temperate (imported) fruits. Such dietary patterns have been associated with the nutrition transition and the growing burden of obesity and non-communicable disease reported in the region" (Thow and Hawkes, 2009). The World Trade Organization (WTO) has recognized health consequences as a legitimate concern for trade policy in relation to access to essential drugs. This suggests that countries should have deliberate policies in relation to the health implications of their international trade. However, the WTO has to date not allowed countries to impose trade barriers against unhealthy foods (Clarke and McKenzie, 2007; Evans et al., 2001).

It is also important to note that agricultural trade will not necessarily worsen diets in developing countries. Diets can also be improved by trade through greater dietary diversification, greater food availability, lower consumer prices, and increases in domestic food production spurred by export demand.

In addition to the effects of agricultural production and trade, specific agriculture and food policies can also be linked to changes in food consumption related to CVD risks. For instance, as part of a broader set of chronic disease prevention approaches in Mauritius, the government implemented policies to change the composition of cooking oil made available to the population by limiting the content of palm oil. After 5 years, there were significant decreases in mean population cholesterol levels (Dowse et al., 1995; Uusitalo et al., 1996). Although this was a promising effect, it is important to note the mixed effects of the broader integrated intervention approach, which is described in more detail later in this chapter. In fact, obesity rose during the same time period and there were no other effects on CVD risk factors, indicating that the overall intervention approach was not sufficient to overcome secular trends (Hodge et al., 1996). Therefore, the Mauritius experience serves as an example of how a middle income country can mobilize governmental policies to achieve future health improvement, but it cannot be used to define the specific tactics that are needed to achieve success, especially without comparison communities (or regions) to control for secular changes. In addition, the specific circumstances of policy implementation and enforcement in a small island nation like Mauritius may not be widely generalizable.

In Poland, changes in economic policy led to reductions in subsidies for animal fat products, and consumption patterns changed, characterized by decreasing amounts of saturated fat and increasing amounts of polyunsaturated fat intake. This was associated with rapid declines in coronary heart disease (CHD) mortality during the same time period (Zatonski and Willett, 2005; Zatonski et al., 1998). However, this is evidence from an unplanned natural experiment using retrospective data, which offers limited lessons on strategic approaches that could be duplicated in other settings. Indeed, in Hungary, Romania, and Bulgaria (neighboring countries with similar political and economic changes) there was little apparent decline in ischemic heart disease mortality.

There is also a history in developing countries of price-based policies to influence nutrition outcomes for their populations—primarily basic food subsidies to reduce undernutrition (Pinstrup-Andersen, 1998). Health goals beyond alleviating undernutrition have not always been a consideration in establishing those policies. Analyses of oil price policies in China (Ng et al., 2008) and staple commodity subsidies in Egypt (Asfaw, 2006) suggest that price policies can influence food choices, in these examples with a negative effect on CVD risk. The consumption of edible oils in China has increased substantially with recent drops in edible oil prices stemming from changes in trade patterns (with especially strong effects on the poor) (Ng et al., 2008). In Egypt, the government subsidizes energy-dense foods, and female body mass index (BMI) appears to be influenced by the availability of those subsidized foods, even as the cost of a high-quality diet is out of reach for many in the population (Asfaw, 2006). This analysis does not establish a causal relationship, but it does suggest that government food price policies are influential and that this potential for price policies to adjust consumer demand for specific food ingredients could be considered as a means to promote consumption of healthier foods. The theoretical argument in support of subsidizing healthy foods responds to the problem of food pricing in which healthier foods (fresh fruits and vegetables) are relatively expensive, and energy-dense foods (sugared and heavily processed) are relatively cheap (Drewnowski, 2004). Preliminary research suggests that a "thin subsidy" to lower the price of healthy foods in the United States would be a cost-effective intervention for CHD and stroke (Cash et al., 2005).

The evidence is not yet available as to the effectiveness of the reverse policy—taxing unhealthy food products. Because tobacco taxation has been a very effective and cost-effective policy tool for reducing CVD risk in a broad range of countries, taxation of other products has been discussed (Brownell and Frieden, 2009) and even tried out on a limited basis in high-income countries. However, there is insufficient evidence on the effectiveness and health impact of this approach (Thow et al., 2010). In addition, for either of these potential price-based policy approaches it should be noted that changing the price of any one category of food or beverage may have impacts on consumption of other categories, which could be for the better or worse of heart health.

There is precedent for strategies to reduce salt in the food supply and in consumption that have been reviewed and documented extensively elsewhere (He and MacGregor, 2009). Salt-reduction strategies in high income countries include public health campaigns to increase consumer awareness of healthy salt intake and to encourage decreased consumption, product labeling legislation, and salt reduction by the food industry (He and MacGregor, 2009). These strategies have the potential to be adapted both to low and middle income country efforts as well as to be scaled up for broader, coordinated global efforts (He and MacGregor, 2009). However, evidence on salt-reduction strategies comes mostly from high income countries, where the majority of salt (80 percent) comes from processed foods (He and MacGregor, 2009; James et al., 1987). Therefore, it is important to note that in many low and middle income countries, even with increasing consumption of processed foods, most of the salt consumed is either added during cooking or in sauces (WHO Forum on Reducing Salt Intake in Populations, 2006). As a result, enhancements to prior policy strategies may be needed when adapting to this context, such as a public health campaign or other efforts to encourage consumers to use less salt. Similarly, precedent for reductions in transfat through policy initiatives, such as the experience in New York City (Angell et al., 2009), offers promise for potential adaptation to a wide range of settings. However, to adapt policy strategies related to the food supply, consideration must be given to the much greater representation of unregulated, informal food sales in most developing countries.

Environmental Policies

There are environmental consequences associated with some of the major CVD drivers that offer an opportunity for shared objectives with the environmental policy sector. Urbanization and increasing air pollution as well as changing global dietary patterns and changing agricultural trends, most notably the rapid increase in meat and palm oil consumption, have implications for CVD risk and also have a significant and often negative impact on the environment (Brown et al., 2005; Langrish et al., 2008; von Schirnding and Yach, 2002; Yach and Beaglehole, 2004).

Agriculture and food production in general is a resource-intensive endeavor, and significant portions of the global workforce, land area, water supply, and energy resources are dedicated to it (Schaffnit-Chatterjee, 2009). Meat and dairy production is particularly resource-intensive. Animal-sourced food requires significantly more energy, water, and land use to produce than do basic crops such as legumes, grain, fruits, and vegetables (Popkin, 2003; Steinfeld et al., 2006). Indeed, it is estimated that the livestock sector is responsible for more than 8 percent of global human water use and accounts for 70 percent of all agricultural land (30 percent of Earth's land surface) (Steinfeld et al., 2006).

Livestock production also erodes topsoil, causes land degradation, pollutes water, and threatens biodiversity. Livestock compact the soil and degrade the land, disrupting the water supply, contributing to erosion and necessitating expansion into new grazing lands. These are often created through deforestation, which destroys the habitat of other animals, threatening biodiversity. The livestock sector is also responsible for an estimated 18 percent of greenhouse gas emissions (a higher share than the transport sector)—a result of poor manure management and methane gas emissions from ruminant species such as cattle, sheep, and goats. Furthermore, manure, fertilizers used for growing feed crops, and waste materials from livestock processing are often dumped into waterways without proper treatment, polluting the water supply (Steinfeld et al., 2006).

The rapid rise in palm oil consumption in some low and middle income countries has also had a significant negative impact on the environment and has strained fragile natural ecosystems. In 2001, Malaysia and Indonesia produced 83 percent of the world's palm oil and were responsible for 89 percent of global palm oil exports. Hundreds of thousands of square miles of rainforest have been cut or burned down to accommodate the growing industry. Palm oil production has also indirectly contributed to further deforestation by displacing local farmers, leading them to expropriate additional rainforest as new land for their subsistence farming. These rainforests are the only habitats for a number of critically endangered species such as the orangutan, the Sumatran tiger, and the Sumatran rhinoceros. Some zoologists believe these species will be pushed into extinction if rainforest destruction continues at its current pace (Brown and Jacobson, 2005; Gooch, 2009).

In addition to contributing to deforestation, palm oil production also contributes to soil and water pollution. As with other crops, extensive use of fertilizers and pesticides on oil palm plantations has led to pollution in the soil and waterways. Additional pollution is caused by oil palm processing, which creates effluent that ends up in rivers and waterways. Indeed, in some Indonesian rivers, pollution from palm oil mill effluent is so severe that fish cannot survive. In the past 6 years, the industry has tried to set standards to ensure that palm oil production is sustainable; however, rainforests continue to be destroyed and effluent continues to be improperly dumped into waterways. While the production of some other oil crops leads to water pollution and rainforest destruction (for example, parts of the Brazilian Amazon are now being cut down to make way for soybean production), the exponential increase in palm oil use combined with the projected future rise in global demand make it a particularly glaring example of potential long-term harmful environmental effects (Brown and Jacobson, 2005; Gooch, 2009).

This opens a door for shared approaches between those trying to promote cardiovascular health and those trying to promote environmentally sustainable development. These shared approaches may include policies to limit overproduction of palm oil production and to encourage shifts in agricultural production from meat and dairy to more fruits and vegetables. Tobacco production, processing, and consumption have also been associated with negative environmental consequences (Bump et al., 2009). This provides an additional rationale for synergistic efforts to overcome the technical, political, and commercial barriers to implementing policy changes in the food and agriculture sectors that both promote health and protect the environment.

Urban Planning Policies and the Built Environment

A broad range of structural factors comprise the "built environment," and many of these factors contribute to health outcomes. They encompass factors such as chemical, physical, and biological agents, as well as physical and social environments, including housing, urban planning, transport, industry, and agriculture (Papas et al., 2007). Thus urbanization is another area for potential synergy between promoting environmentally sustainable development and promoting cardiovascular health.

As described in Chapter 3, trends show that the changes in the built environment due to urbanization are generally associated with several risk factors for CVD, including an increase in tobacco use, obesity, and some aspects of an unhealthful diet, as well as a decline in physical activity and increased exposure to air pollution (Brook, 2008; Gajalakshmi et al., 2003; Goyal and Yusuf, 2006; Langrish et al., 2008; Ng et al., 2009; Steyn et al., 2006; Yang et al., 2008; Yusuf et al., 2001).

Motivated by the growing prevalence of obesity in many developed nations and the potential public health impacts stemming from subsequent CVD and diabetes, studies conducted within the United States, Europe, Australia, and New Zealand over the past three decades have successfully demonstrated the correlation between different aspects of the built environment and physical activity levels (Humpel et al., 2002). These correlations provide a compelling rationale, and reports such as the U.S. Centers for Disease Control and Prevention's Community Guide and the Institute of Medicine's *Local Government Actions to Prevent Childhood Obesity* (2009) have produced guidance for different types of policy initiatives at several levels of jurisdiction, including changes to the built environment.

However, there is a lack of prospective studies investigating the effect of introducing changes to the built environment on individual and population health. These prospective data are much needed as the current cross-sectional analyses have limited ability to demonstrate causality. For example, it is difficult to ascertan if built environments that are more conducive to healthy lifestyles lead to increased physical activity, or whether individuals who are more physically active are more likely to live in a neighborhood that is more conducive to walking, bicycling, or playing sports. It is difficult to obtain prospective data, as there are a wide variety of exogenous variables to interfere with potential findings. In addition, these studies would require a significant financial investment, either on the part of the research funding institution or the local community (Sallis et al., 2009). There has also been little economic analysis of the potential costs associated with modifying an element of the built environment, which could be a barrier in developing countries.

In addition, it is important to note that the majority of data on the correlation of environments and increased physical activity comes from high income countries. With the exception of some work in Latin America described below, there is a lack of evidence from a range of developing country settings, and most guidance documents do not address generalizability or adaptation to low and middle income country settings. While there may be some commonalities between individuals from both urban and rural regions of the developed and developing world, differences in social norms, culture, existing built environment, and local variations in baseline daily activity levels are likely to have a substantial impact on the potential effectiveness of a change in the built environment in leading to behavior change.

On the other hand, low and middle income countries undergoing rapid development and urbanization provide promising opportunities to help fill the evidence gap through future prospective research given the multitude of neighborhoods and cities in the early stages of land use development. The need for investment of resources in this research may be lessened in settings where the intervention is not an alteration of an existing environment but rather an element of design planning where investment has already been committed to future urbanization projects. In fact, prospective studies in the context of planned urbanization in rapidly developing countries could also provide better evidence on the monetary investments required to achieve "successful" future urban design.

A few public health initiatives in middle income countries in Latin America, such as Muévete in Bogota and Agita São Paulo in Brazil, have altered the local built environment as a component of an overall program, but evaluations of their results are limited (Gamez et al., 2006; Matsudo, 2002). The Agita program in Brazil is one of the few programs with an evaluation that uses health outcomes. This was a multicomponent program that included changes in the environment through an increase in the number of walking areas, facilities for bicycling, and recreational facilities. Changes related to the practice of physical activity during the intervention period were observed. An annual survey showed that over 5 years there was a decrease from 14.9 percent to 11.2 percent in the population defined as inactive, a decrease from 30.3 percent to 27 percent in the population deemed irregularly active, and an increase from 54.8 percent to 61.8 percent in the population considered active or very active. Changes were also observed in targeted groups, such as groups of patients suffering from hypertension or diabetes and patients and workers in hospitals and health centers (Matsudo et al., 2006).

In summary, there is limited evidence of the effects on CVD-related outcomes of strategies and investments to alter the existing built environment, and urban planning policies are likely not a CVD priority in many low and middle income countries. However, for policy makers in countries undergoing rapid urbanization, there is a strong evidence-based rationale to take advantage of the opportunity going forward to implement and evaluate strategies to encourage cardiovascular health by making cities walkable, cyclable, safer, and free of air pollution. A more "heart-healthy" approach to growth and urbanization provides opportunities to avoid negative impacts, and possibly to even use the growing investment in new city development for health gains, including CVD prevention and health promotion.

Health Communication Programs

Health communication programs are typically designed to reach a large audience with messages as part of their established exposure to communication sources such as radio, television, billboards, newspapers and other printed material including mass mailings, and the Internet. Such exposure is often passive, relying on routinely accessed sources, rather than requiring the motivation of actively seeking a new communication source by an individual. Communication programs may affect behavior through three paths: (1) by directly educating and persuading individuals to change their behavior (e.g., by changing people's minds and providing skills needed to quit smoking); (2) by changing the expectations of peers in social networks, which in turn influence individual behavior (e.g., by changing friends' willingness to condemn smoking); and (3) by changing public opinion to influence public policy, which then influences individual behavior (e.g., by changing the political climate to permit regulation of secondhand smoke and thus reducing opportunities for individuals to smoke).

The effectiveness of policies and programs can be enhanced if linked to health communication programs targeted to the same objective—for example, to complement lobbying of policy authorities and food manufacturers to restrict salt content with public education about salt reduction. In addition, linking communication programs to policy approaches can make them more likely to gain presence in the public mind and thus gain public support. A communication program may also be designed to precede the policy change to nurture the public support needed for legislative action. Health communication strategies can also be an important complementary component of health systems and community-based approaches. Depending on the infrastructure within a country, communication and health education efforts can occur at multiple levels, from the national government to local authorities and community-based organizations.

The following section describes the evidence and considerations for designing and implementing communication campaigns at scale under the kinds of conditions that would be expected in real-world public health systems rather than research programs. An analysis of the current literature, described in more detail below, indicates that what might be most feasible for short-term implementation, and for coordination with policy approaches, is a focus on reasonably narrowly defined CVD-related targets, rather than trying to change all determinants of CVD at once. This focus can be most effective when using multiple intervention approaches to achieve the same ends, with large-scale communication programs as one important component.

CVD-Related Communication Campaigns in Low and Middle Income Countries

There is currently very limited evidence about the effects of communication interventions on CVD-related behaviors (or morbidity) in low and middle income countries, with few reported examples of communication programs with rigorous evaluations. The evidence is also challenging to interpret because large-scale communication programs tend to be components of multifaceted programs. Even when such multifaceted programs are evaluated, the effects of separate components are difficult to distinguish. In addition, in many reported evaluations no control condition is present, and as a result the effects of secular change can be difficult to discriminate from the effects of intervention efforts.

There are descriptive reports about some programs implemented in middle income countries that incorporate communication elements (Grabowsky et al., 1997). Some of these reports, described below, describe an evaluation and infer effects on CVD-related outcomes, but in some cases these effects are weakly supported, with little evidence of sustained impact.

The Coronary Risk Factor Study (CORIS), conducted in South Africa from 1979 to 1983, was a multilevel, multifactor intervention in which most of its effects were explained by use of a mass media campaign (Rossouw et al., 1993). There were three nonrandomized, matched towns: two treatment and one control. There was a mass media component plus community "events" in one town, and the same with the addition of a high-risk counseling program in a second treatment town. Before-and-after cross-sectional surveys measured knowledge of risk factors, smoking habits, and medical history as well as BMI, blood pressure, and cholesterol. Blood pressure, smoking, and composite risk were lowered compared to the control town, but there was no difference between the two treatment conditions. Thus, this was a replication of a successful use of a mass media strategy and was a test of these methods in a middle income country. However, the program focused only on middle income white South Africans, so the generalizability to other low and middle income countries may be limited. After the initial intervention was implemented, a maintenance program was established and surveyed at 4-year intervals. In a review of the project's 12-year results Steyn et al. (1997) concluded that while the CORIS community intervention was successful in the short term, in the longer term both the control group and one of the two intervention groups showed decreased risk factors. The authors speculate that this can be explained by strong secular trends and local factors. This highlights the challenge of maintaining long-term effects in these interventions.

The Healthy Dubec Project was a single-community, 2-year education campaign in the country that was then Czechoslovakia, with a before-and-after analysis that surveyed height, weight, blood pressure, and cholesterol, as well as sociodemographic variables and behavioral CVD risk factors (Komarek et al., 1995). The education campaign was delivered primarily through print media, including newspaper columns and brochures distributed at community sites and events and to residents' homes. Significant improvements were noted in blood pressure, cholesterol, and saturated fat intake. No effect was observed on smoking or BMI (Albright et al., 2000). This provides another example of some documented effects in a middle income country. Like many of the available examples of evaluated programs, this was a single-community model, which carries less evidentiary weight than studies with one or more control communities. Nonetheless, this study demonstrated the ability to achieve culturally appropriate adaptations of the print materials used in the Stanford Five City Project. This is an important lesson about the potential for transferability of materials tested in high income countries.

In Poland, the Polish Nationwide Physical Activity Campaign "Revitalize Your Heart" had the main goal of promoting an active lifestyle through education via mass media, including large broadcasting stations, public television, popular newspapers, magazines, and leading electronic media. This was accompanied by a country-wide contest and different local interventions (sports events, outdoor family picnics). Questionnaires administered to the participants of the contest and more than 1,000 people in the Polish population showed increased awareness of low physical activity as a problem. In addition, almost 60 percent of participants reported increased frequency and duration of exercise during the campaign (Ruszkowska-Majzel and Drygas, 2005).

Brazil's Agita intervention, described in the previous section, had two main objectives: to increase the population's awareness of how important physical activity is to health and to increase the level of physical activity within the population (Matsudo et al., 2003). To achieve these objectives, the program organized three main types of interventions: mega-events, specific activities with partner institutions, and partnerships with community organizations. The program succeeded in obtaining significant media coverage: 21 million people were reached by means of at least 30 newspapers distributed in the state's various cities, as well as at least 7 national newspapers and 4 broadcasts on national television (Matsudo et al., 2002). As described in the previous section, an annual survey carried out over 4 years showed increased self-reported levels of physical activity (Matsudo et al., 2006).

Potential Lessons from CVD-Related Communication Campaigns in High Income Countries

Although evidence is limited from CVD-related programs in low and middle income countries, there are evaluations of programs in high income countries that offer some lessons for designing and implementing programs in low and middle income countries. This includes those that focused on a single outcome (smoking, physical activity, high blood pressure control, cholesterol reduction, salt consumption) and those that addressed multiple CVD risk factors within a single program. Some of these programs (whether they address a single risk factor or multiple risk factors) make communication a central (or the central) component of the intervention. Others make use of communication as one component of a multicomponent intervention. Even from these high income country programs the evidence is mixed, but a few general conclusions can be drawn.

Tobacco Use There is substantial evidence in support of youth anti-tobacco communication programs, which is described in more detail in

Chapter 6 (Wakefield et al., 2003). There is also some evidence, particularly time-series evidence, supporting the influence of communication on adult smoking (National Cancer Institute, 2008). A detailed synthesis of evidence on the effectiveness of media strategies employed in tobacco control campaigns, including marketing and advertising and news and entertainment media, can be found elsewhere and is not repeated here (National Cancer Institute, 2008).

In addition to tobacco control campaigns, there is good reason to believe that important reductions in tobacco use in part reflect deliberate efforts by the antitobacco movement to shift public opinion to recognize the dangers of secondhand smoke, to publicize the deliberate efforts by the tobacco industry to deceive the public and addict children and young people, and to achieve recognition of the right to restrict the free exercise of individual smoking rights when they affect the health of others. These efforts often included deliberate efforts to shape media coverage of the tobacco issue, and to use that as a path to changing public policy (Shafey et al., 2009). While it is not possible to make definitive attributions of influence, it is reasonable to connect this form of media advocacy to behavior change and to view it as an important model for tobacco control in low and middle income countries as well as for possible extension to other areas of behavior relevant to CVD.

Tobacco also offers an example of how communication can be used in ways that run counter to the promotion of health. For instance, the tobacco industry has used the media to promote tobacco products (Sepe et al., 2002; Shafey et al., 2009; Tye et al., 1987) and has spent billions of dollars a year on marketing initiatives in the United States (Frieden and Bloomberg, 2007). Tobacco advertising has proliferated on the Internet, and pro-tobacco messages are widely available on social networking websites (WHO, 2008). However, the media can also be effectively used for counter advertising, as has been demonstrated in different regions (Emery et al., 2007; Fichtenberg and Glantz, 2000; Goldman and Glantz, 1998; Ma'ayeh, 2002; Pierce, 1994). Moreover, controls on tobacco advertising and marketing can be effective if they are comprehensive, include both direct and indirect advertising and promotion, and are combined with other antitobacco efforts (Frieden and Bloomberg, 2007; Pierce, 1994; Saffer and Chaloupka, 2000).

Other Risk Factors There is some evidence in high income countries of the success of communication efforts in reducing salt consumption (He and MacGregor, 2009) and improving awareness, treatment, and control of hypertension (Roccella and Horan, 1988). There is less evidence for communication efforts alone to influence physical activity outcomes, particularly sustained physical activity changes (Kahn et al., 2002; Taskforce on Community Preventive Services, 2002).

There is also some credible evidence for the effects of communication programs targeted to multiple CVD-related risk factors (Schooler et al., 1997). Six successful community-based, multilevel, multifactor CVD prevention projects in high income countries in the 1970s and 1980s had effects that can be attributed largely to their use of a mass media health communication approach, which is the aspect of these programs discussed here. These projects are also discussed later in this chapter in the section on community-based programs. They were done in the United States, Finland, Australia, Switzerland, and Italy and have been reviewed extensively elsewhere (Schooler et al., 1997).

The North Karelia project in Finland continued for many years and, after its successes on all CVD risk factors during the first 5 years, its methods were applied throughout Finland and culminated in major declines in CVD mortality (Puska et al., 1995). The Stanford Three Community Study showed evidence for effects on important risk factors of smoking, blood pressure, cholesterol, and body weight and a large decrease in total CVD risk (Farquhar et al., 1977; Williams et al., 1981). The Stanford follow-on study (the Five City Project) showed relatively large effects on smoking and blood pressure, with somewhat lesser effects on overall risk than in the previous Three Community Study, and no effect on body weight (Altman et al., 1987; Farquhar et al., 1990; Sallis et al., 1985). The Three Community Study was also the basis for the design of the CORIS project described earlier (Rossouw et al., 1993). Indeed, the North Karelia program and Three Community Study galvanized substantial further major trials and worldwide consideration of community-focused programs to address CVD burdens.

Across the major projects that followed, including CORIS in South Africa, there has been replication of reductions in smoking and blood pressure in all seven projects, cholesterol in three, and body weight in two (Schooler et al., 1997). These replications provide evidence that rather small cities and towns in high income settings appear to have responded well in their risk-factor change to educational programs based largely on mass media.

In contrast, two other large programs that began somewhat later, in the mid-1980s, the Minnesota Heart Health Project and the Pawtucket Heart Health Project in Rhode Island, did not show appreciable effects (Carleton et al., 1995; Luepker et al., 1996). A likely reason for the lack of effect in the latter two programs is their relative lack (Luepker et al., 1996; Mittelmark, 1986) or absence (Carleton et al., 1995) of mass media. Other subsequent studies in Europe also tended to have greater success when extensive broadcast and print media were used (Breckenkamp et al., 1995; Greiser, 1993; Schuit et al., 2006; Weinehall et al., 2001). These programs are also discussed again in the community interventions section below.

Another factor that may affect the success of health communication campaigns is secular trends that influence the novelty and potential effects of the campaign's messages. The earlier studies, done in the 1970s and early 1980s, reflect the possibilities for mass education at that time, when radio and newspapers were a more important news source than at present, and while the trends for risk-factor levels and CVD events were beginning to decline. It was also a time before major changes had occurred in smoking rates, before the messages became more commonplace in the settings where they were implemented, and before the relatively easy changes in diet had occurred for many in the target populations. These studies also preceded the expansion of many of the broad drivers of CVD risk. Therefore, these earlier projects may have faced fewer obstacles to change than might be faced earlier or later in the epidemiological transition cycles.

Potential Lessons from Other Health Communication Programs in Low and Middle Income Countries

Even when communication programs in high income countries have demonstrated success, these programs may be difficult to generalize to developing-country contexts. Because there are so few models of CVD-related communication programs in low and middle income countries, it is worth looking to programs with evidence of effectiveness in these settings that have been targeted to other health-related behaviors for possible models of design and implementation, especially those programs that target outcomes that similarly require sustained behavioral change.

There is a rapidly growing evidence base for communications in low and middle income countries related to a range of health issues. For example, there is credible evidence for communication program effects on child survival-related outcomes including immunization (a repeated behavior requiring parents to bring their children to a clinic or other site), use of rehydration solutions for diarrheal disease (a repeated behavior undertaken at home in response to disease symptoms), and breastfeeding (a behavior already often performed but the campaigns are meant to shape the behavior and extend it in time) (Hornik et al., 2002). In addition, there is support for the effects of communication programs on HIV risk-related behaviors, particularly condom use with "casual" partners, and on family planning behaviors, particularly increasing initial visits to providers of contraceptive services (Bertrand et al., 2006; Hornik and McAnany, 2001).

Principles to Guide Future Design and Implementation of Communication Programs

Health communication campaigns require careful planning, ideally involving professionals with adequate training in health communication. Some of the key principles for designing and implementing these programs are described briefly here; existing resources that have informed communication strategies in developing world settings can provide more thorough guidance for planning CVD-related interventions (see, for example, NCI, 2002; O'Sullivan et al., 2003; Piotrow et al., 2003; Smith, 1999).

Strong communication programs choose messages based on behavior change theory and reflect thorough knowledge of their target audience, in terms of both their structural context—how the old and new behaviors fit into their lives—and their cognitive response to the behavior. Often audiences are heterogeneous and message strategies have to be differentiated by audience segment; formative research to precede widespread launching of a campaign can be used to test prototypes of the campaign's messages with representative subsets of the intended target audience.

From the epidemiological perspective of preventing CVD, it is natural to look at the set of risk factors for CVD as interrelated and to consider how to construct a program that will influence all those factors. However, from the perspective of trying to prioritize and act synergistically with policy interventions to achieve change in risk factors or the behaviors associated with them, it may not be wise to try to address multiple CVD risk factors in one campaign. There may be greater potential to achieve behavior change by constructing independent programs that address each factor by itself (e.g., tobacco use, salt consumption, transfat consumption, saturated fat consumption, physical activity, and obesity). The institutional actors relevant to each of those risk factors are distinct, and the way one might construct communication campaigns for each can be sharply different. For example, there may be different focus audiences; different motivations for adopting new behaviors; and different types of behaviors with regard to timing, difficulty, and opportunity to act. The lack of commonalities among, for example, quitting smoking, maintaining physical activity, or purchasing foods low in saturated fats makes it very difficult to design one communication strategy that will maximally affect all relevant behaviors. However, hybrid campaigns may be preferred in some cases for greater efficiency when, for example, the trained health education staff is already in place.

A communication program can get exposure for the intended message through a number of means. For example, it can be required if the government controls media outlets. However, health authorities may not have access to the media even when it is government controlled. Exposure can also be purchased, although purchasing media time can be expensive especially because the audience needs to be reached repeatedly with the intended messages. If it is necessary to purchase media time, achieving high levels of exposure and maintaining exposure over time could become the most expensive element of communication programs. Low and middle income countries therefore have an economic incentive to seek strategies to ensure the availability of low-cost educational media programming. Another strategy for program exposure is to make news and attract coverage from media outlets (e.g., National Power of Exercise Day in Thailand celebrity endorsement and involvement). However, media coverage may not be reliable and can be biased depending on factors such as whether media outlets are private entities or government agencies, and whether or not they operate within a system that guarantees freedom of the press.

New communications technologies may also provide opportunities to reach people with health-promoting messages and research suggests that channels such as computer programs, websites, and videogames may reach audiences missed by traditional health communication (Barrera et al., 2009; Boberg et al., 1995; Hawkins et al., 1987; Levy and Strombeck, 2002; Walters et al., 2006). However, although programs are emerging that depend on interactive communication technology, there is insufficient evidence at this time to determine if these approaches will be effective in low and middle income countries. One potential disadvantage to these kinds of digital media interventions (at least as they have been implemented up until now) is that they require audiences to seek out, have access to, and make continuing active use of the sources. This is unlike mass media interventions, which assume that the audience can be reached passively through its routine use of media. The requirement for active seeking is likely to limit the proportion of the unreached population who are engaged. This essential weakness runs up against a frequent goal of population-focused programs, which is to involve people who are not substantially motivated to act.

Another critical aspect of effective communication programs, like most behavior change programs, is that they cannot be single, fixed interventions. Rather, they need to evolve in response to changes in their audiences, to changes in the context in which the behavior is to be performed, and to changes in the social expectations of those around the individual. A good program is not defined by its specific communication actions (such as the number of messages on specific channels over a specific time period) but by the methods employed for changing messages and diffusion channels as circumstances change over time. They are more analogous to what a practicing physician might do, ideally, in working with a patient whose symptoms and illness level, readiness to comply with recommendations, and family support change over time.

Finally, capacity is a consideration that cannot be ignored since the capacity to design, implement, and evaluate interventions is generally weak in governments and local nongovernmental organizations in low and middle income countries. Additionally, in local markets the capacity to produce creative executions of messages is often weak. Formally addressing weak capacity must nearly always be an objective, even within the overarching objective of improved health outcomes. Decisions to implement communication campaigns also need to take into account the competition among health communication campaigns for resources, government attention, and target group attention (Smith, 2009).

Conclusion 5.2: Risk for CVD and related chronic diseases is increased by modifiable behavioral factors such as tobacco use; high intake of salt, sugar, saturated and transfats, and unhealthful oils; excessive total caloric intake; lack of consumption of fruits and vegetables; physical inactivity; and excessive alcohol consumption. For some of these risk factors, behavior modification and risk reduction have been successfully achieved through health promotion and prevention policies and communications programs in some countries and communities. However, most policies and programs with evidence of effectiveness have been developed and implemented in high income countries, and even in these settings little population-level progress has been made in some areas, such as reducing total calorie consumption and sedentary behavior. Adaptations to the culture, resources, and capacities of specific settings will be required for population-based interventions to have an impact in low and middle income countries.

Recommendation: Implement Policies to Promote Cardiovascular Health

To expand current or introduce new population-wide efforts to promote cardiovascular health and to reduce risk for CVD and related chronic diseases, national and subnational governments should adapt and implement evidence-based, effective policies based on local priorities. These policies may include laws, regulations, changes to fiscal policy, and incentives to encourage private-sector alignment. To maximize impact, efforts to introduce policies should be accompanied by sustained health communication campaigns focused on the same targets of intervention as the selected policies.

Health Care Delivery

One of the key components in reducing the burden of CVD is an adequate health system to implement the services needed to promote cardiovascular health and control CVD. The need for adequate health care delivery is of course not unique to CVD, although there are aspects of care that need to be disease specific, such as guidelines and training. This section focuses on both areas of health care delivery within which there are specific CVD needs and also touches on broader health systems needs that are relevant for chronic diseases and synergistic with the emerging emphasis on global health systems strengthening and integrated primary care rather than disease-specific clinical programs. Efforts to improve broad health systems functioning are the focus of significant current efforts in global health and have been well described elsewhere (Lewin et al., 2008; Taskforce on Innovative International Financing for Health Systems Working Group 1, 2009; WHO, 2007a).

The World Health Organization (WHO) defines a health system as consisting of "all organizations, people, and actions whose primary intent is to promote, restore, or maintain health" (WHO, 2007a). This encompasses public health approaches such as those described in the preceding sections of this chapter as well as the delivery of clinical health care services to identify and treat patients at high risk and to manage patients with diagnosed disease. Although the definition of health systems is an area of evolving discussions in the global health community, there is emerging consensus around six key building blocks of health systems articulated by WHO: efficient, high-quality health services; equitable access to essential medical products and technologies; financing; the health workforce; information systems (discussed in Chapter 4); and leadership and governance (WHO, 2007a).

There is also agreement that one fundamental goal of a health system is to provide effective, responsive, equitable, and efficient care (Committee on the State of the USA Health Indicators, 2009; Kruk and Freedman, 2008; Liu et al., 2008; Taskforce on Innovative International Financing for Health Systems Working Group 1, 2009). Effective care is timely, safe, improves health outcomes, and continues until a health issue is resolved; or, in the case of chronic diseases, provides ongoing care as needed. This care should also be responsive to the needs of patients through not only the technical competence but also the interpersonal quality of providers. Equity in health systems means that essential health services are accessible to and utilized by all members of society—including those who are disadvantaged or marginalized—and that payment for care is equitable and does not result in catastrophic health care expenditures. This is especially critical for chronic diseases, which require ongoing expenditures on health services. Efficiency means that the health system yields the greatest health gains from the resources that are available and that the system functions productively (Kruk and Freedman, 2008).

There is considerable knowledge of clinical care solutions for treatment of acute cardiovascular events, for management of CVD, and for prevention in high-risk patients that target blood pressure control, blood lipid control, blood glucose control, and smoking cessation. The effectiveness of these clinical solutions themselves, such as pharmacological interventions, are highly generalizable across countries and, as described in more detail below, guidelines and established practices for these clinical solutions, especially pharmacological interventions, are well developed. However, knowing an optimal clinical intervention that works to improve health outcomes is not sufficient. Clinical interventions need to be delivered appropriately to the patients who need them, which requires an effective and equitable system of health care delivery.

In addition to CVD-specific clinical solutions, there are common elements to effective delivery of chronic disease care that have potential to work for many health problems in low and middle income countries (e.g., diabetes, cancer, prenatal care, growth monitoring in children, TB, and HIV). These core elements include first, as a precondition, access and affordability. Other elements include guidelines or established practices that, when followed, lead to clinical success, routine assessment and improvement of quality of care, and monitoring of health status and health outcomes. Ideally, to enhance support for the behavior changes needed to maximize the effectiveness of clinical interventions, these clinical strategies would also be implemented in the context of the broader public health system, including population-based and community-based strategies described elsewhere in this chapter.

Therefore, the work that lies ahead is in improving health care delivery to reduce the burden of CVD in developing countries. There are several challenges that will need to be confronted when building on known, effective interventions in order to adapt and scale up to achieve equitable health care delivery. One challenge is that interventions and delivery mechanisms must be context-specific rather than generic applications of blueprint, uniform approaches. A second is to optimize comprehensive, integrated health programs and greater capacity in a fashion that encourages innovation yet addresses equitable distribution (Victora et al., 2004; WHO Maximizing Positive Synergies Collaborative Group, 2009). It is also critical that the delivery of health care be equitable. Ensuring an equitable health system requires establishing goals specifically for improved coverage for the poor, rather than in entire populations; planning and health interventions directed toward the needs of the disadvantaged; and empowerment of poor stakeholders to be vitally involved in health system design and operation (Gwatkin et al., 2004). Meeting these challenges, although formidable, will go a long way to ensure that the benefits of CVD control programs reach the greatest number of individuals in need.

This section considers in more detail the components of health care delivery that will be crucial to successfully implementing effective clinical prevention and disease management for CVD. These include patient-level interventions, provider-level interventions to improve the quality of care, human resources and workforce, access to care, financing, access to essential medical products and technologies, integration of care delivery, and information technology. For some of these components, there is evidence specific to CVD-related interventions and programs or to approaches that can be generalized to CVD. For others, the discussion focuses on the principles in place in current efforts to strengthen health care delivery in general, which can be inclusive of CVD and related chronic diseases. The tools and strategies described are options for decision makers, managers, and clinicians that can be used to strengthen health care in different country contexts in order to deliver interventions effectively, efficiently, and equitably.

With resource and infrastructure constraints in developing countries, the translation of these strategies into improved health care delivery remains a challenge. However, it is possible to deliver good-quality care, even in resource-poor settings. The best strategies are often incremental and gradual and need to encompass action and motivation at all levels, from national leadership to local support (Jamison et al., 2006). In recent years, infectious disease programs in resource-limited settings have begun to build health care delivery infrastructure, especially in the development of laboratory capacity, supply chain management, quality assurance, and renovation of health centers (Justman et al., 2009). Such developments have brought a growing appreciation for the opportunity to use infectious disease-related systems strengthening to strengthen health systems in general (Jamison et al., 2006). Here, efforts to address chronic disease have the opportunity to build on, rather than duplicate, health systems strengthening efforts. Indeed, as global health begins to shift toward generalized strengthening efforts with a focus on primary care, chronic diseases and models of chronic care and disease management cannot be overlooked.

Patient-Level Interventions

The following section reviews patient-level interventions that are delivered within the health care system to reduce CVD risk and manage disease, including behavior change strategies and clinical interventions for prevention and treatment. Guidelines for delivering clinical interventions are discussed in the section on provider-level interventions, followed by a section on integrated disease management and chronic care strategies. Although different interventions are described in separate categories, they are not intended to be used in isolation from each other but rather as components of a health care provider's services for patients, as well as in synergy with population- and community-based approaches described in other sections of this chapter.

Strategies to Change Behaviors   Provider advice and education are among the interventions delivered to patients as part of health care. There is mixed evidence on the effectiveness of these approaches. In fact, in a review of counseling and education interventions to reduce multiple risk factors for prevention of CHD in settings including primary care, the authors concluded that "[i]t is essential that the current concepts and practices of multiple risk factor intervention . . . through individual risk factor counseling are not exported to poorer countries as the best policy option for dealing with existing and projected burdens of cardiovascular disease" (Ebrahim et al., 2006, p. 23). Therefore, more work is needed to determine the appropriate role and best delivery mechanisms for these intervention approaches.

Economic incentives have also been used to influence consumers' preventive health behaviors. A review by Kane et al. (2004) concluded that economic incentives (including cash, gifts, lotteries, and other free/reduced-price goods or services) appear to be effective in the short run for simple preventive care and distinct, well-defined behavioral goals. According to the review, incentives were effective 73 percent of the time and small incentives produced finite changes. While this is encouraging, the authors recognize that although economic incentives for prevention appear to work, their mechanisms are not well understood. For example, it is not clear what size of incentive is needed to yield a major sustained effect and there is less evidence that economic incentives can sustain the long-term lifestyle changes required for health promotion. In addition, the generalizability of these findings to low and middle income country contexts is not known.

Several randomized trials in high income countries have demonstrated the effectiveness of financial incentives to address tobacco use. Incentives ranged from small amounts of money ($20) for each class attended to an incrementally higher amount for smoking cessation and continued abstinence at 1, 4, and 6 months after the program initiation (Donatelle et al., 2000; Volpp et al., 2006, 2009). A financial incentive for smoking cessation has also been evaluated in the Philippines (Giné et al., 2008). CARES, a voluntary commitment program to help smokers quit smoking, offered smokers a savings account in which they deposited money (a minimum of 50 pesos, or approximately $1) for 6 months without interest. Participants were given a lockbox to aid in daily savings, with a weekly deposit collection service available. Within 1 week of the 6-month maturity date, participants took a urine test for nicotine and its primary metabolite, cotinine. If they passed, their money was returned; otherwise, their money was forfeited to charity. Eleven percent of smokers offered CARES signed a contract, and smokers randomly offered CARES were 3 percentage points more likely to pass the

6-month test than the control group. This effect persisted in surprise tests at 12 months, indicating that CARES produced lasting smoking cessation.

Conditional cash transfers are another strategy to provide incentives to promote adoption of healthy behaviors. In conditional cash transfer programs a cash payment is made to an individual or family contingent upon complying with certain conditions, such as preventive health requirements and nutrition supplementation, education, and monitoring designed to improve health outcomes and promote positive behavior change (Lagarde et al., 2009). Programs of this kind have been implemented by governments or other organizations in low and middle income countries with the goal of improving options for poor families through interventions in health, nutrition, and education. A recent review supports the potential for conditional cash transfer programs to increase the uptake of preventive services and encourage some preventive behaviors (Lagarde et al., 2009). However, mixed results and insufficient evaluations make it difficult to draw conclusions about the potential that these programs have for widescale implementation.

There are few published examples that are directly related to CVD outcomes, but a program in Mexico can be informative for addressing related CVD risk factors, specifically child nutrition and obesity. PROGRESA/ *Oportunidades* examined the effect of conditional cash transfers in 506 rural, low income communities that were randomly assigned to be enrolled immediately or after an 18-month period, allowing for comparison between the two groups during the waiting period. The intervention linked payment to mothers for health behaviors, such as participation in health and nutrition programs including prenatal care, immunization, and nutrition supplementation, and incentives to promote children's school attendance (Rivera et al., 2004).

It was recently evaluated for its impact on several CVD-related outcomes, and the cash transfer component was associated with better outcomes in children (Fernald et al., 2008b). After 5 years, children (n = 2,449) aged 24-68 months who had been enrolled in the program their entire lives were assessed for a range of outcomes related to CVD risk. A doubling of cash transfers was associated with lower body mass index (BMI) for age percentile and lower prevalence of being overweight. Although this is a promising result, the cash component was also negatively associated with adult health outcomes (Fernald et al., 2008a). After 5 years of the program, adults (n = 1,649 early, n = 2,039 late intervention) aged 18-65 years were assessed. A doubling of cumulative cash transfers to the household was associated with higher BMI, higher diastolic blood pressure, and higher prevalence of overweight, grade I obesity, and grade II obesity while controlling for a wide range of covariates, including household composition at baseline.

Clinical Interventions to Reduce Risk and Manage and Treat CVD   There is considerable knowledge of effective clinical solutions to reduce risks for CVD using pharmaceutical interventions to lower blood pressure, blood lipids, and blood glucose and to assist in smoking cessation. There is also considerable technical knowledge on the diagnosis of CVD, treatment of acute cardiovascular events, and post-event treatment and management (Fuster, 2009).

There is particularly strong evidence on the pharmacological management and control of high blood pressure (or hypertension), with a corresponding reduction in cardio- and cerebro-vascular mortalities and morbidities (Fuster, 2009). Low-cost generic blood pressure-lowering medications are in use for controlling hypertension throughout the world (Pereira et al., 2009). As described in more detail in the section on economic analysis in Chapter 7, hypertension control is also one of the interventions with the most potential to be cost-effective in low and middle income countries. Pharmacological interventions to lower blood cholesterol and its main components, such as LDL cholesterol and serum triglycerides, have also proven to be very effective in reducing the cardiovascular mortality and morbidity in populations around the world (Adult Treatment Panel III, 2002; Brugts et al., 2009; Smith, 1997).

Indeed, aspirin, beta-blockers, ACE-inhibitors, and lipid-lowering therapies all have established effectiveness to lower the risk of future vascular events in high-risk patients. The benefits of each of these pharmaceutical interventions appear to be largely independent so that when used together in appropriate patients it is reasonable to expect that about two-thirds to three-quarters of future vascular events could be prevented. Therefore, the potential gains from combined drug therapies are large (Yusuf, 2002). This has led to the development of combination pills, known as "polypills" in an effort to achieve a lower cost, more efficient, and more convenient treatment option for patients at high risk for CVD. The effectiveness and safety of this promising approach is currently being evaluated in a number of trials in both developed and developing countries (Holt, 2009; Xavier et al., 2009).

Adherence to clinical interventions   Lack of adherence to medical treatment is a widespread problem that can lead to worsening health status and increased future treatment costs. Treatment regimens that are easy to administer, accessible, and affordable can help to increase adherence. As described above, improving adherence through simplicity, convenience, and reduced costs is one of the hopes for the emerging "polypill" concept. Affordability and access are discussed in more detail as part of the next section on access to clinical interventions.

Financial incentives are one possible intervention to improve adherence.

In a review of financial incentives to enhance patient compliance, Giuffrida and Torgerson (1997) found that 10 of 11 studies showed improved patient compliance with the use of financial incentives. However, the clinical aim of each study was different and the incentives varied. It is also important to note that all the randomized studies reviewed were carried out in the United States; thus, the results may not translate directly to another country with a different socioeconomic and cultural context.

Adherence to TB treatment is an analogous challenge that is common in developing countries and may provide transferable lessons for pharmaceutical interventions for CVD. In two pilot sites in Tajikistan, Project HOPE used food incentives to enhance adherence to a TB treatment regimen, enable patients to complete treatment without burden on their families, and increase access to directly observed therapy (DOT) for the poor and vulnerable. In this intervention, directly observed therapy was linked with the incentive of a nutritious meal. Among new sputum positive patients who received directly observed therapy, 88 percent of those receiving meal supplements completed treatment and were cured, compared to 63 percent in the non-supplemented patients (Mohr et al., 2005).

Access to clinical interventions An evidence-based, cost-effective primary health care-centered approach that includes targeting screening for high-risk individuals and the provision of treatment for symptom control is critical to ensuring access to appropriate CVD care. Risk-prediction tools that assess risk on the basis of multiple risk factors and CVD history have been developed in the United States and other high income countries (Bannink, 2006; Kannel, 1976), but cannot be assumed to be directly applicable to all populations and settings. For greatest feasibility, screening in resource-limited areas may need to focus on simple methods like family history, medical history and physical measurements such as blood pressure and body mass index or waist-to-hip ratio (Joshi et al., 2008).

As a necessary follow-up to effective screening, access to essential medicines, medical products, and technologies is a critical part of access to care. While one of the Millennium Development Goal targets is to "provide access to affordable essential drugs in developing countries," (United Nations Department of Economic and Social Affairs, 2008, p. 47) recent WHO reports have indicated that essential CVD medicines are largely not available in the public sector in low and middle income countries (Cameron et al., 2009; Mendis et al., 2007a). While there is better availability of these medicines in the private sector, the end-user cost of these private-sector medicines is often quite burdensome to the majority of low and middle income populations. For example, a 1-month course of combined therapy for secondary prevention (aspirin, beta-blocker, ACE-inhibitor, and statin) for patients with established CVD could cost as much as 18 days' wages in

Malawi (Mendis et al., 2007a). In addition, the pharmaceutical component of CVD prevention requires daily, long-term medication treatment, rather than short-course or one-time therapy, which increases the lifetime financial burden. Individuals may not be able to afford continuous treatment for long periods of time. Given that anywhere from 50 to 90 percent of the cost of medicines are financed through individual out-of-pocket payments in low and middle income countries (Quick et al., 2002), the financial burden on individuals and families has the potential to be substantial. Clearly, much needs to be done to ensure a guaranteed supply of affordable CVD medicines to the majority of the low and middle income country population.

Several possible initiatives could potentially help address this problem, although the potential costs of these are difficult to estimate. As described above, the polypill, although not yet evaluated, is an attractive option that could be administered to a broad range of patients, especially if manufactured with generic components. If proven safe and effective, this has the potential to be a pragmatic response to the need for both simplified and affordable treatment regimens in low income countries with weak health systems (Wald and Law, 2003; Yusuf, 2002). Another initiative to help address costs is generic substitution policies, which allow for generic medications to be offered as an alternative to more expensive brand-name medications (Andersson et al., 2007). Elimination of tariffs on medicines, generally a regressive form of taxation, could also increase the equitable access to essential CVD medicines without significant impact on government revenues (Olcay and Laing, 2005). In addition, negotiations with pharmaceutical companies have led to decreases in the price of antiretroviral medications for HIV in low and middle income countries (Borght et al., 2009). New advocacy and private-sector collaboration could lead to improved affordability of medicines for CVD in low and middle income countries. Government-sponsored health insurance schemes can also reduce the end-user cost of both drugs and other health services, as has been done in Rwanda, although this strategy still faces concerns about financial sustainability and availability of services and medicines. Health financing mechanisms are discussed later in this chapter (Twahirwa, 2008).

Finally, improved drug distribution and procurement efficiency has the potential to make drugs more readily available through the public system and affordable through the private system (Joshi et al., 2008). The delivery of drugs, including statins, antihypertensives, nicotine replacement, or a newly created polypill to low-resource settings in a manner timely and reliable enough to maintain individual treatment regimens is an enormous logistical challenge. However, there exists growing expertise in supply chain management in developing countries from both the HIV/AIDS and malaria community as program implementers attempt to scale up their respective initiatives. The Supply Chain Management System was initiated as part of the U.S. President's Emergency Plan for AIDS Relief (PEPFAR) to deliver antiretroviral medications to local implementing partners and programs involved in rapid scale-up efforts (Supply Chain Management System, 2010). The strategies employed by the Supply Chain Management System include combining orders to purchase at wholesale rates, warehousing and distribution through regional distribution centers, preventing product expiration through inventory management that focuses on stock rotation and monitoring, forecasting demand and anticipating country needs, and benefiting from the establishment of long-term contracts (Supply Chain Management System, 2009). These strategies could all potentially be adopted to improve CVD drug delivery.

However, it is important to ensure that CVD-related procurement needs are coordinated with existing efforts in the global health community, so as not to perpetuate the difficulties caused by parallel distribution systems. In HIV/AIDS for example, The Global Fund to Fight AIDS, Tuberculosis and Malaria and PEPFAR each have their own supply chain management protocols, funding streams, and procurement requirements. While each of these agencies expressly endorses coordination wherever possible, local actors still must balance the needs of distinct international funders (The Global Fund, 2009; Partnership for Supply Chain Management Systems, 2010). In order not to compound this problem, it is important for the global CVD community to identify ways to work within or help adapt existing frameworks and supply chains.

In addition to the existing efforts driven by global health organizations, extensive research and efficiency improvement efforts have also been undertaken by the private sector as businesses expand into global markets, and these strategies may offer uncommon insights that can benefit CVD initiatives (Accenture, 2010; Council of Supply Chain Management Professionals, 2010; Kinaxis, 2010). While supply chain systems have grown steadily over the past decade, there is still a great deal of infrastructure and capacity yet to be developed. Ensuring that CVD medications are included during the planning and design phases of these new endeavors is a positive opportunity in which the global CVD community could take an important leadership role.

As with medicines, CVD-related technologies—diagnostics and interventions—have the potential to contribute greatly to the control of global CVD; however, an effort equal in energy and intensity must be made to ensure equitable distribution and access to these technologies as they develop and proliferate. The development of novel diagnostics has accelerated in the area of communicable diseases such as HIV and TB (Houpt and Guerrant, 2008); similar initiatives can be envisioned for CVD. However, for diagnostic technologies to make any noticeable impact on CVD mortality, they need to be suitable to and affordable in the developing world, and there needs to be sufficient provision of health care following diagnosis, or the improved ability to correctly identify patients will be of little use. Some of these new technologies, such as portable electrocardiogram machines, are being produced or are under development in health technology companies in high income countries. They are being rolled out primarily for middle-income developing markets, but are already spreading more widely to poor countries, at least to segments of the population that can afford them (Immelt et al., 2009).

Although the delivery and implementation of the latest, state-of-the-art technologies may have potential to help reduce the burden of disease, in some settings with more developed health systems, a patient's access to the preexisting technologies that are already being used in the local or national health system can have a more profound impact on their survival status than the absolute level of technology in the country or community. For example, it has been shown that poor patients in India suffer higher mortality after acute coronary syndromes, but that this mortality difference is eliminated after controlling for access to treatments (Xavier et al., 2008). Thus, in some countries improving access to essential CVD-related services within broader efforts to improve access and maximize the equitable use of existing health systems infrastructure will likely enhance the role of technology for diagnosis and treatment, even without costly efforts specifically to increase technological capacity within a country.

Provider-Level Interventions to Improve the Quality of Care

Quality of care was defined by the Institute of Medicine (IOM) as "the degree to which health services for individuals and populations increase the likelihood of desired health outcomes and are consistent with current professional knowledge" (IOM, 2001, p. 232). There are three main aspects of quality: process (the actions performed in the delivery of care), outcomes (the observable consequences of care), and structure (the characteristics of health systems, facilities, and staff) (Donabedian, 1988).

Quality improvement strategies that act directly on provider behavior may focus on two aspects of performance—technical and interpersonal. Technical performance refers to the extent to which services are performed according to standards and can be improved through supervision and lifelong training (Taskforce on Innovative International Financing for Health Systems Working Group 1, 2009). Like the patient-level interventions described in the previous section, these approaches need to incorporate sufficient CVD specificity to provide relevant technical knowledge, although the strategies to deliver technical performance improvements can be generalized in a chronic disease model. Interpersonal quality improvement strategies involve meeting users' expectations and values to provide responsive care.

Competence in this area is particularly important for CVD and other diseases that require chronic care and long-term relationships with providers. Establishing norms and codes of conduct, and the provision of supervision and basic amenities, are effective methods for increasing interpersonal performance (Taskforce on Innovative International Financing for Health Systems Working Group 1, 2009).

The strategies to improve quality of care by changing provider behavior described below include guidelines, disease management programs, audit and feedback on performance, public reporting, and performance incentive programs such as pay for performance. This is an area of quality improvement that has become well established in high income countries, but is much less well developed in low and middle income countries. A review of quality improvement intervention studies in low and middle income countries suggests that dissemination of guidelines alone is not effective, but that supervision and audit with feedback show more promise, as well as systems interventions at the level of the hospital or clinic. In addition, interventions with multiple components are likely to be more effective than single components (Rowe et al., 2005). However, the review acknowledged the limited information on strategies to improve performance in low and middle income countries. There is a need for better understanding of the determinants of provider performance, better methods to measure performance, high quality studies to assess long-term effectiveness and costs, and a better understanding of the extent to which results for one setting and area of care can be applied to others (Rowe et al., 2005). This knowledge gap is particularly striking for interventions related to improving CVD-related care in developing countries. Therefore, where evidence is lacking quality improvement on strategies to address CVD and related risk factors in low and middle income countries, there is a discussion in the following sections of evidence that can be generalized from relevant chronic disease-related approaches in high income countries and in some cases, from strategies targeted at other areas of health care in low and middle income countries in order to develop strategies for CVD and related chronic diseases in low and middle income countries.

Guidelines There are multiple national and international guidelines for prevention, treatment, management, and control of CVD and CVD-related risk factors, including hypertension and elevated lipids, many of which have been tailored for a range of high income countries and low and middle income countries. These include, for example, the American Heart Association (AHA) Guidelines (Fuster, 2009); the Joint National Committee on Prevention, Detection, Evaluation, and Treatment of High Blood Pressure (U.S. Department of Health and Human Services, 2004); the European Guidelines on Cardiovascular Disease Prevention in Clinical Practice

(Graham et al., 2007); the Chinese Guidelines on Prevention and Treatment of Hypertension (Committee for Revision of Chinese Guidelines for Prevention and Treatment of Patients with Hypertension, 2005); the Canadian Guidelines for the Diagnosis and Treatment of Dyslipidemia and Prevention of Cardiovascular Disease in the adult (Genest et al., 2005); the Canadian Hypertension Education Program (Canadian Hypertension Education Program, 2009); and the WHO/International Society of Hypertension (ISH) Hypertension Risk Prediction charts (Mendis et al., 2007b).

In principle, these existing, well-established guidelines describe effective care that should be highly transferable across settings. However, this requires that clinicians learn the guidelines and adhere to them in practice, which is not an insignificant barrier. For example, a study of European guidelines for CVD prevention found that guidelines were not being followed. The objectives of the European Action on Secondary Prevention through Intervention to Reduce Events (EUROASPIRE) survey were (1) to determine in patients with CHD whether the European guidelines on CVD prevention were being followed and (2) to determine whether the practice of preventive cardiology in patients with CHD in EUROASPIRE III improved by comparison with the previous surveys, EUROASPIRE I and II, after efforts were implemented to improve adherence to guidelines (Kotseva, 2009b). The study outcomes indicated that most guidelines were not being followed, showing no change in the prevalence of smoking and continued adverse trends in the prevalence of obesity and central obesity. Despite increased use of antihypertensive medications, there was also no change in blood pressure control. An increased prevalence of diabetes, both self-reported and undetected, and deteriorating therapeutic control was found. The study did show an increased use of antiplatelets, beta-blockers, ACE/angiotensin II receptor blockers, and statins along with continued improvement in lipid control (Kotseva, 2009a).

A recent review found that improvements in guideline adherence, as measured by performance indicators, have led to significant reductions in mortality (Mehta et al., 2007). Their findings suggest that improving quality achieves reductions in death in excess of those seen for any new therapy. It is estimated that the use of clinical guidelines for acute myocardial infarction can prevent 80,000 deaths annually in the United States alone (Bahit et al., 2000). Therefore, the potential global implications are significant if effective ways to improve adherence to guidelines can be developed.

Audit and Feedback Audit of performance and feedback have been used in a variety of settings to affect provider behavior and quality of care (Jamtvedt et al., 2006). The potential for an effect on quality of care rests on the general premise that knowledge of one's own performance motivates improvement. With the increased use of electronic medical records, audit and feedback has increasing potential as a measurement tool that can be implemented with greater ease and be linked to performance-based incentives such as pay-for-performance programs (Hysong, 2009).

However, reviews of the literature on audit and feedback have not found consistent evidence of its effectiveness as an intervention to improve quality (Grimshaw et al., 2004; Jamtvedt et al., 2006). A review of 118 randomized trials of audit and feedback reflected these mixed results but concluded that audit and feedback can be effective in improving professional practice. When it is effective, the effects are generally small to moderate. The relative effectiveness of audit and feedback is likely to be greater when baseline adherence to recommended practice is low and when feedback is delivered more intensively (Jamtvedt et al., 2006). A more recent analysis suggests that the effectiveness of audit and feedback is also improved when specific suggestions for improvement are offered along with measurement feedback (Hysong, 2009). However, the vast majority of the studies included in these reviews were conducted in developed countries.

Interest in provider measurement and feedback as a quality-improvement tool in developing countries is growing. For example, studies to date have shown that feedback of health worker performance data on managing childhood diseases in Africa improved compliance with standards of care (Kelley et al., 2001), and audits using a simple checklist of maternal health indicators improved performance in the Philippines (Loevinsohn et al., 1995). Even self-assessment of compliance with standards of care can improve quality, as shown in Mali (Kelley et al., 2003).

Using clinical performance vignettes, the Quality Improvement Demonstration Study (QIDS) in the Philippines provides recent evidence from a middle income country of links between clinical performance feedback and improvements in quality, outcomes, and satisfaction. QIDS was an evaluation to compare the impact of two interventions on physician practices, health behaviors, and health status of children under 5 years: (1) expanded insurance coverage to increase access to care and (2) a pay-for-performance scheme for physicians (Shimkhada et al., 2008). In all sites, randomly selected physicians were administered clinical performance vignettes every 6 months, and their scores were reported back to them individually, along with their rank compared to other physicians. The effects of the pay-for-performance intervention are described in more detail later, but of interest here is that with time—even in the control condition, which had no change to the existing insurance or payment schemes—there were observable quality improvements. This suggests that performance evaluation and dissemination of scores alone affected quality scores (Luck and Shimkhada, 2009; Peabody et al., 2010b; Quimbo et al., 2010).

Public Reporting and Consumer Choice In the United States and other Western nations, public reporting of provider quality data has been employed as a means to support and stimulate quality improvement (Marshall et al., 2000). The ability of public reporting to incite change rests on the assumption that consumers demand and use comparative data in making choices about health care providers. Recent reviews of the literature have sought to assess the impact of public reporting. The results generally point to a limited body of evidence on the effects of provider quality information on consumer choice (Faber et al., 2009; Fung et al., 2008) and weak evidence of provider changes stemming from public reporting (Fung et al., 2008; Robinowitz and Dudley, 2006). Further analysis shows that public reporting of outcomes does appear to have an impact on quality improvements at the hospital level (Fung et al., 2008). However, public reporting appears to have limited impact on quality improvement if consumers have a difficult time understanding the results, particularly when there is little variation among providers (Robinowitz and Dudley, 2006). Poorly constructed report cards do not help consumers in making choices; a summary table of benchmark provider measures may be a better way to communicate provider performance (Devers et al., 2004; Hibbard, 2008).

Shaller et al. (2003, p. 95) have asserted that providing comparative quality information to consumers will drive improvements in health care quality, only if five conditions are met: "(1) consumers are convinced that quality problems are real and consequential and that quality can be improved; (2) purchasers and policymakers make sure that quality reporting is standardized and universal; (3) consumers are given quality information that is relevant and easy to understand and use; (4) the dissemination of quality information is improved; and (5) purchasers reward quality improvements and providers create the information and organizational infrastructure to achieve them."

Work on public reporting in developing countries is limited. However, there have been documented examples of its use. In Uganda, a community-based monitoring system for primary health care providers resulted in improved child outcomes (Bjorkman and Svensson, 2007; McNamara, 2006). In India and the Philippines, provider report cards using data from patient satisfaction surveys have been used (McNamara, 2006). These examples demonstrate feasibility, but more work is needed to assess the value of this type of information on influencing patient behavior and its applicability across other settings.

Performance Incentive Programs Pay-for-performance programs that link financial incentives with quality measures to reward good clinical practice at the level of both providers and institutions have been used extensively in the United States and Europe, with some modest evidence of success

(Campbell et al., 2009; Epstein, 2007; Grossbart, 2006; Lindenauer et al., 2007; Petersen et al., 2006).This approach is gaining popularity in the developing world (Eichler et al., 2009) with substantial donor support, although this support is not necessarily being devoted to CVD care. Pay for performance may confer some unique benefits in a developing-country setting. Namely, in resource-constrained settings, where the quality of care and the health of populations are consistently low and thus targeted by governments and donor agencies alike, the marginal health benefits may be expected to be higher. Providers may be more responsive to incentivized measurement and feedback (Eichler et al., 2009).

There are few rigorous evaluations of pay for performance in developing countries. Taken together, however, efforts in developing countries suggest that an infrastructure for provider measurement, feedback and incentives, can be developed and implemented (McNamara, 2006). QIDS in the Philippines, described earlier, compared the impact on physician practices, health behaviors, and health status of children under 5 years of either expanded insurance coverage to increase access to care or a pay-for-performance scheme in which bonus payments were given to physicians based on quality scores using a randomized design (Shimkhada et al., 2008). Clinical performance vignette scores improved over a period of 2 years in the pay-for-performance sites compared to controls (Peabody et al., 2010b; Solon et al., 2009). Improved access to care and overall system-level reimbursement in the expanded insurance coverage arm also led to changes in quality. In addition, for both intervention arms, there were clinical improvements as measured by the number of children who were not wasted (underweight for height) (Peabody et al., 2010b). Quality improvements were also associated with patient satisfaction (Peabody et al., 2010a).

In another example, in Haiti, incentives for achieving health targets led to significant changes in provider practice such as immunization coverage and attended deliveries (Eichler et al., 2009; McNamara, 2005). In Rwanda, performance-based financing was adopted by the government as a national policy, with performance payments to public and private health facilities (Eichler, 2009; Soeters et al., 2006). The impact on prenatal care utilization, the quality of prenatal care, institutional delivery, and child preventive care utilization was assessed using data produced from a prospective quasi-experimental design nested into a phased program rollout in 165 rural facilities, which allowed for comparisons between first- and second-phase facilities during the 2-year delay in rollout. The incentive effect was isolated from the resource effect by increasing the second-phase facilities' traditional budgets an amount equal to the average pay-for-performance payments to the first-phase facilities. The pay-for-performance program had a large and significant positive impact on some outcomes, including institutional deliveries and young children's preventive care visits. The program also improved the quality of prenatal care as measured by process indicators of the clinical content of care and tetanus toxoid vaccination (Basinga et al., 2009).

Chronic Care and Disease Management Models

Comprehensive models for managing chronic illnesses have been developed with the goal of combining and integrating approaches to increase quality of care by providers, provide appropriate interventions, and improve accompanying behavior change and patient self-management. This is an area where professionals in primary care and in CVD and related chronic diseases have a wealth of experience in developing models that can be offered not only to manage noncommunicable chronic diseases, but also to assist in the evolution of health systems to better address the transition to chronic care needs for patients with chronic infectious diseases such as TB and HIV/AIDS. Multiple models for managing chronic illness have been developed and implemented in high income countries, focusing on improvements in a range of elements such as health systems, clinical decision support, delivery-system redesign, clinical information systems, community resources, and self-management support. These have been described extensively elsewhere (Bodenheimer et al., 2002; CDC, 2003; Feachem et al., 2002; Kane et al., 2003; Klingbeil and Fiedler, 1988; Singh and Ham, 2006; Wagner et al., 1996; WHO Noncommunicable Diseases and Mental Health Cluster, 2002). This is an area of great promise, but it is not always straightforward in its implementation and, although specific components do have a strong evidence base, there have not been many rigorous evaluations of the health impact of the existing overall frameworks. In addition, most available evidence is drawn from the United States, reinforced by recent studies from Europe, Canada, New Zealand, and Australia (Singh and Ham, 2006). Thus evidence from low and middle income countries is sparse and the potential for effective transfer of chronic care models to low and middle income settings remains to be demonstrated (Beaglehole et al., 2008).

A systematic review of randomized clinical trials of disease management programs specifically designed for patients with coronary heart disease showed positive impacts on processes of care and moderate effects on risk-factor profiles (McAlister et al., 2001). However, like most evidence for chronic care models more generally, these trials were all from high income countries, and there has been little implementation or evaluation of care management approaches in low and middle income countries.

A current trial in Shanghai is evaluating a case management model that is intended to be deployed to community hospitals to increase effectiveness of hypertension control through attention to the workflow and process details; an integrated hypertension intervention approach; and intensive education and training to increase the competency of community health providers. The trial initially enrolled 1,442 hypertensive patients randomly assigned to intervention (IG, n = 480) and control (CG, n = 962) groups and was subsequently expanded to 19 districts in Shanghai and a total of 15,200 patients (11,400 in IG/3,800 in CG). The results have not yet been published, but preliminary results have been reported and show promising effects on blood pressure control and quality of life in patients as well as on the knowledge and skill of community hospital physicians. The program has also shown lower costs per mmHg systolic blood pressure or diastolic blood pressure reduction in IG compared to CG over a 12-month period (Lu et al., 2009).

Initiatives to Strengthen Health Systems Capacity and Infrastructure

Human Resources Currently, more than a billion people worldwide have insufficient access to health services (Crisp et al., 2008), which is due in part to a shortage of health workers. The 2006 World Health Report has estimated that there is already a global shortage of more than 4 million health workers, with the greatest shortage being experienced by low income countries (WHO, 2006). With the expected increase in the burden of the global CVD epidemic, it is likely that the shortage in the global health care workforce and leadership will be even more acutely felt in low income countries during the upcoming several decades. Guided by the principles of coverage, motivation, and competence, it will be crucial to meet this challenge with initiatives to increase the health care workforce; to promote task-shifting to less-specialized workers; to provide specialized continuous training at several professional levels of health care worker in clinical, public health, health communications, and behavioral disciplines, as well as health systems and program management; to promote motivation by improving management and providing satisfactory remuneration, adequate resources, appropriate infrastructure, and career development; and to cultivate leadership and innovation (Chen et al., 2004; Lehmann et al., 2009; Willis-Shattuck et al., 2008).

Successful initiatives in this arena will require sustained involvement, leadership, and support of national governments in several realms: (1) to establish a regulatory framework that encourages training, monitoring, and assessment; (2) to implement policies that liberalize resources and create career development and promotion pathways; (3) to guide and support training institutions; (4) to marshal the resources necessary to create incentives for growth in the supply and retention of health care workers; and (5) to secure the support of the multiple stakeholders, including funding sources, educational institutions, practitioners, administrative personnel, and community members (Chen et al., 2004; Crisp et al., 2008; Lehmann et al., 2009). In addition, the input and influence of multilateral organizations will also be of paramount importance in facilitating dialogue and partnership among different stakeholders.

WHO has created the Global Health Workforce Alliance, which is a partnership of national governments, civil society, international agencies, finance institutions, researchers, educators, and professional associations dedicated to working toward solutions for the global health care workforce shortage issue (Global Health Workforce Alliance, no date). Although CVD is not specifically addressed by the Alliance, many of the same principles and proposals apply to the global CVD agenda.

One strategy for increasing the workforce is task-shifting. Examples of successful programs exist. The Integrated Management of Childhood Illnesses recently reported that quality of childcare was equivalent across several categories of health workers irrespective of the duration and level of pre-service training, thus demonstrating that task-shifting to less-specialized workers can yield equivalent results (Huicho et al., 2008). The use of nonphysician clinicians is notable for its lower training costs, shorter training periods, and increased placement in rural resource-deficient communities (Mullan and Frehywot, 2007). In addition, community health workers (CHWs) who are trusted, respected members of the community but do not have formal health training, have been used for decades in several areas of global health, and have proven beneficial in terms of community development, community health education, increased access to basic health services, cultural sensitivity, cost-effectiveness, and improvement in community self-reliance (Berman, 1984; Brownstein et al., 2005; Friedman et al., 2007; Lehman and Sanders, 2007; Prasad and Mulaleedharan, 2007). A review of work in the United States suggests that interventions for prevention and control of CVD can be effectively delivered by community health workers, which suggests that there may be potential for adapting this approach to develop CVD-specific strategies in low and middle income countries (Brownstein et al., 2005). In order to determine the optimal task-shifting policy and use of nonphysician clinicians to meet CVD-specific needs, it will be necessary to determine the optimal mix of specialization and training required to meet the CVD control challenge within individual countries. Successful adoption of such strategies to address the global CVD epidemic would require integrated reconfiguration of health systems with altered scopes of practice at all levels, enhanced training infrastructure, availability of reliable medium- to long-term funding for both training and employment incentives, and community input and participation (Lehmann et al., 2009).

Another strategy is to enhance the cultivation of leadership positions and enhance career development through the creation of academic training partnerships between institutions in high and low income countries. Examples of such successful academic partnerships exist, built upon the following principles: (1) leveraging the institutional resources and credibility of academic medical centers to provide the foundation to build systems of care with long-term sustainability; (2) development of a work environment that inspires personnel to connect with others, make a difference, serve those in great need, provide comprehensive care to restore healthy lives, and grow as a person and as a professional; and (3) training of health care workers at all levels (Einterz et al., 2007; Inui et al., 2007).

The train-the-trainer model is another strategy for increasing workforce capacity. These models have been used extensively for training in the infectious disease field, but the adaptation of chronic disease approaches in this area in developed countries to low and middle income settings remains largely an untapped opportunity. The National Heart, Lung, and Blood Institute (NHLBI), partnering with organizations like the National Council of La Raza and the U.S. Health Resources and Services Administration, has utilized this approach in its Promotora de Salud model for addressing CVD risk factors in high-risk Hispanic communities in the United States (Balcazar et al., 2005, 2009). Based on self-report, trained "promotores" obtained the knowledge and skills to recruit community members to participate, to pass on their knowledge gained, and to support community members in making changes in lifestyle that promote cardiovascular health (Balcazar et al., 2005).

In another example that could be expanded to meet chronic disease needs in developing countries, the U.S. Centers for Disease Control and Prevention (CDC) has developed Field Epidemiology and Lab Training Programs as part of its systems strengthening efforts in developing countries. To establish a training program, the CDC typically provides ministries of health with an in-country resident advisor for 4 to 6 years to help guide training and technical assistance (CDC, 2009b). Since 1992, the CDC's Management for International Public Health course has trained 379 management trainers from 68 countries. Graduates have trained thousands of public health professionals, who subsequently implemented hundreds of management and leadership improvement projects (CDC, 2009a).

A critical issue that will also need to be addressed in order to manage workforce capacity is health worker migration. Several authors have commented that health worker migration contributes to health worker shortages in low income countries and inequity in health care (Agwu and Llewelyn, 2009; O'Brien and Gostin, 2008). In fact, a system of "restitution" has been proposed, in which destination countries (generally high income countries) should compensate or reimburse the source countries (generally low income countries) (Mensah et al., 2005). One proposal to feasibly accomplish this is to shift development assistance toward building health systems in low income countries (O'Brien and Gostin, 2008). If this directed foreign aid assists in the development of sustainable, rewarding, and credible health care-related career pathways in low income countries, this may decrease the supply of migrant health workers. Analogously, in order to decrease the demand for health worker migration, one proposal has been to increase the national self-sufficiency of the high income country health workforce and reduce reliance on recruitment of migrant health workers from low income countries (O'Brien and Gostin, 2008). In the midst of this debate, WHO has drafted a code of practice that addresses the issue of health worker migration, emphasizing that "the development of voluntary international standards and the coordination of national policies on international health worker recruitment are desirable in order to maximize the benefits to and mitigate the potential negative impact on countries and to safeguard the rights of health workers" (WHO, 2008a, p. 1). While there is no current consensus on solutions to this issue, it deserves attention as the global community proceeds to address the global CVD epidemic.

Integration of Care Disease-specific programs have had success in many areas of global health, but as fragmentation occurs, the need for service integration is emerging. Although there are too few evidence-based examples of successful CVD programs in developing countries to be able to assess the effects of fragmentation, it has affected aspects of the management of other chronic diseases such as TB and HIV in some regions. Both fragmentation and duplication of services are likely to be risks if CVD programs are implemented using a similar disease-specific approach (WHO Maximizing Positive Synergies Collaborative Group, 2009).

Integration of different types of service delivery is currently gaining attention in developing countries as health systems capacity needs to be improved to address chronic *infectious* diseases. This has the potential to be valuable for addressing chronic noncommunicable diseases as well. However, the evidence for integrating care is not yet convincing. Operational research is needed to provide information about the relative costs and benefits of vertical versus integrated health delivery. A move toward integration of care delivery should recognize the benefits of starting with a strong delivery system and the compatibility of the intervention protocols being integrated (Wallace et al., 2009). This is the basis on which economies of scale have a higher probability of being realized.

Integration approaches need to be selected according to the health issues being addressed, the population being targeted, the urgency of the need for services, the capability of the health systems and other contextual factors. Necessary to the success of integrating programs is the support of government officials and key stakeholders; the avoidance of overburdening existing services; sufficient staff training to implement integration; staff workloads that can be managed to incorporate new responsibilities; overcoming discrimination; and factoring in initial costs (Taskforce on Innovative International Financing for Health Systems Working Group 1, 2009).

Also of important consideration when planning for integration of services are the needs for scale-up to the national level. These include political commitment, human resources, financing, coordinated program management, and effective decentralization (Taskforce on Innovative International Financing for Health Systems Working Group 1, 2009). Before the decision to expand programs is even made, the strength of the existing system and supports must be considered. After the existing system has been assessed, service integration can be phased in beginning with limited services at the community level and expanding gradually as services strengthen (Taskforce on Innovative International Financing for Health Systems Working Group 1, 2009).

Even though chronic disease prevention and treatment is becoming an increasingly important component of primary health care and primary health care is a growing area of emphasis on the global health agenda, there is limited evidence about how to effectively integrate care for chronic diseases into developing primary care systems (Beaglehole et al., 2008). Therefore, while integration is compelling in principle, there is still a need to develop and evaluate interventions to better integrate CVD with other care delivery programs, including maternal and child health programs and programs for prevention and management of chronic infectious diseases such as HIV/AIDS and TB.

In one example of an integrated care approach for chronic diseases, Médecins Sans Frontières (MSF) initiated an outpatient program in collaboration with the ministry of health of Cambodia that integrated diabetic and hypertension care in two hospital-based chronic disease clinics in rural high-prevalence, low-resource settings. The program featured standardized diagnosis and treatment protocols, multidisciplinary teams, and heavily subsidized care (Raguenaud et al., 2009). Compared to baseline values in the patient population, there were significant and clinically important mean improvements in glycemia and blood pressure that were sustained over the 5-year study period; however, a relatively low proportion of patients reached optimal treatment targets for diabetes control (Raguenaud et al., 2009). These results and the high loss to follow-up rate highlight the challenges of delivering diabetic care in rural, resource-limited settings.

Strategies to Change Structural Conditions Health care delivery can also be affected by changes in structural conditions. The Taskforce on Innovative International Financing for Health Systems (2009) recently considered potential mechanisms for structural changes as part of its review of approaches to support health systems strengthening. These changes can include approaches such as contracting, decentralization, adjusting the ratio of public and private provision of care and services, and innovative use of the private sector such as tailoring interventions to be implemented in non-health settings (Taskforce on Innovative International Financing for Health Systems Working Group 1, 2009).

Contracting can be employed by governments to, for example, subsidize the services of faith-based and other civil society providers or to contract with NGOs for their services. Government contracting with for-profit organizations has not been as extensively explored, although for-profits have been contracted for hospital and clinic management. Contracts can extend services quickly and to previously underserved areas and are often financed based on results. However, a contracting approach requires that governments must have the capacity to manage contracts and provide supervision. In addition, further study should be considered to explore the capacity of nonstate entities to provide large-scale, long-term services; the effects of introducing private contracts where public services already exist; the sustainability of contracts that depend on outside funding; and the implications of contracting out what might be regarded as core functions of the state (Taskforce on Innovative International Financing for Health Systems Working Group 1, 2009).

In one example in Cambodia, management of government health services was contracted out to NGOs in five selected districts that had randomly been made eligible for contracts that specified targets for improving maternal and child health services. The contracted services increased the availability of 24-hour service, reduced provider absence, and increased supervisory visits. The targeted outcomes improved relative to comparison districts, but changes in non-targeted outcomes were small. CVD-related health care activities were not measured in either set of outcomes. The program required increased public health funding, but this was roughly offset by reductions in private expenditure as residents in districts managed by the NGOs switched from unlicensed drug sellers and traditional healers to the provided clinics (Bloom et al., 2006).

Information Technology and E-Health[2]

Information is crucial for both clinical and public health practice. As described in Chapter 4, the use of electronic and mobile technologies is emerging in a range of global health contexts with the potential to be adapted or expanded to include chronic diseases. Investment in information and communication technology is an important potential component

---

[2] This section is based in part on a paper written for the committee by Alejandro Jadad.

of health care delivery for CVD and related chronic diseases. Electronic records are the focus of attention in industrialized countries and best practices are beginning to emerge (Fraser et al., 2005). Although challenging to implement, they hold potential for developing countries (Williams and Boren, 2008). In addition, communication technologies, such as mobile phones, are becoming increasingly common in developing countries (ITU, 2009) and are a potential mechanism to reach a wide representation of the population.

The importance of organized, efficient, and up-to-date information-gathering systems is illustrated by the experience of global HIV programs. Given the shared importance of long-term patient follow-up, the principles underlying successful developing country implementation of electronic records for HIV and TB care (Fraser et al., 2007) are quite relevant to CVD. OpenMRS, one example of an electronic medical records system for HIV/AIDS care in several countries in Sub-Saharan Africa, demonstrates the use of information technology for clinical care, treatment adherence optimization, coordination with laboratory results, strategic planning, reports to national and donor agencies, and research (Allen et al., 2007; OpenMRS, 2010). This type of platform and information architecture can be expanded to include data for CVD care (Braitstein et al., 2009). The OpenMRS experience also illustrats potential benefits to be gained from sharing intellectual and human resources across universities, institutions, and countries. Such types of open formats and open-source software will be crucial elements of the information and communication technology-related aspects of future public health programs (Reidpath and Allotey, 2009).

In addition to better management of information, communications technology offers new mechanisms to deliver interventions. A recent review aimed to determine the effectiveness of telehealth in CHD management (Neubeck et al., 2009). Eleven studies were reviewed that evaluated telephone, videoconference, or web-based interventions and provided objective measurements of mortality, changes in multiple risk-factor levels, or quality of life. Telehealth interventions were associated with significantly lower total cholesterol and systolic blood pressure, and fewer smokers. These results support the potential for telehealth interventions to be adapted for use to address CVD in developing-country settings.

There have been some examples of intervention approaches using mobile health (m-health) technology in low and middle income countries, in some cases with applications for chronic diseases. UKIERI's Mobile Disease Management System is a joint effort by engineers at universities in the United Kingdom and India. A monitoring system was developed that uses a mobile phone to collect up to four different physiological measures from patients, including electrocardiogram (ECG), blood pressure, oxygen saturation, and blood glucose level. These are relayed to health professionals for remote assessment (Jadad, 2009).

MDNet creates free mobile phone networks to facilitate communication among physicians within countries in Africa. MDNet Ghana created the first country-wide mobile network of doctors. This made the first country-wide directory of physicians available, allowing for the delivery of bulk text messages to all physicians in Ghana and improving country-wide emergency response capabilities and communication. MDNet Liberia was subsequently launched as a partnership among the Liberian Ministry of Health, the Liberian Medical & Dental Association, and the Liberian Medical Board. After less than a year, the free communication network already linked 100 percent of physicians in the country (Jadad, 2009).

FrontlineSMS is a free open-source software application that allows a laptop and a mobile phone to be used to create a central communications hub. The program, which has been successfully tested in Malawi, enables text messages to be sent and received among large groups of users through mobile phones, without an Internet connection or need for additional training. This communication allows for timely remote support among health care professionals. FrontlineSMS:Medic works with any existing plan on all Global System for Mobile Communications (GSM) phones, modems, and networks and can be used anywhere in the world simply by switching the cell phone's Subscriber Identity Module (SIM) card. Recently, FrontlineSMS:Medic has created a collaboration with Hope Phones, a U.S.-based nation-wide mobile phone collection campaign that supports m-health programs at medical clinics in more than 30 countries (Jadad, 2009).

Health Care Financing

The scope of financing health care delivery involves the following four components: (1) raising money, or raising revenue for health systems through general taxation and social insurance; community-based insurance; and private insurance; (2) pooling risk, which is the accumulation and management of revenue so that the risk of paying for health care is borne by all members of the pool (out-of-pocket payments are the least desirable method of pooling risk, yet are often a significant source of funding in low income countries); (3) purchasing services, which is how funds are allocated to lower levels of the health system, and how health providers are paid for the services they provide. This can be done through global budgets, capitation, fee-for-service, and specific incentive payments; and (4) financing the institutional framework of the health system (Taskforce on Innovative International Financing for Health Systems Working Group 1, 2009).

Health care financing in developing countries has some significant differences that make it less equitable, less efficient, and less certain than health financing in developed countries (Schieber et al., 2007; Taskforce on Innovative International Financing for Health Systems Working Group 1, 2009). Combining all sources, relatively little is spent on health in developing countries, far less than in richer countries. Taking into account variations in national data due to limitations in availability, reliability, and validity, WHO-standardized National Health Expenditure account data show that in 2006 low income countries spent, on average, 4.3 percent of gross domestic product (GDP) on health-related expenditures, lower-middle income countries 4.5 percent of GDP, upper-middle income countries 6.3 percent of GDP, and high income countries 11.2 percent of GDP (WHO, 2006). Instead of the social or private insurance systems or tax-funded systems of health care that prevail in developed countries, people in developing countries pay the bulk of their own health care expenses, and generally receive care from a mix of public and private settings—depending on their ability to pay and access. This section describes the sources of health care funding in developing countries, including donors, national governments, and individuals and households.

Global Donors Donor financing of health care is a significant share of total health expenditures in low income countries, much more so than in middle and high income countries. WHO reported that 17.2 percent of total health spending in low income countries came from external sources in 2006, an increase from 11.1 percent in 2000 (Figure 5.2) (WHO, 2006). This change over time reflects the rapidly rising amounts of external resources for health in recent years (Ravishankar et al., 2009).

National Governments and Health Systems National governments are fundamentally responsible for the health of their citizens and are the primary decision makers regarding health policy and resource allocations to health. However, national governments are not the primary financiers of health in poor countries. In low income countries, the public sector finances only 36.8 percent of all health care, compared to 61.6 percent in high income countries (WHO, 2006). Taxpayer-financed health care programs are more progressive than privately financed systems. A number of middle income developing countries—Chile, Mexico, Thailand, and others (Bastias et al., 2008; Frenk et al., 2009; Hu, 2010)—have created universal health insurance in part to help manage the financing needs of chronic conditions equitably.

The percentage of national health spending that goes to prevention, treatment, and care of CVD and related chronic diseases is not documented across countries. According to WHO's Global Survey on the Progress in National Chronic Disease Prevention and Control, 68 percent of responding countries reported having a specific budget for chronic disease pre-

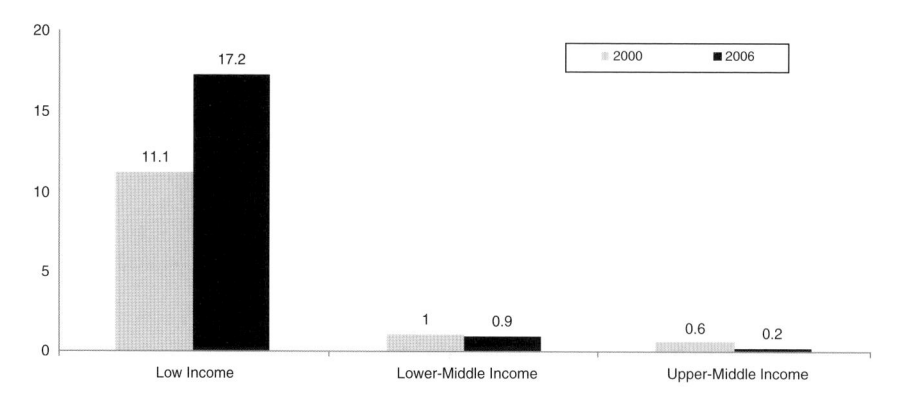

FIGURE 5.2 External resources as percentage of total expenditure on health.
SOURCE: World Health Organization National Health Accounts.

vention and control, ranging from a high of 83 percent in the South-East Asian region to a low of 58 percent in the African region (WHO, 2007b). Unfortunately, however, most developing countries do not maintain a sufficiently detailed national health account to allow national spending on CVD to be estimated.

Individuals and Households In developing-country settings, individual households bear the primary burden of financing health care needs beyond primary care because out-of-pocket spending is the predominant way that health care is financed. In a recent analysis of global health financing the average share of total health spending from out-of-pocket payments was 70 percent for low income countries, 43 percent for low-middle income countries, and 30 percent for upper-middle income countries. This was compared to 15 percent for high income countries (Scheiber et al., 2007).

The proportion of individual/household income spent on health care also varies markedly across low and middle income countries. In Nepal, on average, individuals spent 5.5 percent of their total per-capita expenditures on health (Hotchkiss et al., 1998), while in Guatemala, health expenditures are 16 percent of household income (McIntyre et al., 2006). Unofficial or "under the table" costs are an additional financial requirement placed on individuals in many low and middle income settings. In Bulgaria, unofficial payments were found to be common, averaging 21 percent of the minimum monthly salary for the country (Balabanova and McKee, 2002). In addition, lower income households generally pay more out-of-pocket for health care than wealthier households.

Knowledge is limited on the share of household health care costs spent specifically on cardiovascular disease in low and middle income countries, but it is known that costs to the patient and caregivers are very high for chronic and long-term illness. Much of the data about household health expenditures for chronic illness comes from studies of spending related to malaria and HIV/AIDS (Babu et al., 2002; Goudge et al., 2009a, 2009b; Hansen et al., 1998).

Chapter 3 described the economic effects on households and frequent impoverishment that results from health spending. The consistency of this finding across very disparate countries suggests a need for health financing to pay for persistent health expenditures (Somkotra et al., 2009). An example is Seguro Popular in Mexico, which has succeeded in improving access to health services and improving blood glucose levels for poor diabetics (Sosa-Rubi et al., 2009). Another informative example for the design of health financing schemes for CVD is the Philippines health insurance plan (PhilHealth). The plan does not cover outpatient medicines and is spending more than $56 million annually on inpatient care for hypertension. Most households cannot afford the repeated expense of pharmacologic therapy. An outpatient medicines benefit could be a very cost-effective option to reduce intensive treatment for hypertension and relieve the burden on households of choosing between antihypertensives and other essential needs (Wagner et al., 2008).

> ***Conclusion 5.3:*** *Reduction of biological risk factors such as elevated blood pressure, blood lipids, and blood glucose can reduce individual risk for CVD. However, implementation of these approaches requires an adequate health systems infrastructure, including a trained workforce and sufficient supplies with equitable access to affordable essential medicines and diagnostic, preventive, and treatment technologies. Many countries do not currently have sufficient infrastructural capacity. Current efforts to strengthen health systems in many low and middle income countries provide an opportunity to improve delivery of high-quality care to prevent and manage CVD, including chronic care approaches that are applicable to other chronic diseases and infectious diseases requiring chronic management, such as HIV/AIDS.*

Recommendation: Include Chronic Diseases in Health Systems Strengthening

Current and future efforts to strengthen health systems and health care delivery funded and implemented by multilateral agencies, bilateral public health and development agencies, leading international nongovernmental organizations, and national and subnational health authorities should include attention to evidence-based prevention, di-

agnosis, and management of CVD. This should include developing and evaluating approaches to build local workforce capacity and to implement services for CVD that are integrated with primary health care services, management of chronic infectious diseases, and maternal and child health.

Community-Based Intervention Approaches

Health behaviors and health status are influenced by many nonbiological factors, including economic, political, cultural, and socioeconomic factors (Schooler et al., 1997; Stokols, 1992, 1996). Health care focusing on the individual and relying primarily on clinical services provided by physicians can neither prevent most chronic disease nor reach the entire population in need. Therefore, efforts to change behavior and improve health will be more successful if they go beyond the individual to include family, social, and cultural contexts. A primary tenet of community prevention programs is the opportunity to intervene in multiple settings and domains, focusing on the interdependencies among environmental, social, and individual factors and the potential for public health strategies to interact with individual-level therapeutic and medical strategies (Farquhar and Fortmann, 2007; Kasl, 1980; Schooler et al., 1997; Shea and Basch, 1990a).

Community-based programs offer an opportunity to approximate the ideal multicomponent approach described at the beginning of this chapter by coordinating population-based policy and health communication and education strategies with intervention programs in local communities. Social norms and community attributes have an important impact on health. Governmental and private institutions in the community influence health behaviors by controlling, for example, health, recreational, and transportation services and youth access to tobacco. The health and safety policies and worksite health promotion practices of businesses can also affect health. Stores and restaurants also shape health when they determine what types of food to sell (Schooler et al., 1997).

Thus, the ideal program design would include programs established through worksites, schools, recreation sites, libraries, churches, local business organizations, and other sites in order to supplement and expand the effects of policy and health education approaches and appropriate delivery of health care. This broad reach into the community is advantageous because nearly all people in a community are at some level of risk for CVD and may benefit from interventions to encourage and reinforce healthful behavior, leading to potential population impact on highly prevalent risk factors. In fact, most CVD does not occur among the relatively few adults at highest risk, but rather than among the many at modeeate risk (Blackburn, 1983; Kottke et al., 1985; Puska et al., 1985; Schooler et al., 1997). Therefore, promotion of cardiovascular health has to happen at a population level and among people who may not be engaged with the health system or particularly motivated to reduce a possible distant risk of CVD.

While some behavior change reflects only an individual recognizing risk and deciding to reduce that risk, a population-wide impact may be more than the accumulation of individual risk assessments; rather, diffusion of behavior change may reflect a social process—individuals learning about new behaviors from neighbors, or individuals being encouraged to adopt new behaviors by people important to them in their social networks. This sort of social diffusion will likely result best from increasing opportunities to learn about and implement new behaviors, with an accompanying increase in social expectations for doing so. This requires building a surrounding environment that coherently and consistently favors behavior change. In addition to the policy changes and large-scale communications campaigns described earlier in this chapter, this total environmental change may be accomplished through the work of entrepreneurs recognizing a growing market and developing new products to accelerate behavior change, through workplaces that fund wellness programs, through schools that modify food available to children and require physical activity, and through programs in other settings in the community. Thus, the goal is to create a cascade of behavior change, and that may come from the synergistic interactive effects that can occur when individual components are embedded in a total community-based program campaign that encourages institutional change, leaves space for entrepreneurs, and includes mass media and environmental change (Schooler et al., 1997).

A multifactor community intervention approach also has the potential to act synergistically with clinical services rendered by physicians and other health professionals. Adherence to dietary and exercise advice from health care professionals may be easier to follow when family members, friends, and colleagues are aware of and are practicing some of the same principles. Motivation to adhere to medication regimens may also be easier when others in the patient's social network have also learned the importance, for example, of controlling blood pressure and blood lipids. Health professionals, and the sites of their practices, have the potential to contribute to the "total push" for better health by, for example, making print materials on health available and publicizing forthcoming health fairs and other events. Classes can be made available in hospital and other clinical settings. The local media can call upon local health professionals to speak and to contribute to the "health news."

In summary, comprehensive community-based efforts that include multiple types of interventions can be designed to modify the environment in ways that support healthy or inhibit unhealthy individual actions, to create organizational and institutional support for programs, and to influence the knowledge, attitudes, and behaviors of individuals (Schooler et al., 1997). However, it is important to take a pragmatic view on implementing community-based programs. There is good reason to be skeptical about investing in programs that rely on institutions for whom reducing the CVD burden is not central to their primary missions. For workplaces, schools, and community organizations the advantages may be abstractly logical as a way to reach people and provide needed services, but implementing these approaches is often not logical in practice, especially for long-term viability.

Community-level organizations may not be able to commit limited resources to programs over the long term if the incentives for doing so are weak and the interventions are complex to implement, manage, and maintain. The programs may dissipate even if there is early enthusiasm, and there is very little knowledge about what it will take to put such programs together and diffuse them on a large scale in low and middle income countries. For example, businesses that have insurance incentives to reduce smoking and obesity might invest in CVD prevention programs, but there is not a lot of precedent for long-term sustainability and effectiveness in high income countries—and the potential incentives for businesses in low and middle income countries are even less clear. Similarly, physical activity may be central in some schools, but schools may not be able to stay engaged if there is competition for limited resources with their primary academic mission. The infrastructure and capacity may be even more fragile in other less formalized community organizations.

CVD-Related Community-Based Programs in Low and Middle Income Countries

Although the evidence for successful implementation of multicomponent programs in community settings is reasonably strong in high income countries, it is weak in middle income countries and nearly absent in low income countries. Some community programs in middle income countries, because their efforts relied heavily on the use of mass media, were described earlier in this chapter, including programs in South Africa (Rossouw et al., 1993), Brazil (Matsudo, 2002), the Czech Republic (Komarek, 1995), and Poland (Ruszkowsk-Majzel and Drygas, 2005).

Another example of a "total country" effort in Mauritius, a middle income country, was also described previously because the effect was mainly due to a change in agriculture and food policy. Multiple approaches were organized with the goal of combating rising CVD risk factors, including mass media; fiscal and legislative measures; and widespread community, school, and workplace health education activities (Dowse et al., 1995; Hodge et al., 1996; Uusitalo et al., 1996). Total cholesterol fell due to a government-sponsored switch from palm to soybean oil. However, body weights rose and there were no other effects on CVD risk factors (Uusitalo et al., 1996). This is testimony to the fact that secular trends can overcome educational and organizational efforts to combat obesity and hypertension. The Mauritian investigators described their findings as highlighting "the difficulty of reversing the adverse effects of lifestyle change in rapidly modernizing countries" (Hodge et al., 1996, p. 137). This may be an example of the difficulty that many low and middle income countries will face during economic development, while CVD risk factors and CVD events are rising.

Potential Lessons from CVD-Related Community Trials in High Income Countries

The evidence for effective community-based programs in high income countries is mixed, and the reasons for success and failure can provide some useful lessons to inform the design of future efforts to adapt these programs for trials in low and middle income settings. A wave of successful community trials in the 1970s and 1980s in the United States, Finland, Australia, Switzerland, and Italy were described earlier in this chapter because, although they involved a number of intervention components, a dominance of broadcast and print mass media underlied their success in reducing smoking, blood pressure, and body weight. These were followed by five later high income country studies in the United States, Sweden, Holland, Denmark, and Germany that demonstrated only limited success. These studies included intervention components such as broadcast and print media, classes, clinical screening, community events, policy changes, school programs, and close involvement of civic and business leaders. These programs have all been described extensively elsewhere (Schooler et al., 1997) and therefore are not described in detail here. Rather this discussion focuses on the potential lessons learned that could inform the design of future interventions in low and middle income countries.

A key factor of success was the extent of the use of broadcast and print mass media. Indeed, one of the possible reasons for the lack of robust results in the Minnesota Heart Health Project and the Pawtucket Heart Health Project in Rhode Island (Carleton et al., 1995; Luepker et al., 1996) was the diversion of resources for education efforts into community events, school programs, and clinical screening, resulting in a relatively low use of broadcast media compared to the more successful Stanford and North Karelia projects (Farquhar et al., 1977; Puska et al., 1995). This reinforces an emphasis on health communications campaigns as a greater priority for intervention strategies to address CVD than other kinds of community programs, especially in the short term. In addition, the overall community effects were not materially improved with the addition of a high-risk component in the Three Community Study, the Australian study, nor the CORIS project in South Africa (Schooler et al., 1997).

Another factor of success is local community participation and support, which was exemplified in the Stanford Five City Project (Farquhar et al., 1990; Flora et al., 1993; Mittelmark et al., 1993). This may indicate that affinity and cooperation with local health and education resources is a predictor of both initial success and longer-term maintenance of an intervention. The successful Norsjo project in Sweden (Weinehall et al., 2001) and Hartslag-Limburg project in the Netherlands (Schuit et al., 2006), both of which made efforts to target low income residents, also show that local community support is important. Another important factor in these two projects was linkage to their excellent health care systems, which unfortunately in many low and middle income countries is not available.

Another characteristic of successful programs in high income countries is the length of the intervention. The Slangerup project in Denmark was of 1-year duration and led to no differences in classical risk factors between the intervention and control area (Osler and Jespersen, 1993), perhaps to be expected from the brevity and relatively low intensity of the interventions.

The "dose" and the likely cost of community interventions are especially important to consider in determining the feasibility of replicating an intervention design. However, there are many country-specific determinants for both so the information may have limited generalizability, and in any case it is rare for either of these to be reported except in very general terms. For the Stanford Five City Project, there were about 100 exposures per year for each adult from all varieties of educational experience for an intervention dose of about 5 hours of exposure for each adult per year (Farquhar et al., 1990). Of these, about 70 per year were from broadcast media, for less than 1 hour per year. In comparison, each adult's exposure to television advertising of all types during the early 1980s was estimated at 292 hours per year, of which one-third contained often misleading health-related content (Farquhar et al., 1990; Schooler et al., 1997). The yearly delivery cost during 5 years at the time, excluding research, was found to be close to $4 per capita per year (Farquhar et al., 1990). Therefore, both delivery costs and message exposure are relatively low for the result achieved, which was a 16 percent fall in total CHD risk (Farquhar et al., 1990). The previous Stanford Three Community Study also had a quite low-cost broadcast and print mass media approach, with a 23 percent net reduction in overall CVD risk (Schooler et al., 1997; Shea and Basch, 1990b).

These levels of estimated CVD risk reduction were comparable to that found in the first 5 years of the Finnish North Karelia project, which was later translated into a very large decrease in CVD events, including mortality. An assessment of the cost savings from the first 20 years of the project offers some sense of the potential for monetary returns from investments in well-designed and well-implemented community-based interventions (Puska et al., 2009). Given the very large drop in CVD in North Karelia, the proportional reduction in CVD-related costs within the province itself, a population of about 180,000, was estimated to be about $30 million for the 20th year (1992) alone (Puska et al., 2009). Although the Finnish authors warn that this is a "crude estimate," this would translate into a much larger total over all 20 years.

To determine feasibility for adaptation and replication it is also eminently desirable that maintenance and dissemination should follow the major effort of a demonstration project or intervention trial. Unfortunately, in high income countries it has been uncommon for health promotion to continue in force after the main research phase of CVD community-based interventions. Two major exceptions to this are found in the Stanford Five City Project and the NKP. In the former, the health department of Monterey County in Northern California, where the project occurred, was the major continuation force, and the county's political leadership was a critical supporter of this expansion. In the later years of the research phase, the health department began to support project activities, indicating a trend toward maintenance by the community. Thereafter, county activities moved into health promotion for all residents, with attention to chronic disease prevention needs and of the growing Hispanic population (Flora et al., 1993; Monterey County Health Department, 2007). A recent activity enlisted the local Mexican-American owners of 35 Taquerias to include healthier items on their menus, including a switch from lard to vegetable oils in their cooking (Hanni et al., 2009). Successes in the initial and subsequent health promotion activities have engendered continued support by the county's government, its residents, the voluntary health agencies, and the health system.

In the case of North Karelia, the ministry of health of Finland adopted and augmented the methods in a remarkable expansion throughout Finland, so both maintenance and dissemination occurred (Puska et al., 1995, 2009). Expansion began in earnest after the first 5 years of the project, when the national health authorities adopted the education methods and added major policy changes in agriculture (e.g., a switch to margarine from butter and from dairying to berry farming) and public health policy. The public enthusiasm in the province was also disseminated nation-wide (e.g., through the powerful housewives association "Martta"). The expansion was successful because the effects of the NKP in reducing CVD mortality were seen within 5 years, the economic benefits became clear to the nation's leaders, and the international acceptance of the lessons of North Karelia reinforced the Finnish government's support.

Therefore, maintenance is achieved in settings where public health institutions and their political leadership adopt and support continuation of health promotion methods. Such support is founded on demonstrated success in changing health patterns and in a common understanding of the science behind the need for change. Initiation by respected academic institutions, public awareness of the health problems being addressed, and enlightened leadership are essential.

Potential Lessons from Community-Based Programs Targeting HIV/AIDS in Low and Middle Income Countries

Community-based methods analogous to those used in high and middle income countries to target CVD have been used to target other outcomes in low and middle income countries, such as HIV/AIDS; this provides some reason for optimism regarding transferability of these approaches. These methods include community organizing and mobilizing, use of mass media for social marketing to total community populations, policy interventions, and reliance on the concept of diffusion of innovation.

As an example, after widespread media-based social marketing, condom sales in Zaire increased from fewer than 1 million per year in 1987 to more than 18 million in 1991 (Auerbach and Coates, 2000). Policy interventions also can effectively change social norms and behaviors to promote HIV prevention, as shown in the "100% Condom Program" initiated by the government of Thailand in 1990. This program made condom use mandatory in all brothels and was implemented in the community through partnerships among brothel owners, police, and public health clinics. Among sex workers there was a 90 percent increase in consistent condom use and a 75 percent decrease in sexually transmitted diseases. In addition, among military recruits, who frequent brothels, the prevalence of HIV infection declined from about 11 percent before to 6.7 percent after the policy change was enacted (Auerbach and Coates, 2000). The strategy of community organizing and mass media to mobilize at the community level has been effective in increasing condom sales and distribution in a variety of populations in Sub-Saharan Africa including truckers, urban and peri-urban adults, male miners, adolescents, and men and women seeking services for sexually transmitted infections. "Project Accept" used community mobilization to increase counseling and testing, thus increasing the rate of HIV testing, knowledge of status, and frequency of discussions about HIV. They did so through social marketing that increased adoption of needed innovations and fit the criteria of "diffusion theory" (Rogers, 1962). In one aspect of this type of intervention, Project Accept recruited indigenous opinion leaders as change agents to use their social networks to increase adoption (Khumalo-Sakutukwa et al., 2008).

As described in these examples, the community intervention strategies that have been important to the success of CVD community-based interventions in high income countries have been used successfully in HIV/AIDS interventions in developing countries. This is a strong indication that these strategies will be transferable to the design of CVD interventions that are appropriate to the culture present in any particular country.

Intervention Components Implemented in Community Settings in Low and Middle Income Countries

Although very few multicomponent community-based approaches have been reported in low and middle income countries, there have been some documented interventions that have been implemented and evaluated in trials in community facilities or in community settings in low and middle income countries. These are not comprehensive, multicomponent, community-based programs, but they are discussed here for their potential to offer lessons learned and to be considered as components or rationale for the design of future community-based programs.

A project in China targeted sodium intake, hypertension, and other CVD risk factors in the city of Tianjin (Nissinen et al., 2001; Tian et al., 1995; Yu et al., 1999, 2000). The intervention included activities such as health education and a community-based hypertensive management system with local health worker visits. Population surveys at a 7-year interval showed mixed effects on CVD risk factors, including blood pressure, smoking, and obesity (Yu et al., 1999, 2000). A specific sodium reduction project was also carried out within the Tianjin project. In collaboration with local health workers, lay people were trained to implement health education efforts, which included the door-to-door dissemination of nutrition information leaflets, posters and stickers at food retail stores, and health exhibitions. Other interventions included the distribution of smaller teaspoons to measure salt used in cooking and the availability of mineral salt in retail stores in the intervention areas. A comparison of geographically defined intervention areas to reference areas showed significant reductions over the 3-year project period in sodium intake in men and in systolic blood pressure in the total population (Tian et al., 1995).

Randomized trials in a rural community in China (The China Salt Substitute Study Collaborative Group, 2007) and in retirement homes in Taiwan (Chang et al., 2006) have also demonstrated effectiveness in salt reduction efforts. In the China Salt Substitute Study, participants were randomly assigned to replace their household salt with either the study salt substitute or normal salt for a 12-month period. At follow-up, systolic blood pressure was significantly lower in the salt-substitute group than in the normal salt group, with no differences in diastolic blood pressure (The China Salt Substitute Study Collaborative Group, 2007). In Taiwan, five kitchens of a veteran retirement home were randomized into two groups, and veterans assigned to those kitchens were given either potassium-enriched salt or regular salt for 31 months. The substitution of potassium-enriched salt reduced the CVD mortality hazard ratio to 60 percent that of the control group, and the experimental group had a longer life expectancy than did the control group. However, the authors note that the effect may primarily be due to the increase in potassium intake, because the sodium reduction achieved was moderate (Chang et al., 2006).

A small double-blind controlled trial in South Africa determined that the modification of salt in commonly consumed foods significantly lowered blood pressure in hypertensive participants of low socioeconomic status. In this 8-week study among 80 Cape Town residents aged 50-75 years with mild to moderate hypertension, the intervention group had five commonly consumed food items (brown bread, margarine, stock cubes, soup mixes, and flavor enhancer) with reduced sodium content and modified potassium, magnesium, and calcium content delivered to them. The control group was provided the same foods, but of standard commercial composition (Charlton et al., 2008). Results showed a significantly gre0ater reduction in blood pressure from baseline to post intervention in the intervention group compared to the control group (Charlton et al., 2008). The results of this study further support the positive effects of blood pressure reduction through consumption of products with modified salt contents. However, the short duration and small sample size of this study warrant considerations when generalizing results. In addition, the direct provision of food in this study is not likely to be feasible to replicate on a large scale.

A project on salt reduction from Ghana provides important lessons on intervention approaches delivered in community settings in a low income country (Cappuccio et al., 2006). The Ghana Salt Reduction Study was a project in which 12 villages were randomized into intervention and control. In each condition, half were rural and half semi-urban. Education was provided by indigenous health workers in 1-hour meetings in communal areas, weekly for 6 months. A small but significant reduction in diastolic blood pressure occurred, but without a between-group urinary sodium difference. However, an anticipated correlation was shown within all samples between urinary sodium and systolic blood pressure. Also, a significant difference between the rural and semi-urban samples occurred, with lower blood pressures in the rural villages. The major lesson is that in Sub-Saharan villages, including those without electricity or piped water, a moderately successful intervention can be mounted, probably at reasonably low cost. Initial commitment made through tribal leaders and village elders represented successful use of a method analogous to one of the initial steps in any successful high income country's community-based intervention. The results, although not robust, represent an example of successfully carrying out a community-based intervention trial that may have applicability in many Sub-Saharan locales and in other low income countries.

Another small randomized cross-over trial recently evaluated an education-based intervention in Jamaica and Nigeria. Individuals were allocated to either a low-salt diet or a high-salt diet with additional salt added to the participants' normal diet. This was followed by a washout period and a cross-over phase. During the low-salt phase, individuals were given case managers to provide information and counseling. Jamaican participants were also provided with low-sodium spices and were offered the option of purchasing specially prepared low-sodium food at their own expense (Forrester et al., 2005). The trial showed reductions in sodium intake and systolic blood pressure of an average of 5 mmHg in normotensive adults. However, this was a very brief and small study of only 114 participants with only 3 weeks on the low-sodium diet in the cross-over design (Forrester et al., 2005). Therefore, it is difficult to determine the feasibility of delivering the intervention more widely and the likelihood of longer-term adherence to the low-salt diet.

Principles to Guide Future Design and Evaluation of Community-Based Programs

Despite the strong rationale for the approach, there is very limited evidence demonstrating effectiveness and successful implementation of broad multicomponent community-based approaches to reduce CVD or risk for CVD in developing countries. The capacity for planned community organizing that favors reduction in CVD risk has been demonstrated, on a very limited scale, in middle income settings in China, Mauritius, and South Africa and in low income settings in Ghana, Jamaica, and Nigeria, although evidence for effectiveness was limited in these programs. In addition, mass media-based community interventions with community-level organization have succeeded in middle income countries, as described earlier in this chapter. However, these are diverse examples that make it difficult to extract any comprehensive findings to apply broadly. Lifestyles, such as tobacco use, dietary habits, and exercise patterns, are strongly influenced by custom and culture. In addition, resources and capacity can be quite limited and varied in developing-country communities. Therefore, based on the available documented evidence, multifactor community-based prevention approaches for CVD are not ready to be implemented widely at scale in developing countries.

However, three decades of trials of the "total community" health promotion approach for CVD prevention in high income settings support the potential feasibility of these approaches and the potential to result in significant changes in health habits of populations. Therefore, these approaches hold promise as a potential component of comprehensive approaches to address global CVD, and the critical next step is better setting-specific design and evaluation of demonstration projects and subsequent dissemination of these approaches. Transferability of the methods and components used in high income countries is not assured. However, theories of self-efficacy and common biological attributes, such as responses to nutrients and to nicotine, allow some prediction of transferability. The use of similar principles in successful HIV/AIDS interventions in developing countries is also a strong indication that these strategies will be transferable to the design of CVD interventions, with attention to message design and appropriateness to the culture specific to any particular country.

The methods for the design of the approaches in high income countries have been reviewed extensively elsewhere (Farquhar and Fortmann, 2007), and only a few key messages that relate to transferability to low and middle income country settings are repeated here. The steps needed to design and evaluate community-based programs include problem identification; organizing the community; planning, design, and implementation; evaluation; changes based on evaluation results; maintenance; and dissemination. Organizing and educating communities requires advocacy, activism, coalition building, and leadership. Regulatory change can enhance the success of community efforts. In addition, community-level efficacy that can result when the population gains self-efficacy through education can enhance capacity to change institutional policy and practice, thus maintaining community change. Theory and intervention methods matter, an adequate reach and duration of health communication is needed, and use of well-designed electronic and print media can provide education that is more cost-effective than that provided by more intensive classroom approaches. Intervention effectiveness requires formative evaluation, both before onset and during the intervention period. This ensures cultural appropriateness through tailoring and adapting messages to a particular community. A strong evaluation design is also critical, including assessments not only of outcomes but also of economic feasibility and implementation strategies, such as mobilizing communities and training interventionists.

Schools and Worksites

Schools and worksites have received particular attention as settings that offer an opportunity to implement prevention programs, whether implemented individually or as a synergistic part of the integrated approach described above. Therefore, these specific components are discussed separately here.

School-Based Interventions Schools provide one possible setting for delivering interventions to promote healthful eating and exercise in children. Health education programs that are integrated into academic curricula have a greater potential to be accepted by school administrators, teachers, parents, and students. School-based programs can also be readily incorporated into family-based and community-based chronic disease prevention projects that target a wide range of chronic disease risk factors in children and adults. Many schools have limited access to healthful foods and inadequate physical education facilities and hours. Thus, school-based programs can potentially have synergistic effects if physical education and classroom health education are implemented alongside broader changes in physical environment, food services, and policies.

School-based and other programs targeted to children and adolescents are discussed in full in Chapter 6. In summary, intensive, longer-term social influence-oriented programs have been effective to reduce tobacco use in youth. There is some evidence to support physical education-based approaches, school-environmental approaches, and integrated multicomponent approaches to increase physical activity and physical fitness among children. In addition, school-environment changes and policy-oriented approaches to improve diet and physical activity and reduce childhood obesity have been studied. Reducing sugar-sweetened beverages has promise to prevent childhood obesity, and reduction of screen time, especially TV watching, is a potential avenue to reduce childhood obesity, improve diet, and increase physical activity. There is little evidence that school-based programs significantly affect intermediate CVD risk factors such as blood pressure, blood lipids, or blood glucose.

Like many of the intervention components discussed in this chapter, it is very important to note that the vast majority of these studies were conducted in high income countries, with very little evidence from low and middle income countries. In addition, a number of methodological problems have hindered the interpretation of the results and the development of best practice recommendations in school-based interventions. These include small sample sizes, short duration, nonrandomized design, high attrition rate, lack of theoretical framework, low intervention intensity, inadequate assessment tools for diet, physical activity, and adiposity in children. There have also been no economic analyses of these intervention programs. Many of the interventions do not seem to have high resource requirements if a sufficient school infrastructure is already in place, so there is some potential for successful adaptation in settings that are analogous to the high income country settings in which these programs have been evaluated. However, evaluations of interventions adapted to local contexts are needed to inform future implementation of school-based approaches.

Workplace Interventions The workplace has historically been a common site of public health interventions. It will continue to be an important site for CVD prevention and health promotion activities in the context of the global spread of CVD. Several large corporations in developed countries, recognizing both the economic and social responsibility rationales, have initiated programs aimed at improving the health behaviors of their employees. In addition, several corporations in a variety of industries have instituted tobacco-free workplace policies, independent of local and state tobacco regulations. The World Economic Forum (WEF) and WHO (WHO and WEF, 2008) jointly produced a report that reviewed wellness-in-the-workplace programs targeting chronic disease risk factors.

The WEF/WHO report identified the following elements as critical to the success of workplace interventions: (1) establishing clear goals and objectives and linking health promotion programs to business objectives; (2) clear and strong support of the management; (3) adopting a multistakeholder approach and securing the involvement of government agencies and ministries, NGOs, trade unions, and employees at all levels of the corporation; (4) creating supportive environments; (5) adapting the intervention to social norms and building social support; and (6) considering incentives to foster adherence to the programs and improving self-efficacy of the participants.

The report found that such programs improve health, increase productivity, and reduce health care costs. Indeed, workplace interventions in diet, physical activity, and tobacco cessation are beneficial to both the employee and the employer. Such programs have been shown to reduce absenteeism, workers' compensation, and job stress and increase worker health and job satisfaction. In a review of worksite health promotion studies, Chapman (2003) reported a 27 percent average reduction in sick leave absenteeism, a 26 percent average reduction in health care costs, and a 32 percent average reduction in workers' compensation and disability claim costs. However, it should be noted that the majority of studies that have examined the effectiveness and the economic impact of workplace interventions have occurred in high income countries, and cost-effectiveness data for workplace interventions are still not largely available.

Muévete Bogotá is one of only a few examples of a well-documented program implemented in workplaces in a developing-country setting. This program seeks to increase physical activity by means of a media campaign coupled with programs aimed at changing behavior tied to physical activity (Gamez et al., 2006). The interventions within the program take place in various settings, but workplace interventions to promote physical activity are the program's main focus (Bauman et al., 2005). Muévete has been successful in gaining strong support of workplace managers through regular training and capacity-building sessions. Additionally, the program draws in and prepares partner companies for program implementation through advisory services. This approach has garnered the involvement of stakeholders such as the Secretary of Health of Bogotá, the Colombian Heart Association, the Colombian Diabetes Association, university departments, the Fundación FES Social/Bogotá, the U.S. Centers for Disease Control and Prevention, and the Pan American Health Organization (Gamez et al., 2006). Although process measures indicate successful implementation of the program, there has been little analysis of effects on levels of physical activity or on health outcomes (Bauman et al., 2005; Gamez et al., 2006). In addition, it is worth noting that although the program has been a model for programs throughout Latin America, considerations for transferability need to include the availability of adequate human resources and funding for interventions carried out by companies (Bauman et al., 2005).

Another example of a successful worksite intervention was recently described in India (Prabhakaran et al., 2009). A combination of individual- and population-based intervention activities, as well as health fairs and group motivational sessions, yielded superior results with respect to risk-factor control such as lipids, blood pressure, and waist circumference. Health-related behaviors such as tobacco use, fruit consumption, salt consumption, and physical activity all were better among the industrial groups who received the workplace intervention. Another workplace intervention in China's Capital Steel and Iron Company demonstrated benefits in health-related knowledge, salt intake, blood pressure, and stroke mortality. The intervention included strategies for health education and promotion as well as strategies for individual detection and management of hypertension (Chen et al., 2008).

In Malaysia, a quasi-experimental study was conducted among Malay-Muslim male security guards working in a public university in Kuala Lumpur (intervention group) and men working in the teaching hospital of the same university (comparison group). The intervention group members received intensive individual and group counseling on diet, physical activity, and quitting smoking and showed a significant reduction in their mean total cholesterol levels as compared with the comparison group at a 2-year follow-up. The intervention group also reported a reduction in the amount of cigarettes smoked (Moy et al., 2006). Although implemented in a limited population, this example is useful in demonstrating how the adoption of healthy behaviors can be incorporated into workplace policies.

There remain gaps in the current knowledge about the optimum workplace intervention characteristics, especially in low income countries. These include data on effectiveness of programs on risk-factor control, cost–benefit analysis of various programs and models, whether healthful behavior in the workplace translates into healthful behavior at home, and the impact on health outcomes such as myocardial infarction and stroke. In addition, practical issues still need to be clarified and resolved, such as the incorporation of diet and physical activity interventions in the workplace, development of validated instruments for diet and physical activity evaluation, cost-sharing agreements between government agencies and the private sector, and taking into account local cultural factors, size of businesses, and informal worksites (Leurent et al., 2008).

CONCLUSION

Risk for CVD can be modified through a combination of individual-level and population-level interventions. For some of these risk factors, reductions have been successfully achieved through health promotion and prevention programs in some countries and communities. Because of its broad determinants, it is clear that the prevention of CVD extends beyond the realm of the health sector. A coordinated approach at the governmental level is required so that policies in non-health sectors of government can be developed synergistically to promote, or at least not adversely affect, cardiovascular health. This is especially important for those sectors involved in agriculture, urban development, transportation, education, and in the private sector.

However, most policies and programs with evidence of effectiveness have been developed and implemented in high income countries. Even in high income countries little population-level progress has been made in some areas, such as obesity-related risk factors including total calorie consumption and reduction of sedentary behavior. Adaptations to the culture, resources, and capacities of specific settings are required for interventions to have an impact in low and middle income countries.

Reduction of risk for CVD through clinical interventions requires an adequate health systems infrastructure, including a trained workforce and sufficient supplies with equitable access to affordable essential medicines and diagnostic, preventive, and treatment technologies. Many countries do not currently have sufficient infrastructural capacity. Current efforts to strengthen health systems in many low and middle income countries provide an opportunity to improve delivery of high-quality care to prevent and manage CVD, including chronic care approaches that are applicable to other chronic diseases and infectious diseases requiring chronic management, such as HIV/AIDS.

Conclusion 5.4: Developing countries will want to focus efforts on goals that promise to be economically feasible, have the highest likelihood of intervention success, and have the largest morbidity impact. While priorities will vary across countries, the evidence suggests that substantial progress in reducing CVD can be made in the near term through a prioritized subset of goals and intervention approaches, including tobacco control, reduction of salt in the food supply and in consumption, and improved delivery of clinical prevention using pharmaceutical interventions in high-risk patients. Many countries will want to focus their efforts on achieving these goals on the grounds that they have limited financial and human resources and political energy to allocate to CVD programming, that the evidence for lowered CVD morbidity associated with achieving these goals is credible, and that there are examples of successful implementation of programs in each of these focus areas with the potential to be adapted for low and middle income countries.

Local context matters enormously for the planning and implementation of any of the approaches to prevent and manage CVD described in this chapter. Context also influences the effectiveness of these approaches. While there are common needs and priorities across settings, each site has its own specific needs that require evaluation. Knowledge needs to be developed on how to implement programs with proven effectiveness in settings where resources of all types are scarce, where priorities remain fixed on other health and development agendas, and where there might be cultural and influences vary. Implementation and translational research will be critical to develop and evaluate interventions in the settings in which they are intended to be implemented.

REFERENCES

Accenture. 2010. *High performance in a volatile world: Seven imperatives for acheiving dynamic supply chains.* https://microsite.accenture.com/management_consulting/dynamic-supply-chains/Pages/default.aspx (accessed February 3, 2010).
Adult Treatment Panel III. 2002. *Detection, evaluation, and treatment of high blood cholesterol in adults: Final report.* Bethesda, MD: National Institutes of Health.
Agwu, K., and M. Llewelyn. 2009. Compensation for the brain drain from developing countries. *Lancet* 373(9676):1665-1666.
Allen, C., D. Jazayeri, J. Miranda, P. G. Biondich, B. W. Mamlin, B. A. Wolfe, C. Seebregts, N. Lesh, W. M. Tierney, and H. S. Fraser. 2007. Experience in implementing the OpenMRS medical record system to support HIV treatment in Rwanda. *Studies in Health Technology and Informatics* 129(Pt 1):382-386.
Altman, D. G., J. A. Flora, S. P. Fortmann, and J. W. Farquhar. 1987. The cost-effectiveness of three smoking cessation programs. *American Journal of Public Health* 77(2):162-165.
Andersson, K., G. Bergstrom, M. G. Petzold, and A. Carlsten. 2007. Impact of a generic substitution reform on patients' and society's expenditure for pharmaceuticals. *Health Policy* 81(2-3):376-384.
Angell, S. Y., L. D. Silver, G. P. Goldstein, C. M. Johnson, D. R. Deitcher, T. R. Frieden, and M. T. Bassett. 2009. Cholesterol control beyond the clinic: New York City's trans fat restriction. *Annals of Internal Medicine* 151(2):129-134.

Asfaw, A. 2006. Do government food prices affect the prevalence of obesity? Empirical evidence from Egypt. *World Development* 35(4):687-701.
Auerbach, J., and T. Coates. 2000. HIV prevention research: Accomplishments and challenges for the third decade of AIDS. *American Journal of Public Health* 90(7):1029-1032.
Babu, B. V., A. N. Nayak, K. Dhal, A. S. Acharya, P. K. Jangid, and G. Mallick. 2002. The economic loss due to treatment costs and work loss to individuals with chronic lymphatic filariasis in rural communities of Orissa, India. *Acta Tropica* 82(1):31-38.
Bahit, M., C. Granger, K. Alexander, J. Kramer, et al. 2000. Applying the evidence: Opportunity in U.S. for 80,000 additional lives saved per year (abstract). *Circulation* 102(Suppl 2).
Balabanova, D., and M. McKee. 2002. Understanding informal payments for health care: The example of Bulgaria. *Health Policy* 62(3):243-273.
Balcazar, H., M. Alvarado, M. L. Hollen, Y. Gonzalez-Cruz, and V. Pedregon. 2005. Evaluation of salud para su corazon (health for your heart)—national council of La Raza promotora outreach program. *Preventing Chronic Disease* 2(3):A09.
Balcazar, H., M. Alvarado, F. Cantu, V. Pedregon, and R. Fulwood. 2009. A promotora de salud model for addressing cardiovascular disease risk factors in the U.S.-Mexico border region. *Preventing Chronic Disease* 6(1):A02.
Bandura, A., D. Ross, and S. A. Ross. 1963. Imitation of film-mediated agressive models. *Journal of Abnormal and Social Psychology* 66:3-11.
Bannink, L., S. Wells, J. Broad, T. Riddell, and R. Jackson. 2006. Web-based assessment of cardiovascular disease risk in routine primary care practice in New Zealand: The first 18,000 patients (predict CVD-1). *New Zealand Medical Journal* 119(1245):U2313.
Barrera, A. Z., E. J. Pérez-Stable, K. L. Delucchi, and R. F. Muñoz. 2009. Global reach of an internet smoking cessation intervention among spanish- and english-speaking smokers from 157 countries. *International Journal of Environmental Research and Public Health* 6(3):927-940.
Basinga, P., P. Gertler, A. Binagwaho, A. Soucat, J. Sturdy, and C. Vermeersch. 2009. Impact of paying primary health care centers for performance in Rwanda. Washington, DC: World Bank.
Bastias, G., T. Pantoja, T. Leisewitz, and V. Zárate. 2008. Health care reform in Chile. *Canadian Medical Association Journal* 179(12):1289-1292.
Bauman, A., S. Schoeppe, and M. Lewicka. 2005. Review of best practice in interventions to promote physical activity in developing countries: Background document prepared for the WHO workshop on physical activity and public health. Edited by T. Armstrong, V. Candeias, and J. Richards. Geneva: World Health Organization.
Beaglehole, R., J. Epping-Jordan, V. Patel, M. Chopra, S. Ebrahim, M. Kidd, and A. Haines. 2008. Improving the prevention and management of chronic disease in low-income and middle-income countries: A priority for primary health care. *Lancet* 372(9642): 940-949.
Berman, P. A. 1984. Village health workers in Java, Indonesia: Coverage and equity. *Social Science and Medicine* 19(4):411-422.
Bertrand, J. T., K. O'Reilly, J. Denison, R. Anhang, and M. Sweat. 2006. Systematic review of the effectiveness of mass communication programs to change HIV/AIDS-related behaviors in developing countries. *Health Education Research* 21(4):567-597.
Bjorkman, M., and J. Svensson. 2007. *Power to the people: Evidence from a randomized field experiment of a community-based monitoring project in Uganda*. Washington, DC: World Bank.
Blackburn, H. 1983. Research and demonstration projects in community cardiovascular disease prevention. *Journal of Public Health Policy* 4(4):398-421.

Bloom, E., E. King, I. Bhushan, M. Kremer, D. Clingingsmith, B. Loevinsohn, R. Hong, and J. B. Schwartz. 2006. Contracting for health: Evidence from Cambodia. Unpublished working paper. Washington, DC: Brookings Institution.

Boberg, E. W., D. H. Gustafson, R. P. Hawkins, C.-L. Chan, E. Bricker, S. Pingree, H. Berhe, and A. Peressini. 1995. Development, acceptance, and use patterns of a computer-based education and social support system for people living with AIDS/HIV infection. *Computers in Human Behavior* 11(2):289-311.

Bodenheimer, T., E. H. Wagner, and K. Grumbach. 2002. Improving primary care for patients with chronic illness. *JAMA* 288(14):1775-1779.

Borght, S. V. D., V. Janssens, M. S. V. D. Loeff, A. Kajemba, H. Rijckborst, J. Lange, and T. R. D. Wit. 2009. The accelerating access initiative: Experience with a multinational workplace programme in Africa. *Bulletin of the World Health Organization* 87:794-798.

Braitstein, P., R. M. Einterz, J. E. Sidle, S. Kimaiyo, W. Tierney, P. Braitstein, R. M. Einterz, J. E. Sidle, S. Kimaiyo, and W. Tierney. 2009. "Talkin' about a revolution": How electronic health records can facilitate the scale-up of HIV care and treatment and catalyze primary care in resource-constrained settings. *Journal of Acquired Immune Deficiency Syndromes* 52(Suppl 1):S54-S57.

Breckenkamp, J., U. Laaser, and S. Meyer. 1995. The German cardiovascular prevention study: Social gradient for the net effects in the prevention of hypercholesterolemia. *Zeitschrift fur Kardiologie* 84(9):694-699.

Breslow, L., and M. Johnson. 1993. California's Proposition 99 on tobacco, and its impact. *Annual Review of Public Health* 14:585-604.

Brook, R. D. 2008. Cardiovascular effects of air pollution. *Clinical Science* 115(5-6):175-187.

Brown, E., and M. Jacobson. 2005. *Cruel oil: How palm oil harms health, rainforest & wildlife*. Washington, DC: Center for Science in the Public Interest.

Brownell, K. D., and T. R. Frieden. 2009. Ounces of prevention: The public policy case for taxes on sugared beverages. *New England Journal of Medicine* 860(18):1805-1808.

Brownstein, J. N., L. R. Bone, C. R. Dennison, M. N. Hill, M. T. Kim, and D. M. Levine. 2005. Community health workers as interventionists in the prevention and control of heart disease and stroke. *American Journal of Prevention* 29(551):128-133.

Brugts, J. J., T. Yetgin, S. E. Hoeks, A. M. Gotto, J. Shepherd, R. G. J. Westendorp, A. J. M. de Craen, R. H. Knopp, H. Nakamura, P. Ridker, R. van Domburg, and J. W. Deckers. 2009. The benefits of statins in people without established cardiovascular disease but with cardiovascular risk factors: Meta-analysis of randomised controlled trials. *British Medical Journal* 338:b2376.

Bump, J. B., M. R. Reich, O. Adeyi, and S. Khetrapal. 2009. *Towards a political economy of tobacco control in low- and middle-income countries*. Washington, DC: World Bank.

Cameron, A., M. Ewen, D. Ross-Degnan, D. Ball, and R. Laing. 2009. Medicine prices, availability, and affordability in 36 developing and middle-income countries: A secondary analysis. *Lancet* 373(9659):240-249.

Campbell, S. M., D. Reeves, E. Kontopantelis, B. Sibbald, and M. Roland. 2009. Effects of pay for performance on the quality of primary care in England. *New England Journal of Medicine* 361(4):368-378.

Canadian Hypertension Education Program. 2009. *2009 CHEP recommendations for the management of hypertension* http://hypertension.ca/chep/wp-content/uploads/2009/04/09-complete-recs.pdf (accessed December 10, 2009).

Cappuccio, F. P., S. M. Kerry, F. B. Micah, J. Plange-Rhule, and J. B. Eastwood. 2006. A community programme to reduce salt intake and blood pressure in Ghana. *BMC Public Health* 6:13.

Carleton, R. A., T. M. Lasater, A. R. Assaf, H. A. Feldman, and S. McKinlay. 1995. The Pawtucket heart health program: Community changes in cardiovascular risk factors and projected disease risk. *American Journal of Public Health* 85(6):777-785.

Cash, S., D. Sunding, and D. Zilberman. 2005. Fat taxes and thin subsidies: Prices, diet, and health outcomes. *Acta Agriculturae Scandinavica, Section C—Economy* 2:167-174.

CDC (U.S. Centers for Disease Control and Prevention). 2003. *Promising practices in chronic disease prevention and control: A public health framework for action*. Atlanta, GA: Department of Health and Human Services.

CDC. 2009a. *Capacity and development news: Working together for a healthier world*. Spring 2009 Newsletter. Atlanta, GA: CDC.

CDC. 2009b. *Division of Global Public Health and Capacity Development 2008 Field Epidemiology Training Program*. Atlanta, GA. Washington, DC: U.S. Department of Health and Human Services.

Chang, H.-Y., Y.-W. Hu, C.-S. J. Yue, Y.-W. Wen, W.-T. Yeh, L.-S. Hsu, S.-Y. Tsai, and W.-H. Pan. 2006. Effect of potassium-enriched salt on cardiovascular mortality and medical expenses of elderly men. *American Journal of Clinical Nutrition* 83(6):1289-1296.

Chapman, L. 2003. Meta evaluation of worksite health promotion economic return studies. *Art of Health Promotion* 6(5):1-16.

Charlton, K. E., K. Steyn, N. S. Levitt, N. Peer, D. Jonathan, T. Gogela, K. Rossouw, N. Gwebushe, and C. J. Lombard. 2008. A food-based dietary strategy lowers blood pressure in a low socio-economic setting: A randomised study in South Africa. *Public Health Nutrition* 11(12):1397-1406.

Chen, C., and F. C. Lu. 2004. The guidelines for prevention and control of overweight and obesity in Chinese adults. *Biomedical and Environmental Sciences* 17 Suppl:1-36.

Chen, J., X. Wu, and D. Gu. 2008. Hypertension and cardiovascular diseases intervention in the Capital Steel and Iron Company and Beijing Fangshan community. *Obesity Review* 9 (Suppl 1):142-145.

Chen, L., T. Evans, S. Anand, J. I. Boufford, H. Brown, M. Chowdhury, M. Cueto, L. Dare, G. Dussault, G. Elzinga, E. Fee, D. Habte, P. Hanvoravongchai, M. Jacobs, C. Kurowski, S. Michael, A. Pablos-Mendez, N. Sewankambo, G. Solimano, B. Stilwell, A. de Waal, and S. Wibulpolprasert. 2004. Human resources for health: Overcoming the crisis. *Lancet* 364(9449):1984-1990.

The China Salt Substitute Study Collaborative Group. 2007. Salt substitution: A low-cost strategy for blood pressure control among rural Chinese. A randomized, controlled trial. *Journal of Hypertension* 25(10):2011-2018.

Clarke, D., and T. McKenzie. 2007. *Legislative interventions to prevent and decrease obesity in Pacific Island countries: Report prepared for WHO Western Pacific Regional Office*. Geneva: WHO.

Committee for Revision of Chinese Guidelines for Prevention and Treatment of Patients with Hypertension. 2005. Chinese guidelines for prevention and treatment of patients with hypertension [in Chinese]. *Chinese Journal of Hypertension* 134:2-41.

Committee on the State of the USA Health Indicators. 2009. *State of the USA Health Indicators: Letter report*. Washington, DC: The National Academies Press.

Cooper, R. S., C. N. Rotimi, J. S. Kaufman, W. F. Muna, and G. A. Mensah. 1998. Hypertension treatment and control in Sub-Saharan Africa: The epidemiological basis for policy. *British Medical Journal* 316(7131):614-617.

Council of Supply Chain Management Professionals. 2010. *Council of Supply Chain Management Professionals*. http://cscmp.org/ (accessed February 3, 2010).

Crisp, N., B. Gawanas, and I. Sharp. 2008. Training the health workforce: Scaling up, saving lives. *Lancet* 371(9613):689-691.

da Costa, L. M., and S. Goldfarb. 2003. Government Leadership in Tobacco Control: Brazil's Experience. In *Tobacco control policy: Strategies, successes, and setbacks*, edited by J. de Beyer and L. W. Brigden. Washington, DC: The World Bank and The International Development Research Centre.

de Beyer, J., and L. W. Brigden, eds. 2003. *Tobacco control policy: Strategies, successes, and setbacks*. Washington, DC: World Bank and International Development Research Centre.

Devers, K. J., H. H. Pham, and G. Liu. 2004. What is driving hospitals' patient-safety efforts? *Health Affairs* 23(2):103-115.

Donabedian, A. 1988. The quality of care: how can it be assessed? *Journal of the American Medical Association* 260(12):1743-1748.

Donatelle, R. J., S. L. Prows, D. Champeau, and D. Hudson. 2000. Randomised controlled trial using social support and financial incentives for high risk pregnant smokers: Significant other supporter (SOS) program. *Tobacco Control* 9(90003):67-69.

Dowse, G. K., H. Gareeboo, K. G. Alberti, P. Zimmet, J. Tuomilehto, A. Purran, D. Fareed, P. Chitson, and V. R. Collins. 1995. Changes in population cholesterol concentrations and other cardiovascular risk factor levels after five years of the non-communicable disease intervention programme in Mauritius. Mauritius Non-communicable Disease Study Group. *British Medical Journal* 311(7015):1255-1259.

Drewnowski, A. 2004. Obesity and the food environment: Dietary energy density and diet costs. *American Journal of Preventive Medicine* 27(3 Suppl):154-162.

Ebrahim, S., A. Beswick, M. Burke, and G. Davey Smith. 2006. Multiple risk factor interventions for primary prevention of coronary heart disease. *Cochrane Database of Systematic Reviews* (4):CD001561.

Efroymson, D., and S. Ahmed. 2003. Building momentum for tobacco control: The case of Bangladesh. In *Tobacco control policy: Strategies, successes, and setbacks*, edited by J. de Beyer and L. W. Brigden. Washington, DC: The World Bank and The International Development Research Center.

Eichler, R., R. Levine, and the Performance-Based Incentives Working Group. 2009. *Performance incentives for global health: Potential and pitfalls*. Washington, DC: Center for Global Development.

Einterz, R. M., S. Kimaiyo, H. N. Mengech, B. O. Khwa-Otsyula, F. Esamai, F. Quigley, and J. J. Mamlin. 2007. Responding to the HIV pandemic: The power of an academic medical partnership. *Academic Medicine* 82(8):812-818.

Emery, S. L., G. Szczypka, L. M. Powell, and F. J. Chaloupka. 2007. Public health obesity-related T.V. advertising: Lessons learned from tobacco. *American Journal of Preventive Medicine* 33(4 Suppl):S257-S263.

Epstein, A. M. 2007. Pay for performance at the tipping point. *New England Journal of Medicine* 356(5):515-517.

Evans, M., R. C. Sinclair, C. Fusimalohi, and V. Liava'a. 2001. Globalization, diet, and health: An example from Tonga. *Bulletin of the World Health Organization* 79:856-862.

Faber, M. P., M. M. Bosch, H. M. D. P. Wollersheim, S. P. Leatherman, and R. P. Grol. 2009. Public reporting in health care: How do consumers use quality-of-care information?: A systematic review. *Medical Care* 47(1):1-8.

Faeh, D., J. William, L. Tappy, E. Ravussin, and P. Bovet. 2007. Prevalence, awareness and control of diabetes in the Seychelles and relationship with excess body weight. *BMC Public Health* 7:163.

Farquhar, J., and S. Fortmann. 2007. Community-based health promotion. In *Handbook of epidemiology*. Vol. 11. Edited by W. Ahrens and I. Peugot. Berlin Heidelberg: Springer-Verlag. Pp. 1306-1321.

Farquhar, J. W., N. Maccoby, P. D. Wood, J. K. Alexander, H. Breitrose, B. W. Brown, Jr., W. L. Haskell, A. L. McAlister, A. J. Meyer, J. D. Nash, and M. P. Stern. 1977. Community education for cardiovascular health. *Lancet* 1(8023):1192-1195.

Farquhar, J. W., S. P. Fortmann, J. A. Flora, C. B. Taylor, W. L. Haskell, P. T. Williams, N. Maccoby, and P. D. Wood. 1990. Effects of communitywide education on cardiovascular disease risk factors. The Stanford Five-City Project. *Journal of the American Medical Association* 264(3):359-365.

Feachem, R. G., N. K. Sekhri, and K. L. White. 2002. Getting more for their dollar: A comparison of the NHS with California's Kaiser Permanente. *British Medical Journal* 324(7330):135-141.

Fernald, L. C., P. J. Gertler, and X. Hou. 2008a. Cash component of conditional cash transfer program is associated with higher body mass index and blood pressure in adults. *Journal of Nutrition* 138(11):2250-2257.

Fernald, L. C. H., P. J. Gertler, and L. M. Neufeld. 2008b. Role of cash in conditional cash transfer programmes for child health, growth, and development: An analysis of Mexicos oportunidades. *Lancet* 371(9615):828-837.

Fichtenberg, C. M., and S. A. Glantz. 2000. Association of the California tobacco control program with declines in cigarette consumption and mortality from heart disease. *New England Journal of Medicine* 343(24):1772-1777.

Flora, J. A., R. C. Lefebvre, D. M. Murray, E. J. Stone, A. Assaf, M. B. Mittelmark, and J. R. Finnegan, Jr. 1993. A community education monitoring system: Methods from the Stanford Five-City Project, the Minnesota Heart Health Program and the Pawtucket Heart Health Program. *Health Education Research* 8(1):81-95.

Forrester, T., A. Adeyemo, S. Soarres-Wynter, L. Sargent, F. Bennett, R. Wilks, A. Luke, E. Prewitt, H. Kramer, and R. S. Cooper. 2005. A randomized trial on sodium reduction in two developing countries. *Journal of Human Hypertension* 19(1):55-60.

Fraser, H., P. Biondich, B. Mamlin, et al. 2005. Deploying electronic medical record systems in developing countries. *Primary Care Informatics* 13:88-95.

Fraser, H., C. Allen, C. Bailey, G. Douglas, S. Shin, and J. Blaya. 2007. Information systems for patient follow-up and chronic management of HIV and tuberculosis: A life-saving technology in resource-poor areas. *Journal of Medical Internet Research* 9(4):e29.

Frenk, J., O. Gomez-Dantes, and F. M. Knaul. 2009. The democratization of health in Mexico: Financial innovations for universal coverage. *Bulletin of the World Health Organization* 87(7):542-548.

Frieden, T. R., and M. R. Bloomberg. 2007. How to prevent 100 million deaths from tobacco. *Lancet* 369(9574):1758-1761.

Fung, C. H., Y.-W. Lim, S. Mattke, C. Damberg, and P. G. Shekelle. 2008. Systematic review: The evidence that publishing patient care performance data improves quality of care. *Annals of Internal Medicine* 148(2):111-123.

Fuster, V., ed. 2009. *The AHA guidelines and scientific statements handbook*. Sussex, UK: Wiley-Blackwell.

Gajalakshmi, V., R. Peto, T. S. Kanaka, P. Jha, V. Gajalakshmi, R. Peto, T. S. Kanaka, and P. Jha. 2003. Smoking and mortality from tuberculosis and other diseases in India: Retrospective study of 43,000 adult male deaths and 35,000 controls.[see comment]. *Lancet* 362(9383):507-515.

Gamez, R., D. Parra, M. Pratt, and T. L. Schmid. 2006. Muévete Bogotá: Promoting physical activity with a network of partner companies. *Promotion et Education* 13(2):138-143, 164-169.

Genest, J., R. McPherson, J. Frohlich, T. Anderson, N. Campbell, A. Carpentier, P. Couture, R. Dufour, G. Fodor, G. A. Francis, S. Grover, M. Gupta, R. A. Hegele, D. C. Lau, L. Leiter, G. F. Lewis, E. Lonn, G. B. Mancini, D. Ng, G. J. Pearson, A. Sniderman, J. A. Stone, and E. Ur. 2009. 2009 Canadian Cardiovascular Society/Canadian guidelines for the diagnosis and treatment of dyslipidemia and prevention of cardiovascular disease in the adult—2009 recommendations. *Canadian Journal of Cardiology* 25(10):567-579.

Giné, X., D. Karlan, and J. Zinman. 2008. Put your money where your butt is: A commitment contract for smoking cessation. Washington, DC: World Bank.

Giuffrida, A., and D. J. Torgerson. 1997. Should we pay the patient? Review of financial incentives to enhance patient compliance. *British Medical Journal* 315(7110):703-707.

The Global Fund (The Global Fund to Fight AIDS, Tuberculosis and Malaria). 2009. *Guidelines to the Global Fund's policies on procurement and supply management*. Geneva: The Global Fund to Fight AIDS, Tuberculosis and Malaria.

Global Health Workforce Alliance. no date. Highlights. http://www.who.int/workforcealliance/en/ (accessed August 27, 2009).

Goldman, L., and S. Glantz. 1998. Evaluation of antismoking advertising campaigns. *Journal of the American Medical Association* 279(10):772-777.

Gooch, L. 2009. Success of palm oil brings plantations under pressure to preserve habitats. *The New York Times*, September 18.

Goudge, J., L. Gilson, S. Russell, T. Gumede, and A. Mills. 2009a. Affordability, availability and acceptability barriers to health care for the chronically ill: Longitudinal case studies from South Africa. *BMC Health Services Research* 9:75.

Goudge, J., L. Gilson, S. Russell, T. Gumede, and A. Mills. 2009b. The household costs of health care in rural South Africa with free public primary care and hospital exemptions for the poor. *Tropical Medicine and International Health* 14(4):458-467.

Goyal, A., and S. Yusuf. 2006. The burden of cardiovascular disease in the Indian subcontinent. *Indian Journal of Medical Research* 124(3):235-244.

Grabowsky, T. A., J. W. Farquhar, K. R. Sunnarborg, V. S. Bales, and Stanford University School of Medicine. 1997. *Worldwide efforts to improve heart health: A follow-up to the Catalonia Declaration—selected program descriptions*. http://www.international hearthealth.org/Publications/catalonia.pdf (accessed February 5, 2009).

Graham, I., D. Atar, K. Borch-Johnsen, G. Boysen, G. Burell, R. Cifkova, J. Dallongeville, G. D. Backer, S. Ebrahim, B. Gjelsvikg, C. Herrmann-Lingen, A. Hoes, S. Humphries, M. Knapton, J. Perk, S. G. Priori, K. Pyorala, Z. Reiner, L. Ruilope, S. Sans-Menendez, W. S. O. Reimer, P. Weissberg, D. Woods, J. Yarnell, and J. L. Zamorano. 2007. European guidelines on cardiovascular disease prevention in clinical practice: Fourth joint task force of the European Society of Cardiology and other societies on cardiovascular disease prevention in clinical practice. *European Journal of Cardiovascular Prevention and Rehabilitation* 14(Suppl 2):S1-S113.

Greiser, E. 1993. Risk factor trends and cardiovascular mortality risk after 3.5 years of community-based intervention in the German cardiovascular prevention study. *Annals of Epidemiology* 3:S13-S27.

Grimshaw, J. M., R. E. Thomas, G. MacLennan, C. Fraser, C. R. Ramsay, L. Vale, P. Whitty, M. P. Eccles, L. Matowe, L. Shirran, M. Wensing, R. Dijkstra, and C. Donaldson. 2004. Effectiveness and efficiency of guideline dissemination and implementation strategies. *Health Technology Assessment* 8(6):iii-iv, 1-72.

Grossbart, S. R. 2006. What's the return? Assessing the effect of "pay-for-performance" initiatives on the quality of care delivery. *Medical Care Research and Review* 63(Suppl 1):29S-48S.

Gwatkin, D. R., A. Bhuiya, and C. G. Victora. 2004. Making health systems more equitable. *Lancet* 364(9441):1273-1280.

Hanni, K. D., E. Garcia, C. Ellemberg, and M. Winkleby. 2009. Steps to a healthier Salinas: Targeting the taqueria: Implementing healthy food options at Mexican American restaurants. *Health Promotion Practice* 10(Suppl 2):91S-99S.

Hansen, K., G. Woelk, H. Jackson, R. Kerkhoven, N. Manjonjori, P. Maramba, J. Mutambirwa, E. Ndimande, and E. Vera. 1998. The cost of home-based care for HIV/AIDS patients in Zimbabwe. *AIDS Care* 10(6):751-759.

Hawkes, C. 2006. Agricultural and food policy for cardiovascular health in Latin America. *Prevention and Control* 2(3):137-147.

Hawkins, R. P., D. H. Gustafson, P. M. Day, B. Chewning, and K. Bosworth. 1987. Interactive computer programs as public information campaigns for hard-to-reach populations: The barn project example. *Journal of Communication* 37(2):8-28.

He, F. J., and G. A. MacGregor. 2009. A comprehensive review on salt and health and current experience of worldwide salt reduction programmes. *Journal of Human Hypertension* 23(6):363-384.

Hibbard, J. H. 2008. What can we say about the impact of public reporting? Inconsistent execution yields variable results. *Annals of Internal Medicine* 148(2):160-161.

Hodge, A. M., G. K. Dowse, H. Gareeboo, J. Tuomilehto, K. G. Alberti, and P. Z. Zimmet. 1996. Incidence, increasing prevalence, and predictors of change in obesity and fat distribution over 5 years in the rapidly developing population of Mauritius. *International Journal of Obesity and Related Metabolic Disorders* 20(2):137-146.

Holt, S. 2009. Time to implement the polypill approach. *New Zealand Medical Journal* 122(1296):88-89.

Hornik, R., and E. McAnany. 2001. Mass media and fertility change. In *Diffusion processes and fertility transition*. Edited by J. Casterline. Washington, DC: National Academy Press. Pp. 208-239.

Hornik, R., J. McDivitt, S. Zimicki, P. S. Yoder, E. C. Budge, J. McDowell, and M. Rasmuson. 2002. Communication in support of child survival: Evidence and explanations from eight countries. In *Public health communication: Evidence for behavior change*. Mahwah, NJ: Lawrence Erlbaum.

Hotchkiss, D. R., J. J. Rous, K. Karmacharya, and P. Sangraula. 1998. Household health expenditures in Nepal: Implications for health care financing reform. *Health Policy and Planning* 13(4):371-383.

Houpt, E. R., and R. L. Guerrant. 2008. Technology in global health: The need for essential diagnostics. *Lancet* 372(9642):873-874.

Hu, J. 2010. The role of health insurance in improving health services use by thais and ethnic minority migrants. *Asia-Pacific Journal of Public Health* 22(1):42-50.

Huicho, L., R. W. Scherpbier, A. M. Nkowane, and C. G. Victora. 2008. How much does quality of child care vary between health workers with differing durations of training? An observational multicountry study. *Lancet* 372(9642):910-916.

Humpel, N., N. Owen, and E. Leslie. 2002. Environmental factors associated with adults' participation in physical activity: A review. *Am J Prev Med* 22(3):188-199.

Hysong, S. J. P. 2009. Meta-analysis: Audit and feedback features impact effectiveness on care quality. *Medical Care* 47(3):356-363.

Ibrahim, M. M., H. Rizk, L. J. Appel, W. E. Aroussy, S. Helmy, Y. Sharaf, Z. Ashour, H. Kandil, E. Roccella, and P. K. Whelton. 1995. Hypertension prevalence, awareness, treatment, and control in Egypt: Results from the Egyptian national hypertension project (NHP). *Hypertension* 26(6):886-890.

Immelt, J., V. Govindarajan, and C. Trimble. 2009. How GE is disrupting itself. *Harvard Business Review*. October 2009.

Inui, T. S., W. M. Nyandiko, S. N. Kimaiyo, R. M. Frankel, T. Muriuki, J. J. Mamlin, R. M. Einterz, and J. E. Sidle. 2007. Ampath: Living proof that no one has to die from HIV. *Journal of General Internal Medicine* 22(12):1745-1750.

IOM (Institute of Medicine). 2001. *Crossing the quality chasm: A new health system for the 21st century.* Washington, DC: National Academy Press.

IOM. 2009. *Local government actions to prevent childhood obesity.* Washington, DC: The National Academies Press.

IOM. 2010. *Secondhand smoke exposure and cardiovascular effects: Making sense of the evidence.* Washington, DC: The National Academies Press.

ITU (International Telecommunications Union). 2009. *Key global telecom indicators for the world telecommunication service sector.* http://www.itu.int/ITU-D/ict/statistics/at_glance/KeyTelecom99.html (accessed March 12, 2010).

Jadad, A. 2009. Preventing and managing cardiovascular diseases in the age of mHealth and global telecommunications: Lessons from low- and middle-income countries. Prepared for the Institute of Medicine Committee on Preventing the Global Epidemic of Cardiovascular Disease in Developing Countries. Toronto, Canada.

James, W. P., A. Ralph, and C. P. Sanchez-Castillo. 1987. The dominance of salt in manufactured food in the sodium intake of affluent societies. *Lancet* 1(8530):426-429.

Jamison, D. 2006. Effective strategies for noncommunicable diseases, risk factors, and behaviors. In *Priorities in health.* Edited by D. Jamison, J. Breman, A. Measham, G. Alleyne, M. Claeson, D. Evans, P. Jha, A. Mills, and P. Musgrove. New York: Oxford University Press. Chapter 5.

Jamtvedt, G., J. M. Young, D. T. Kristoffersen, M. A. O'Brien, and A. D. Oxman. 2006. Does telling people what they have been doing change what they do? A systematic review of the effects of audit and feedback. *Quality & Safety in Health Care* 15(6):433-436.

Jean, M.-C., and L. St-Pierre. 2009. Applicability of the success factors for intersectorality in developing countries. France: IUHPE. Background paper commissioned by the Committee.

Jha, P., F. J. Chaloupka, M. Corrao, and B. Jacob. 2006. Reducing the burden of smoking world-wide: Effectiveness of interventions and their coverage. *Drug and Alcohol Review* 25(6):597-609.

Joshi, R., S. Jan, Y. Wu, and S. MacMahon. 2008. Global inequalities in access to cardiovascular health care: Our greatest challenge. *Journal of the American College of Cardiology* 52(23):1817-1825.

Justman, J., S. P. Koblavi-Deme, A. Tanuri, A. B. A. Goldberg, L. F. Gonzalez, and C. R. P. Gwynn. 2009. Developing laboratory systems and infrastructure for HIV scale-up: A tool for health systems strengthening in resource-limited settings. *Journal of Acquired Immune Deficiency Syndromes* 52(Suppl 1):S30-S33.

Kahn, E. B., L. T. Ramsey, R. Brownson, et al. 2002. The effectiveness of interventions to increase physical activity: a systematic review. *American Journal of Preventive Medicine* 22(4S):73-107.

Kane, R. L., G. Keckhafer, S. Flood, B. Bershadsky, and M. S. Siadaty. 2003. The effect of evercare on hospital use. *Journal of the American Geriatrics Society* 51(10):1427-1434.

Kane, R. L., P. E. Johnson, R. J. Town, and M. Butler. 2004. A structured review of the effect of economic incentives on consumers' preventive behavior. *American Journal of Preventive Medicine* 27(4):327-352.

Kannel, W. B., D. McGee, and T. Gordon. 1976. A general cardiovascular risk profile: The Framingham study. *American Journal of Cardiology* 38(1):46-51.

Kasl, S. V. 1980. Cardiovascular risk reduction in a community setting: Some comments. *Journal of Consulting and Clinical Psychology* 48(2):143-149.

Kelley, E., C. Geslin, S. Djibrina, and M. Boucar. 2001. Improving performance with clinical standards: The impact of feedback on compliance with the integrated management of childhood illness algorithm in Niger, West Africa. *The International Journal of Health Planning and Management* 16(3):195-205.

Kelley, E., A. G. Kelley, C. H. T. Simpara, O. Sidibé, and M. Makinen. 2003. The impact of self-assessment on provider performance in Mali. *The International Journal of Health Planning and Management* 18(1):41-48.

Khumalo-Sakutukwa, G., S. F. Morin, K. Fritz, E. D. Charlebois, H. van Rooyen, A. Chingono, P. Modiba, K. Mrumbi, S. Visrutaratna, B. Singh, M. Sweat, D. D. Celentano, and T. J. Coates. 2008. Project Accept (hptn 043): A community-based intervention to reduce HIV incidence in populations at risk for HIV in Sub-Saharan Africa and Thailand. *Journal of Acquired Immune Deficiency Syndromes* 49(4):422-431.

Kinaxis. 2010. *Four essential requirements for today's global supply chain management.* http://www.kinaxis.com/whitepapers/Four-Essential-Supply-Chain-Management-Requirements.cfm (accessed February 3, 2010).

Klingbeil, G. E., and I. G. Fiedler. 1988. Continuity of care. A teaching model. *American Journal of Physical Medicine and Rehabilitation* 67(2):77-81.

Komarek, L., V. Kebza, L. Lhotska, K. Osancova, J. Janovska, J. Okenkova, Z. Roth, J. Vignerova, J. Potockova, R. J. Havel, C. L. Albright, J. W. Farquhar, R. Poledne, M. Andel, J. Malkova, P. Kraml, H. Bartakova, D. Herman, S. Palmer, and I. Stankova. 1995. "Healthy Dubec" design of a joint Czech-American community project for the reduction of cardiovascular and cerebrovascular disease (adapted from American experience). *Central European Journal of Public Health* 3(4):230-233.

Kotseva, K., D. Wood, G. De Backer, D. De Bacquer, K. Pyorala, and U. Keil. 2009a. Cardiovascular prevention guidelines in daily practice: A comparison of EUROASPIRE I, II, and III surveys in eight European countries. *Lancet* 373(9667):929-940.

Kotseva, K., D. Wood, G. De Backer, D. De Bacquer, K. Pyorala, U. Keil, and Euroaspire Study Group. 2009b. EUROASPIRE III: A survey on the lifestyle, risk factors and use of cardioprotective drug therapies in coronary patients from 22 European countries. *European Journal of Cardiovascular Prevention & Rehabilitation* 16(2):121-137.

Kottke, T., P. Puska, J. T. Salonen, J. Tuomilehto, and A. Nissinen. 1985. Projected effects of high-risk versus population-based prevention strategies in coronary heart disease. *American Journal of Epidemiology* 121(5):697-704.

Kruk, M. E., and L. P. Freedman. 2008. Assessing health system performance in developing countries: A review of the literature. *Health Policy* 85(3):263-276.

Lagarde, M., A. Haines, and N. Palmer. 2009. The impact of conditional cash transfers on health outcomes and use of health services in low and middle income countries. Cochrane Database of Systematic Reviews. http://www.mrw.interscience.wiley.com/cochrane/clsysrev/articles/CD008137/frame.html (accessed November 10, 2009).

Langrish, J. P., N. L. Mills, and D. E. Newby. 2008. Air pollution: The new cardiovascular risk factor. *Internal Medicine Journal* 38(12):875-878.

Lehman, U., and D. A. Sanders. 2007. *Community health workers: What do we know about them? The state of the evidence on programmes, activities, costs, and impact on health outcomes of using community health workers.* Geneva: World Health Organization.

Lehman, U., I. Friedman, and D. Sanders. 2004. Review of the utilisation and effectiveness of community-based health workers in Africa: Joint Learning Initiative on Human Resources for Health and Development working paper.

Lehmann, U., W. Van Damme, F. Barten, and D. Sanders. 2009. Task shifting: The answer to the human resources crisis in Africa? *Human Resources for Health* 7(1):49.

Leurent, H., K. S. Reddy, J. Voute, and D. Yach. 2008. Wellness in the workplace: A multistakeholder health-promoting initiative of the World Economic Forum. *American Journal of Health Promotion* 22(6):379-380, ii.

Levy, J. A., and R. Strombeck. 2002. Health benefits and risks of the internet. *Journal of Medical Systems* 26(6):495-510.
Lewin, S., J. N. Lavis, A. D. Oxman, G. Bastias, M. Chopra, A. Ciapponi, S. Flottorp, S. G. Marti, T. Pantoja, G. Rada, N. Souza, S. Treweek, C. S. Wiysonge, and A. Haines. 2008. Supporting the delivery of cost-effective interventions in primary health-care systems in low-income and middle-income countries: An overview of systematic reviews. *Lancet* 372(9642):928-939.
Lindenauer, P. K., D. Remus, S. Roman, M. B. Rothberg, E. M. Benjamin, A. Ma, and D. W. Bratzler. 2007. Public reporting and pay for performance in hospital quality improvement. *New England Journal of Medicine* 356(5):486-496.
Liu, Y., K. Rao, J. Wu, and E. Gakidou. 2008. China's health system performance. *Lancet* 372(9653):1914-1923.
Loevinsohn, B. P., E. T. Guerrero, and S. P. Gregorio. 1995. Improving primary health care through systematic supervision: A controlled field trial. *Health Policy and Planning* 10(2):144-153.
Lu, W., X. Li, M. Chen, Y. Zhang, Y. Qian, S. Chen, and D. Zhu. 2009. Clinical study for disease management of hypertension in Shanghai community hospitals: DMaP-Shanghai. PowerPoint Presentation. Shanghai: Shanghai Municipal Center for Disease Control and Prevention.
Luck, J., and R. Shimkhada. 2009. The Effectiveness and Impact of Measurement to Improve Health. Prepared for the Institute of Medicine Committee on Preventing the Global Epidemic of Cardiovascular Disease in Developing Countries. Los Angeles, CA.
Luepker, R. V., L. Rastam, P. J. Hannan, D. M. Murray, C. Gray, W. L. Baker, R. Crow, D. R. Jacobs, Jr., P. L. Pirie, S. R. Mascioli, M. B. Mittelmark, and H. Blackburn. 1996. Community education for cardiovascular disease prevention. Morbidity and mortality results from the Minnesota Heart Health Program. *American Journal of Epidemiology* 144(4):351-362.
Ma'ayeh, S. 2002. *Jordan: Mass media campaign combating smoking requires serious commitment and not just words.* http://www.who.int/tobacco/training/success_stories/en/best_practices_jordan_media.pdf (accessed June 20, 2009).
Maibach, E., J. A. Flora, and C. Nass. 1991. Changes in self-efficacy and health behavior in response to a minimal contact community health campaign. *Health Communication* 3(1):1-15.
Malan, M., and R. Leaver. 2003. Political Change in South Africa: New Tobacco Control and Public Health Policies. In *Tobacco control policy: Strategies, successes, and setbacks*, edited by J. de Beyer and L. W. Brigden. Washington, DC: The World Bank and The International Development Research Center.
Marshall, M. N., P. G. Shekelle, S. Leatherman, and R. H. Brook. 2000. The public release of performance data: What do we expect to gain? A review of the evidence. *Journal of the American Medical Association* 283(14):1866-1874.
Matsudo, S. M., and V. R. Matsudo. 2006. Coalitions and networks: Facilitating global physical activity promotion. *Promotion and Education* 13(2):133-138, 158-163.
Matsudo, S. M., V. R. Matsudo, T. L. Araujo, D. R. Andrade, E. L. Andrade, L. C. de Oliveira, and G. F. Braggion. 2003. The agita São Paulo program as a model for using physical activity to promote health. *Revista Panamericana de Salud Publica* 14(4):265-272.
Matsudo, S. M., V. R. Matsudo, D. R. Andrade, T. L. Araújo, E. Andrade, L. d. Oliveira, and G. Braggion. 2004. Physical activity promotion: Experiences and evaluation of the agita São Paulo program using the ecological mobile model. *Journal of Physical Activity and Health* 1(2):81-94.
Matsudo, V. 2002. The agita São Paulo experience in promoting physical activity. *West Indian Medical Journal* 51(Suppl 1):48-50.

Matsudo, V., S. Matsudo, D. Andrade, T. Araujo, E. Andrade, L. C. de Oliveira, and G. Braggion. 2002. Promotion of physical activity in a developing country: The agita São Paulo experience. *Public Health and Nutrition* 5(1A):253-261.

McAlister, F. A., F. M. Lawson, K. K. Teo, and P. W. Armstrong. 2001. Randomised trials of secondary prevention programmes in coronary heart disease: Systematic review. *British Medical Journal* 323(7319):957-962.

McIntyre, D., M. Thiede, G. Dahlgren, M. Whitehead, D. McIntyre, M. Thiede, G. Dahlgren, and M. Whitehead. 2006. What are the economic consequences for households of illness and of paying for health care in low- and middle-income country contexts? *Social Science and Medicine* 62(4):858-865.

McNamara, P. 2005. Quality-based payment: Six case examples. *International Journal for Quality in Health Care* 17(4):357-362.

McNamara, P. 2006. Provider-specific report cards: A tool for health sector accountability in developing countries. *Health Policy and Planning* 21(2):101-109.

Mehta, R. H., E. D. Peterson, and R. M. Califf. 2007. Performance measures have a major effect on cardiovascular outcomes: A review. *American Journal of Medicine* 120(5):398-402.

Mendis, S., K. Fukino, A. Cameron, R. Laing, A. F. Jr., O. Khatib, J. Leowski, and M. Ewen. 2007a. The availability and affordability of selected essential medicines for chronic diseases in six low- and middle-income countries. *Bulletin of the World Health Organization* 85(4):279-288.

Mendis, S., L. H. Lindholm, G. Mancia, J. Whitworth, M. Alderman, S. Lim, and T. Heagerty. 2007b. World Health Organization (WHO) and International Society of Hypertension (ISH) risk prediction charts: Assessment of cardiovascular risk for prevention and control of cardiovascular disease in low and middle-income countries. *Journal of Hypertension* 25(8):1578-1582.

Mensah, K., M. Mackintosh, and L. Henry. 2005. The "skills drain" of health professionals from the developing world: A framework for policy formulation. http//:www.medact.org/content/Skills%20drain/Mensah%20et%20al.%202005.pdf (accessed June 28, 2009).

Mittelmark, M. B., R. V. Luepker, D. R. Jacobs, et al. 1986. Communitywide prevention of cardiovascular disease: education strategies of the Minnesota Heart Health Program. *Preventive Medicine* 15:1-17.

Mittelmark, M. B., M. K. Hunt, G. W. Heath, and T. L. Schmid. 1993. Realistic outcomes: Lessons from community-based research and demonstration programs for the prevention of cardiovascular diseases. *Journal of Public Health Policy* 14(4):437-462.

Mohr, T., O. Rajobov, Z. Maksumova, and R. Northrup. 2005. Using incentives to improve tuberculosis treatment results: lessons from Tajikistan. Washington, DC: The Core Group.

Monterey County Health Department. 2007. *Health profile 2007: Conditions and behaviors.* http://www.co.ca/us/health/publications (accessed December 16, 2009).

Moy, F., A. A. Sallam, and M. Wong. 2006. The results of a worksite health promotion programme in Kuala Lumpur, Malaysia. *Health Promotion International* 21(4):301-310.

Mullan, F., and S. Frehywot. 2007. Non-physician clinicians in 47 Sub-Saharan African countries. *Lancet* 370(9605):2158-2163.

NCI (National Cancer Institute). 2002. Making health communication programs work. Bethesda, MD: National Institutes of Health, U.S. Department of Health and Human Services.

NCI. 2008. *The role of the media in promoting and reducing tobacco use. NCI tobacco control monograph 19.* Bethesda, MD: National Institutes of Health, U.S. Department of Health and Human Services.

Neubeck, L., J. Redfern, R. Fernandez, T. Briffa, A. Bauman, and S. B. Freedman. 2009. Telehealth interventions for the secondary prevention of coronary heart disease: A systematic review. *European Journal of Cardiovascular Prevention and Rehabilitation* 16(3):281-289.

Ng, S. W., F. Zhai, and B. M. Popkin. 2008. Impacts of China's edible oil pricing policy on nutrition. *Social Science and Medicine* 66(2):414-426.

Ng, S. W., E. C. Norton, et al. 2009. Why have physical activity levels declined among Chinese adults? Findings from the 1991-2006 China health and nutrition surveys. *Social Science & Medicine* 68(7): 1305-1314.

Nissinen, A., X. Berrios, and P. Puska. 2001. Community-based noncommunicable disease interventions: Lessons from developed countries for developing ones. *Bulletin of the World Health Organization* 79(10):963-970.

O'Brien, P., and L. Gostin. 2008. Health worker shortages and inequalities: The reform of United States policy. *Global Health Governance* 2(2):1-29.

Olcay, M., and R. Laing. 2005. *Pharmaceutical tariffs: What is their effect on prices, protection of local industry and revenue generation?* Geneva: WHO Commission on Intellectual Property Rights, Innovation and Public Health.

OpenMRS. 2010. OpenMRS. http://openmrs.org/ (accessed February 1, 2010).

Osler, M., and N. B. Jespersen. 1993. The effect of a community-based cardiovascular-disease prevention project in a Danish municipality. *Danish Medical Bulletin* 40(4):485-485.

O'Sullivan, G. A., J. A. Yonkler, W. Morgan, and A. P. Merritt. 2003. *A field guide to designing a health communication strategy*. Baltimore, MD: Johns Hopkins Bloomberg School of Public Health/Center for Communication Programs.

Papas, M. A., A. J. Alberg, R. Ewing, K. J. Helzlsouer, T. L. Gary, and A. C. Klassen. 2007. The built environment and obesity. *Epidemiologic Reviews* 29:129-143.

Partnership for Supply Chain Management Systems. 2010. http://www.pfscm.org (accessed February 3, 2010).

Peabody, J. W., P. J. Gertler, and A. Leibowitz. 1998. The policy implications of better structure and process on birth outcomes in Jamaica. *Health Policy* 43(1):1-13.

Peabody, J. W., J. Florentino, R. Shimkhada, O. Solon, and S. Quimbo. 2010a. Quality variation and its impact on costs and satisfaction: Evidence from the QIDS study. *Medical Care* 48(1):25-30.10.1097/MLR.1090b1013e3181bd1047b1092.

Peabody, J. W., S. Quimbo, J. Florentino, M. F. Bacate, K. Woo, R. Shimkhada, and O. Solon. 2010b. A randomized experiment introducing incentives to improve quality of care. *Health Affairs*.

Pereira, M., N. Lunet, A. Azevedo, and H. Barros. 2009. Differences in prevalence, awareness, treatment and control of hypertension between developing and developed countries. *Journal of Hypertension* 27(5):963-975.

Petersen, L. A., L. D. Woodard, T. Urech, C. Daw, and S. Sookanan. 2006. Does pay-for-performance improve the quality of health care? *Annals of Internal Medicine* 145(4): 265-272.

Pierce, J., N. Evans, A. J. Farkas, S. W. Cavin, C. Berry, M. Kramer, et al. 1994. *Tobacco use in California: An evaluation of the tobacco control program, 1989-1993. A report to the California Department of Health Services*. http://www.escholarship.org/uc/item/3c7259dj (accessed January 11, 2010).

Pinstrup-Andersen, P., ed. 1988. *Food subsidies in developing countries: Costs, benefits, and policy options*. London and Baltimore: The Johns Hopkins University Press (for the International Food Policy Research Institute).

Piotrow, P. T., J. G. I. Rimon, A. Payne Merritt, and G. Saffitz. 2003. Advancing health communication: The PCS experience in the field. Baltimore, MD: Johns Hopkins Bloomberg School of Public Health/Center for Communication Programs.

Popkin, B. M. 2003. Dynamics of the nutrition transition and its implications for the developing world. *Forum on Nutrition* 56:262-264.

Prabhakaran, D., P. Jeemon, S. Goenka, R. Lakshmy, K. R. Thankappan, F. Ahmed, P. P. Joshi, B. V. Mohan, R. Meera, M. S. Das, R. C. Ahuja, R. K. Saran, V. Chaturvedi, and K. S. Reddy. 2009. Impact of a worksite intervention program on cardiovascular risk factors: A demonstration project in an Indian industrial population. *Journal of the American College of Cardiology* 53(18):1718-1728.

Prasad, B., and Y. Mulaleedharan. 2007. Community health workers: A review of concepts, practice, and policy concerns. HRH Global Resource Center.

Puska, P., A. Nissinen, J. Tuomilehto, J. T. Salonen, K. Koskela, A. McAlister, T. E. Kottke, N. Maccoby, and J. W. Farquhar. 1985. The community-based strategy to prevent coronary heart disease: Conclusions from the ten years of the North Karelia project. *Annual Review of Public Health* 6:147-193.

Puska, P., J. Tuomilehto, A. Nissinen, et al. 1995. *The North Karelia project. 20 year results and experiences*. Helsinki: The National Public Health Institute (KTL).

Puska, P., E. Vartiainen, T. Laatinkainen, P. Jousilahti, and M. Paavola, eds. 2009. *The North Karelia project: From North Karelia to national action*. Helsinki: Helsinki University Printing House.

Quick, J. D., H. V. Hogerzeil, G. Velasquez, and L. Rago. 2002. Twenty-five years of essential medicines. *Bulletin of the World Health Organization* 80(11):913-914.

Quimbo, S., J. W. Peabody, R. Shimkhada, and O. Solon. Evidence of a causal link between health outcomes, insurance coverage and a policy to expand access: experimental data from children in the Philippines. *Health Economics*.

Raguenaud, M.-E., P. Isaakidis, T. Reid, S. Chy, L. Keuky, G. Arellano, and W. Van Damme. 2009. Treating 4,000 diabetic patients in Cambodia, a high-prevalence but resource-limited setting: A 5-year study. *BMC Medicine* 7(1):33.

Ravishankar, N., P. Gubbins, R. J. Cooley, K. Leach-Kemon, C. M. Michaud, D. T. Jamison, and C. J. Murray. 2009. Financing of global health: Tracking development assistance for health from 1990 to 2007. *Lancet* 373(9681):2113-2124.

Reidpath, D. D., and P. Allotey. 2009. Opening up public health: A strategy of information and communication technology to support population health. *Lancet* 373(9668):1050-1051.

Rivera, J. A., D. Sotres-Alvarez, J. P. Habicht, T. Shamah, and S. Villalpando. 2004. Impact of the Mexican program for education, health, and nutrition (progresa) on rates of growth and anemia in infants and young children: A randomized effectiveness study. *Journal of the American Medical Association* 291(21):2563-2570.

Robinowitz, D. L., and R. A. Dudley. 2006. Public reporting of provider performance: Can its impact be made greater? *Annual Review of Public Health* 27(1):517-536.

Roccella, E. J., and M. J. Horan. 1988. The national high blood pressure education program: Measuring progress and assessing its impact. *Health Psychology* 7:297-303.

Rogers, E. M. 1983. *Diffusion of Innovations*. New York: Free Press.

Rossouw, J. E., P. L. Jooste, D. O. Chalton, E. R. Jordaan, M. L. Langenhoven, P. C. Jordaan, M. Steyn, A. S. Swanepoel, and L. J. Rossouw. 1993. Community-based intervention: The coronary risk factor study (CORIS). *International Journal of Epidemiology* 22(3):428-438.

Rowe, A. K., D. de Savigny, C. F. Lanata, and C. G. Victora. 2005. How can we achieve and maintain high-quality performance of health workers in low-resource settings? *Lancet* 366(9490):1026-1035.

Ruszkowska-Majzel, J., and W. Drygas. 2005. The great nationwide physical activity campaign "revitalize your heart" as an effective method to promote active lifestyle in Poland. *Przeglad Lekarski* 62(Suppl 3):23-26.

Saffer, H., and F. Chaloupka. 2000. The effect of tobacco advertising bans on tobacco consumption. *Journal of Health Economics* 19(6):1117-1137.

Sallis, J. F., J. A. Flora, S. P. Fortmann, C. B. Taylor, and N. Maccoby. 1985. Mediated smoking cessation programs in the Stanford Five-City Project. *Addictive Behaviors* 10(4):441-443.

Sallis, J. F., M. Story, and D. Lou. 2009. Study designs and analytic strategies for environmental and policy research on obesity, physical activity, and diet: Recommendations from a meeting of experts. *American Journal of Preventive Medicine* 36(Suppl 2):S72-S77.

Schaffnit-Chatterjee, C. 2009. *The global food equation: Food security in an environment of increasing scarcity.* Frankfurt, Germany: Deutsche Bank Research.

Schieber, G., C. Baeza, D. Kress, and M. Maier. 2006. Financing health systems in the 21st century. In *Disease control priorities in developing countries.* 2nd ed, edited by D. T. Jamison, J. G. Breman, A. R. Measham, G. Alleyne, M. Claeson, D. B. Evans, P. Jha, A. Mills and P. Musgrove. New York: Oxford University Press. Pp. 225-242.

Schieber, G. J., P. Gottret, L. K. Fleisher, and A. A. Leive. 2007. Financing global health: Mission unaccomplished. *Health Affairs* 26(4):921-934.

Schooler, C., J. W. Farquhar, S. P. Fortmann, and J. A. Flora. 1997. Synthesis of findings and issues from community prevention trials. *Annals of Epidemiology* 7(Suppl 1):S54-S68.

Schuit, A. J., G. C. W. Wendel-Vos, W. M. M. Verschuren, E. T. Ronckers, A. Ament, P. Van Assema, J. Van Ree, and E. C. Ruland. 2006. Effect of 5-year community intervention Hartslag Limburg on cardiovascular risk factors. *American Journal of Preventive Medicine* 30(3):237-242.

Sepe, E., and S. A. Glantz. 2002. Bar and club tobacco promotions in the alternative press: targeting young adults. *American Journal of Public Health* 92(1):75-78.

Shafey, O., M. Eriksen, H. Ross, and J. Mackay. 2009. *The tobacco atlas.* 3rd ed. Atlanta: American Cancer Society.

Shaller, D., S. Sofaer, S. D. Findlay, J. H. Hibbard, D. Lansky, and S. Delbanco. 2003. Consumers and quality-driven health care: A call to action. *Health Affairs* 22(2):95-101.

Shea, S., and C. Basch. 1990a. A review of five major community-based cardiovascular disease prevention programs. Part II: Intervention strategies, evaluation methods, and results. *American Journal of Health Promotion* 4(4):279-287.

Shea, S. and C. Basch. 1990b. A review of five major community-based cardiovascular disease prevention programs. Part I: Rationale, design, and theoretical framework. *American Journal of Health Promotion* 4(3):203-213.

Shimkhada, R., J. Peabody, S. Quimbo, and O. Solon. 2008. The quality improvement demonstration study: An example of evidence-based policy-making in practice. *Health Research Policy and Systems* 6(1):5.

Singh, D., and C. Ham. 2006. *Improving care for people with long-term conditions: A review of UK and international frameworks.* Birmingham, UK: University of Birmingham.

Smith, B. 2009. Social marketing programs in health in developing countries. Presentation at Public Information Gathering Session for the Institute of Medicine Committee on Preventing the Global Epidemic of Cardiovascular Disease, Washington, DC.

Smith, S. C. 1997. Review of recent clinical trials of lipid lowering in coronary artery disease. *American Journal of Cardiology* 80(Suppl 2):10H-13H.

Smith, W. A., ed. 1999. *Social marketing lite: Ideas for folks with small budgets and big problems.* Washington, DC: AED (Academy for Educational Development).

Soeters, R., C. Habineza, and P. B. Peerenboom. 2006. Performance-based financing and changing the district health system: Experience from Rwanda. *Bulletin of the World Health Organization* 84(11):884-889.

Solon, O., K. Woo, S. A. Quimbo, R. Shimkhada, J. Florentino, and J. W. Peabody. 2009. A novel method for measuring health care system performance: Experience from QIDS in the Philippines. *Health Policy and Planning* 24(3):167-174.

Somkotra, T., L. P. Lagrada, T. Somkotra, and L. P. Lagrada. 2009. Which households are at risk of catastrophic health spending: Experience in Thailand after universal coverage. *Health Affairs* 28(3):w467-w478.

Sosa-Rubi, S. G., O. Galarraga, and J. E. Harris. 2009. Heterogeneous impact of the "Seguro Popular" Program on the utilization of obstetrical services in Mexico, 2001-2006: A multinomial probit model with a discrete endogenous variable. *Journal of Health Economics* 28(1):20-34.

Steinfeld, H., Food and Agriculture Organization of the United Nations Livestock, Environment, and Development Initiative. 2006. *Livestock's long shadow: Environmental issues and options*. Rome: Food and Agriculture Organization of the United Nations.

Steyn, K., M. Steyn, A. S. Swanepoel, P. C. Jordaan, P. L. Jooste, J. M. Fourie, and J. E. Rossouw. 1997. Twelve-year results of the coronary risk factor study (CORIS). *International Journal of Epidemiology* 26(5):964-971.

Steyn, N. P., D. Bradshaw, R. Norman, J. Joubert, M. Schneider, and K. Steyn. 2006. *Dietary changes and the health transition in South Africa: Implications for health policy*. Cape Town: South African Medical Research Council.

Stokols, D. 1992. Establishing and maintaining healthy environments. Toward a social ecology of health promotion. *American Psychologist* 47(1):6-22.

Supply Chain Management System. 2009. *Three years of saving lives through stronger HIV/AIDS supply chains: A report on the global impacts of SCMS*. Arlington, VA: Supply Chain Management System.

Supply Chain Management System. no date. http://scms.pfscm.org/scms/about (accessed February 3, 2010).

Task Force on Community Preventive Services. 2002. Recommendations to increase physical activity in communities. *American Journal of Preventive Medicine* 22(4S):67-72.

Taskforce on Innovative International Financing for Health Systems Working Group 1. 2009. *Constraints to scaling up and costs: Working group 1 report*. Geneva: International Health Partnership.

Thow, A. M., and C. Hawkes. 2009. The implications of trade liberalization for diet and health: A case study from Central America. *Globalization and Health* 5(1):5.

Thow, A. M., S. Jan, S. Leeder, and B. Swinburn. 2010. The effect of fiscal policy on diet, obesity and chronic disease: A systematic review. *Bulletin of the World Health Organization*.

Tian, H. G., Z. Y. Guo, G. Hu, S. J. Yu, W. Sun, P. Pietinen, and A. Nissinen. 1995. Changes in sodium intake and blood pressure in a community-based intervention project in China. *Journal of Human Hypertension* 9(12):959-968.

Twahirwa, A. 2008. Sharing the burden of sickness: Mutual health insurance in Rwanda. *Bulletin of the World Health Organization* 86(11):823-824.

Tye, J. B., K. E. Warner, et al. 1987. Tobacco advertising and consumption: Evidence of a causal relationship. *Journal of Public Health Policy* 8(4):492-508.

United Nations Department of Economic and Social Affairs. 2008. *The millennium development goals report*. Geneva: United Nations.

United Nations Statistics Division. 2008. Millenium development goals indicators. http://unstats.un.org/unsd/mdg/Host.aspx?Content=Indicators/OfficialList.htm (accessed May 21, 2010).

U.S. Department of Health and Human Services. 2004. *Seventh report of the Joint National Committee on Prevention, Detection, Evaluation, and Treatment of High Blood Pressure*. Bethesda, MD: National Institutes of Health.

Uusitalo, U., E. J. Feskens, J. Tuomilehto, G. Dowse, U. Haw, D. Fareed, F. Hemraj, H. Gareeboo, K. G. Alberti, and P. Zimmet. 1996. Fall in total cholesterol concentration over five years in association with changes in fatty acid composition of cooking oil in Mauritius: Cross sectional survey. *British Medical Journal* 313(7064):1044-1046.

Vateesatokit, P. 2003. Tailoring Tobacco Control Efforts to the Country: The Example of Thailand. In *Tobacco control policy: Strategies, successes, and setbacks*, edited by J. de Beyer and L. W. Brigden. Washington, DC: The World Bank and The International Development Research Centre.

Victora, C. G., K. Hanson, J. Bryce, and J. P. Vaughan. 2004. Achieving universal coverage with health interventions. *Lancet* 364(9444):1541-1548.

Volpp, K. G., A. Gurmankin Levy, D. A. Asch, J. A. Berlin, J. J. Murphy, A. Gomez, H. Sox, J. Zhu, and C. Lerman. 2006. A randomized controlled trial of financial incentives for smoking cessation. *Cancer Epidemiology Biomarkers & Prevention* 15(1):12-18.

Volpp, K. G., A. B. Troxel, M. V. Pauly, H. A. Glick, A. Puig, D. A. Asch, R. Galvin, J. Zhu, F. Wan, J. DeGuzman, E. Corbett, J. Weiner, and J. Audrain-McGovern. 2009. A randomized, controlled trial of financial incentives for smoking cessation. *New England Journal of Medicine* 360(7):699-709.

von Schirnding, Y., and D. Yach. 2002. Unhealthy consumption threatens sustainable development. *Revista de Saude Publica* 36(4):379-382.

Wagner, A. K., M. Valera, A. J. Graves, S. Lavina, and D. Ross-Degnan. 2008. Costs of hospital care for hypertension in an insured population without an outpatient medicines benefit: An observational study in the Philippines. *BMC Health Services Research* 8(161).

Wagner, E. H., B. T. Austin, and K. Michael Von. 1996. Organizing care for patients with chronic illness. *The Milbank Quarterly* 74(4):511-544.

Wakefield, M., B. Flay, M. Nichter, and G. Giovino. 2003. Effects of anti-smoking advertising on youth smoking: A review. *Journal of Health Communication* 8(3):229-247.

Wald, N. J., and M. R. Law. 2003. A strategy to reduce cardiovascular disease by more than 80%. *British Medical Journal* 326(7404):1419.

Wallace, A., V. Dietz, and K. L. Cairns. 2009. Integration of immunization services with other health interventions in the developing world: What works and why? Systematic literature review. *Tropical Medicine and International Health* 14(1):11-19.

Walters, S. T., J. A. Wright, J. and R. Shegog. 2006. A review of computer and internet-based interventions for smoking behavior. *Addictive Behaviors* 3(2):264-277.

Weinehall, L., G. Hellsten, K. Boman, and G. Hallmans. 2001. Prevention of cardiovascular disease in Sweden: The Norsjo community intervention programme—motives, methods and intervention components. *Scandinavian Journal of Public Health* 29(Suppl 56):13-20.

WHO (World Health Organization). 2003. *WHO framework convention on tobacco control*. Geneva: World Health Organization.

WHO. 2006. *WHO country health information*. http://www.who.int/nha/country/en/ (accessed February 17, 2010).

WHO. 2007a. *Everybody's business—strengthening health systems to improve health outcomes: WHO's framework for action*. Geneva: World Health Organization.

WHO. 2007b. *Report of the global survey on the progress in national chronic diseases prevention and control*. Geneva: World Health Organization.

WHO. 2008a. *Draft: The WHO code of practice on the international recruitment of health personnel*. http://www.who.int/hrh/migration/code/draft_code_en.pdf (accessed December 16, 2009).

WHO. 2008b. *Mpower: A policy package to reverse the tobacco epidemic*. Geneva: World Health Organization.

WHO. 2008c. WHO report on the global tobacco epidemic, 2008: The MPOWER package. Geneva: World Health Organization.

WHO and WEF (World Economic Forum). 2008. *Preventing noncommunicable diseases in the workplace through diet and physical activity: WHO/World Economic Forum report of a joint event.* http://www.weforum.org/pdf/Wellness/WHOWEF_report.pdf (accessed April 11, 2009).

WHO Forum on Reducing Salt Intake in Populations. October 2006. *Reducing salt intake in populations: Report of a WHO forum and technical meeting.* Paris: World Health Organization.

WHO Maximizing Positive Synergies Collaborative Group. 2009. An assessment of interactions between global health initiatives and country health systems. *Lancet* 373(9681): 2137-2169.

WHO Noncommunicable Diseases and Mental Health Cluster. 2002. *Innovative care for chronic conditions: Building blocks for actions: Global report.* Geneva: World Health Organization.

Williams, F., and S. Boren. 2008. The role of the electronic medical record (EMR) in care delivery in developing countries: Case study, Ghana. *International Journal of Information Management* 16(2):139-145.

Williams, P. T., S. P. Fortmann, J. W. Farquhar, A. Varady, and S. Mellen. 1981. A comparison of statistical methods for evaluating risk factor changes in community-based studies: An example from the Stanford Three-Community Study. *Journal of Chronic Diseases* 34(11):565-571.

Willis-Shattuck, M., P. Bidwell, S. Thomas, L. Wyness, D. Blaauw, and P. Ditlopo. 2008. Motivation and retention of health workers in developing countries: A systematic review. *BMC Health Services Research* 8:247.

Xavier, D., P. Pais, P. J. Devereaux, C. Xie, D. Prabhakaran, K. S. Reddy, R. Gupta, P. Joshi, P. Kerkar, S. Thanikachalam, K. K. Haridas, T. M. Jaison, S. Naik, A. K. Maity, and S. Yusuf. 2008. Treatment and outcomes of acute coronary syndromes in India (CREATE): A prospective analysis of registry data. *Lancet* 371(9622):1435-1442.

Xavier, D., P. Pais, A. Sigamani, J. Pogue, R. Afzal, and S. Yusuf. 2009. The need to test the theories behind the polypill: Rationale behind the Indian polycap study. *Nature Clinical Practice Cardiovascular Medicine* 6(2):96-97.

Yach, D., and R. Beaglehole. 2004. Globalization of risks for chronic diseases demands global solutions. *Perspectives on Global Development and Technology* 3(1):213-233.

Yang, G., L. Kong, W. Zhao, X. Wan, Y. Zhai, L. C. Chen, and J. P. Koplan. 2008. Emergence of chronic non-communicable diseases in China. *Lancet* 372(9650):1697-1705.

Yu, Z., G. Song, Z. Guo, G. Zheng, H. Tian, E. Vartiainen, P. Puska, and A. Nissinen. 1999. Changes in blood pressure, body mass index, and salt consumption in a Chinese population. *Preventive Medicine* 29(3):165-172.

Yu, Z., A. Nissinen, E. Vartiainen, G. Song, Z. Guo, and H. Tian. 2000. Changes in cardiovascular risk factors in different socioeconomic groups: Seven year trends in a Chinese urban population. *Journal of Epidemiology and Community Health* 54(9):692-696.

Yusuf, S. 2002. Two decades of progress in preventing vascular disease. *Lancet* 360(9326): 2-3.

Yusuf, S., S. Reddy, S. Ounpuu, and S. Anand. 2001. Global burden of cardiovascular diseases: Part I: General considerations, the epidemiologic transition, risk factors, and impact of urbanization. *Circulation* 104(22):2746-2753.

Zatonski, W. A., and W. Willett. 2005. Changes in dietary fat and declining coronary heart disease in Poland: Population based study. *British Medical Journal* 331(7510):187-188.

Zatonski, W. A., A. J. McMichael, and J. W. Powles. 1998. Ecological study of reasons for sharp decline in mortality from ischaemic heart disease in Poland since 1991. *British Medical Journal* 316(7137):1047-1051.

6

Cardiovascular Health Promotion Early in Life

The risk factors for cardiovascular disease (CVD) in adults are now well established. However, emerging evidence highlights the importance of exposures and experiences throughout the life course, beginning as early as the prenatal period, on the subsequent development of CVD. As a result, there are opportunities for intervention during the early years of life that can form a crucial component of the global effort to reduce the burden of CVD. This chapter describes the determinants of CVD that have origins early in life, followed by a discussion of the effects of childhood health promotion and prevention initiatives on later CVD risk.

This chapter, consistent with the scope of this report as described in Chapter 1, focuses on the accumulation starting early in life of risk for coronary heart disease and stroke This is not intended to underemphasize the importance of treating and preventing congenital heart diseases and other cardiovascular diseases in childhood, including prevention and treatment of streptococcal infections to prevent rheumatic heart disease, which exacts a high toll on children in low and middle income countries and was discussed in more detail in Chapter 2.

In addition, although the emerging epidemiological evidence is compelling for the importance of childhood and adolescence in the development of risk for CVD, this chapter is not intended to imply that attention should be drawn away from much-needed intervention approaches to reduce risk in adults. Indeed, there is not sufficient low and middle income country evidence on intervention effectiveness, health impact, or cost-effectiveness analyses to conclude that childhood prevention alone is a top priority for widespread implementation.

Rather, the aim of this chapter is to highlight several important messages. First, although evidence has not fully elucidated the onset of risk in early childhood, well-documented trends on youth tobacco use and childhood obesity present an immediate obstacle to achieving future reductions in CVD disease burden. Second, those already working in child health globally should take chronic disease prevention into consideration where there are relatively feasible and evidence-based interventions available in order to achieve not only short-term child outcomes but also to promote lifelong health. Third, the impact of health promotion and health education in children on adult CVD outcomes as well as the effectiveness of active CVD prevention programs in early childhood, youth, and adolescence in low and middle income countries are areas to be emphasized for further intervention research.

A summary framework of opportunities to promote lifelong heart health during development and to engage the next generation in the fight against CVD and related chronic diseases is illustrated in Figure 6.1.

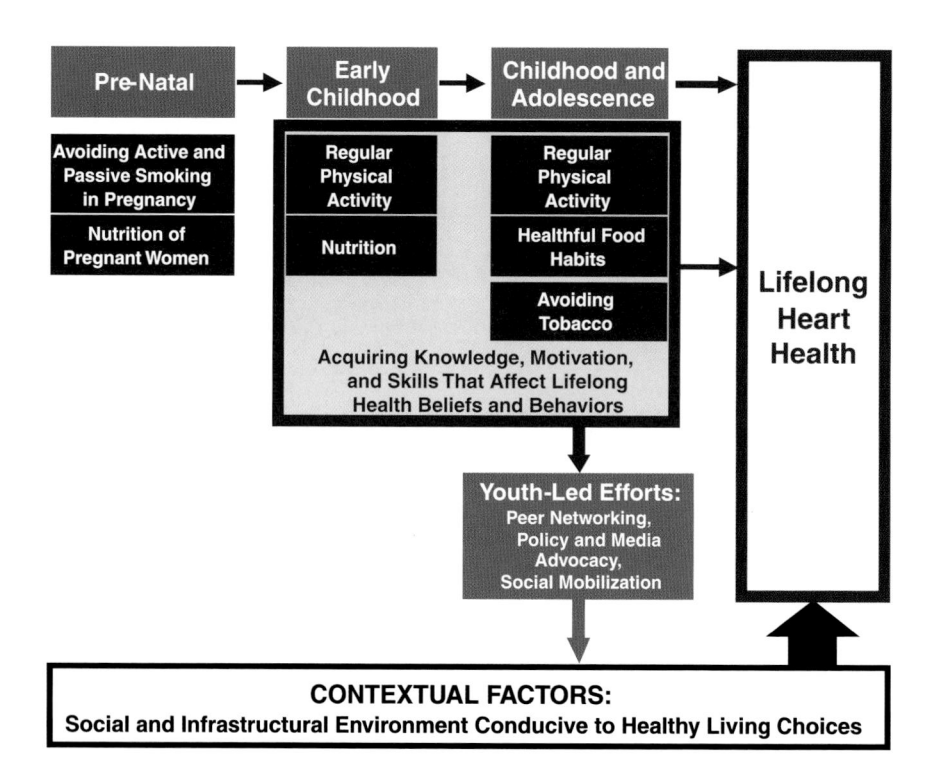

FIGURE 6.1 Growing toward heart health: Influences and opportunities into adulthood.

ASSOCIATION BETWEEN EARLY LIFE FACTORS AND SUBSEQUENT RISK FOR CVD

Prenatal, Infancy, and Early Childhood

There is growing recognition in developing and developed countries, based on recent data emanating from prospective cohort studies, of the importance of the fetal and early childhood periods in the onset of CVD later in life (Aboderin et al., 2002; Victora et al., 2008; Walker and George, 2007; WHO, 2009). The influences during this period include maternal factors during pregnancy, such as smoking, obesity, and malnutrition, and factors in infancy and early childhood, such as breastfeeding, low birth weight, and undernutrition, especially when coupled with rapid weight gain later in childhood.

Maternal smoking during pregnancy has been linked to CVD-related risk factors. It has been consistently associated with increased childhood obesity independent of other risk factors (Oken et al., 2008). This raises the concern that the increasing trend of smoking among young women in the developing world, described in Chapter 2, could contribute to increased prevalence of childhood obesity and obesity-related diseases in those populations.

A number of studies have examined the effects of maternal obesity on the body weight of their children; however, the evidence is inconsistent. Two cohort studies in the United States found that excessive weight gain or maternal obesity during pregnancy was associated with overweight and obesity in the children at ages 3 and 4 years (Gillman et al., 2008; Whitaker, 2004). Similarly, a cohort study in Finland found that mothers' body mass index (BMI) was positively associated with their sons' BMI in childhood (Eriksson et al., 1999). However, the recent Avon Longitudinal Study of Parents and Children (ALSPAC) study in the United Kingdom found no association between maternal BMI and child BMI (Davey Smith, 2008; Davey Smith et al., 2007). Furthermore, several researchers have expressed methodological concerns about the retrospective cohort studies that have been used thus far to assess the relationship between maternal and child BMI, asserting that such studies cannot account for confounding variables such as postnatal eating habits of children with obese parents (Davey Smith, 2008).

Another factor that appears to influence risk for long-term cardiovascular health is breastfeeding. Breastfeeding has been found to not only reduce childhood morbidity and mortality but also to be weakly protective against obesity later in life (Bhutta et al., 2008; Gluckman et al., 2008). However, the promotion of breastfeeding must be considered in coordination with other global health efforts so as not to encourage the spread of some infectious diseases, including HIV, which can be transmitted through breast milk.

A link to adult CVD risk has also been made for maternal malnutrition, low birth weight, and undernutrition in infancy, especially when followed by rapid weight gain. These have been associated with increased risk of CVD and diabetes in adulthood (Barker and Bagby, 2005; Caballero, 2005; Gluckman et al., 2008; Prentice and Moore, 2005). In what is known as the developmental origins theory of CVD, disruptions to the nutritional, metabolic, and hormonal environment at critical stages of development (in utero and in the first years of life) are hypothesized to lead to permanent "programming" of the body's structure, physiology, and metabolism that translate into pathology and disease, including CVD, later in life (Barker, 1997, 1998, 2007). The exact physiological mechanisms through which this programming occurs are not yet fully elucidated; however, there is evidence that fetal and early postnatal undernutrition can cause metabolic, anatomic, and endocrine adaptations that affect the hypothalamic-pituitary-adrenal axis, lipoprotein profiles, and end organ glucose uptake, among other processes (Prentice and Moore, 2005).

Support for the developmental origins theory of CVD comes from a number of retrospective, and more recently prospective, cohort studies in various populations. Studies in the United Kingdom, the United States, Finland, and India found that fetal undernutrition (as measured by low birth weight, small birth size, ratio of birth length to weight, or ratio of head circumference to weight at birth), followed by a rapid catch-up growth from childhood to early adolescence was significantly associated with the later development of CVD in both men and women (Barker et al., 2005; Eriksson et al., 1999; Forsen et al., 1999; Osmond and Barker, 2000; Stein et al., 1996). Early undernutrition followed by catch-up growth during childhood has also been associated with subsequent hypertension and type 2 diabetes (Barker, 1998; Osmond and Barker, 2000). More recently, Stein et al. (2005) reviewed nutritional studies from China, India, Guatemala, Brazil, and the Philippines and found that growth failure between conception and age 2 years and accelerated weight gain from childhood to adolescence were associated with significantly increased risk of diabetes and CVD in adulthood. In another developing country cohort, a longitudinal study of more than 3,000 children in South Africa also found that the combination of low birth weight and rapid growth in childhood was associated with an increased risk of obesity and risk factors for type 2 diabetes (Crowther et al., 1998; Richter et al., 2007). This emerging data on the effects of rapid weight gain after early undernutrition have prompted some researchers to suggest a shift from the original "fetal origins" hypothesis to an "accelerated postnatal growth hypothesis" of CVD (Singhal et al., 2003, 2004).

Some researchers have expressed reservations about interpreting the available data in this area due to concerns that much of the research to date has not sufficiently accounted for the confounding impact of the social and economic environment during early childhood (Davey Smith, 2007, 2008). In addition, although there is a growing body of evidence exploring the effects of undernutrition in infancy followed by rapid catch-up growth later in childhood on CVD, diabetes, obesity, and metabolic disease in adulthood, evidence is mixed on the effects of rapid growth between birth and age 2 years (Victora et al., 2008). Singhal et al. (2004) found that rapid weight gain within the first 2 weeks after birth was associated with adverse cardiovascular effects later in life. On the other hand, several recent reviews and meta-analyses of studies examining early undernutrition found rapid weight gain between birth and age 2 years was associated with lower morbidity and mortality in low and middle income countries (Black et al., 2008; Victora et al., 2008).

The emerging evidence on the association between low birth weight followed by rapid growth in childhood and subsequent risk for CVD raises important considerations for addressing global CVD because low birth weight and exposure to undernutrition in utero and in infancy are common in many developing countries (Caballero, 2009; Kelishadi, 2007). For example, the 2005-2006 National Family Health International Survey in India found that more than 40 percent of children under age 3 were underweight (International Institute of Population Studies, 2005-2006). In addition, the coexistence of these high rates of undernutrition in utero and early childhood with the potential for overnutrition in later childhood and adulthood may accelerate the epidemics of obesity and CVD in populations that undergo rapid nutrition transitions (Victora et al., 2008). Identifying the most prudent strategy for nourishing low birth weight and stunted infants while neither compromising their childhood health nor increasing their risk for cardiovascular and metabolic complications later in life will be an important area of future research.

Childhood and Adolescence

The acquisition and accumulation of risk for CVD continues in childhood and adolescence (Celermajer and Ayer, 2006; Freedman et al., 2001; Strong et al., 1999). Unhealthful lifestyle practices such as consumption of high calorie and high fat foods, tobacco use, and physical inactivity begin in childhood, introducing major behavioral risks for CVD. Childhood adversity also influences adult cardiovascular health. In addition, there is also an emerging body of evidence on the presence of biological risk factors in children and youth, including pathophysiological processes associated with heart disease that can be seen as early as childhood.

Childhood Obesity and CVD Risk

Childhood obesity is associated with multiple risk factors for CVD, which are amplified in the presence of overweight and persist from childhood into adulthood. These risk factors include hyperlipidemia, high blood pressure, impaired glucose tolerance and high insulin levels, as well as metabolic syndrome. It has been estimated that 60 percent of overweight children possess at least one of these risk factors that can lead to CVD in adulthood (Freedman et al., 1999). This is especially important in terms of implications for global CVD because, as will be described later in this chapter, the prevalence of childhood obesity is increasing in developing countries (WHO, 2008b).

The Bogalusa Heart Study, conducted in the United States in a community near New Orleans, examined the natural history of CVD among children and young adults (Berenson, 2002; Freedman et al., 2001). Repeated cross-sectional and longitudinal studies with participants aged 5 to 38 years suggested that overweight children and adolescents are more likely to become obese adults. A large prospective cohort study from Denmark also found that higher BMI during childhood is associated with an increased risk of coronary heart disease (CHD) in adulthood and that the elevated risk associated with childhood obesity increases with the age of the child (Baker et al., 2007).

Several studies in developed countries have reported that the prevalence of hypertension is significantly higher in obese children as compared to normal-weight children (Guillaume et al., 1996; Rosner et al., 2000; Sorof and Daniels, 2002). Obese children are at a three-fold higher risk of developing hypertension compared to nonobese children, and the risk continues to increase with higher BMI values (Sorof and Daniels, 2002). Similar findings have been reported in studies across developing countries. Verma et al. (1994) found that the prevalence of hypertension was 13.7 percent in obese children as compared to 0.4 percent in nonobese children in Punjab, India.

Childhood obesity is associated with impaired glucose tolerance (Sinaiko et al., 2001) and diabetes mellitus (Rocchini, 2002; Sinha et al., 2002) among children and adolescents. Over the years it has been observed that the upsurge in the prevalence of obesity among children and adolescents has been paralleled by an increasing prevalence of diabetes mellitus. This finding is significant, especially in developing countries such as India and China, which have the highest number of persons with diabetes in the world (Hossain et al., 2007). Sinha et al. (2002) found 25 percent of children (4-10 years) and 21 percent of adolescents (11-18 years) to have impaired glucose tolerance in the United States.

Metabolic syndrome is associated with childhood obesity, as established by several studies in developed (Cook et al., 2003; Cruz et al., 2004) as well as developing countries (Agirbasli et al., 2006; Csabi et al., 2000; Kelishadi, 2007). Singh et al. (2007) estimated the prevalence of metabolic syndrome using the National Cholesterol Education Program Adult Treatment Panel III (NCEP ATP III) criterion in adolescents aged 12-17 years in Chandigarh, India, to be 4.2 percent with no gender differences. Moreover, the study also estimated that 11.5 percent of the overweight adolescents and 1.9 percent of those who were of normal weight met the criterion of metabolic syndrome, suggesting a significant difference. Similar findings have been noted in studies conducted in other low and middle income countries (Agirbasli et al., 2006; Csabi et al., 2000; Kelishadi, 2007).

Childhood Adversity and CVD Risk

Stressful or traumatic circumstances in childhood also appear to increase the risk of CVD later in life. The Adverse Childhood Experiences study found that adults exposed to adversities such as abuse, household dysfunction (defined as the presence of alcohol or substance abuse, mental illness, or criminal behavior in the house), or neglect during childhood were significantly more likely to smoke, be physically inactive, be severely obese, and be depressed or angry, all risk factors for CVD. There was a dose–response relationship between the number of childhood exposures to adverse experiences and the number of risk factors for chronic disease later in life (Dong et al., 2004; Felitti et al., 1998). In a further analysis of the study data, Dong et al. (2004) found a similar graded relationship between the number of childhood adverse experiences and risk of ischemic heart disease in adulthood.

In addition to adverse experiences, growing up poor has also been linked to an increased risk of developing and dying from CVD. A review of prospective and cross-sectional studies in high income countries reported that the vast majority found an association between poor socioeconomic circumstances in childhood and greater risk of CHD, angina, stroke, and atherosclerosis in adulthood. This association was independent of the economic circumstances of study participants in adulthood (Galobardes et al., 2006).

Initiation of Tobacco Use

Tobacco use initiated in childhood or adolescence is another factor that leads to early vascular dysfunction and later adult CVD. There are an array of biological, social, environmental, and interpersonal factors that influence experimentation and maintenance of tobacco use among youth. Nicotine is a highly addictive substance. Cigarettes and other forms of tobacco act as carriers of nicotine, which affects the brain by reinforcing behavior, altering mood and creating a need that did not exist prior to drug exposure (Oates et al., 1988). Once youth start using tobacco, many of them become addicted to nicotine. After reaching the brain, nicotine stimulates the reward pathways in the brain and stimulates the release of dopamine, which is a neurotransmitter associated with addiction (Glover et al., 2003). The brains of children and adolescents, which are still in developmental stages, are highly susceptible to nicotine addiction (Difranza et al., 2002). The number of cigarettes and the duration of smoking that is necessary for making a person addicted are lower in adolescents than in adults. A study by Difranza et al. (2002) showed that some adolescents begin to experience loss of control over their smoking within weeks of smoking the first cigarette.

The U.S. Surgeon General's report of 1994, *Preventing Tobacco Use Among Young People*, described four broad categories of psychosocial risk factors that are linked to the initiation of the habit of smoking: sociodemographic, behavioral, personal, and environmental (U.S. Department of Health and Human Services, 1994). The specific sociodemographic factors associated with tobacco use are low socioeconomic status, male gender, low parental education, and single-parent households (Buttross and Kastner, 2003; Tyas and Pederson, 1998). Various behavioral and personal factors are poor academic achievement, low self-esteem, and peer influences (Buttross and Kastner, 2003; Tyas and Pederson, 1998). Environmental influences include smoking by parents, siblings, and peers; absence of rules prohibiting smoking at home (Buttross and Kastner, 2003; Tyas and Pederson, 1998); and the influence of films, television, and media campaigns (Prokhorov et al., 2006). Although these factors leading to initiation of tobacco use have been widely studied in developed countries, the evidence from youth in developing countries remains relatively sparse.

Early CVD Pathology in Childhood

Many of the risk factors described above have been shown to be related to surrogates for CVD pathophysiology that can already be observed in childhood, such as increased left ventricular mass, left ventricular systolic dysfunction, and higher arterial thickness in overweight children (Johnson et al., 1999; Laird and Fixler, 1981; Sorof et al., 2003). Although the predictive value of elevated C-reactive protein (CRP) and raised intima media thickness (IMT) are still under debate, it is worth noting that these have been demonstrated in obese children, along with impaired endothelial function of arteries as well as arterial stiffness and calcification (Celermajer and Ayer, 2006). BMI measured in childhood has been shown to be significantly associated with carotid IMT measured in adulthood. The Bogalusa Heart

Study suggested that low-density lipoprotein (LDL) cholesterol and BMI in childhood are independent risk factors for increased carotid IMT in young adulthood, whereas the Cardiovascular Risk in Young Finns study suggested that systolic blood pressure, LDL cholesterol, smoking, and BMI measured at 12-18 years predict adult IMT (Li et al., 2003; Raitakari, 2003).

The Pathobiological Determinants of Atherosclerosis in Youth Study study also suggested that atherosclerosis, which is a major pathological cause of coronary artery disease, has its origins in childhood (Strong et al., 1999). Fatty streaks in children are associated with risk factors such as dyslipidemia, hypertension, cigarette smoking, and diabetes mellitus (Celermajer and Ayer, 2006). Berenson (2002) suggested that fatty streaks start appearing in the aorta and other arteries as early as 3 years of age, and high maternal cholesterol levels in the ante-natal period contribute to their formation. Fatty streaks and raised lesions in the arteries, especially the aorta and coronary and carotid arteries, increase rapidly in prevalence and extent during the 15- to 34-year age span.

In summary, the evidence cited here clearly suggests that the behavioral and biological risk factors for CVD in adulthood frequently start appearing in childhood and adolescence. The risk factors are genetic, environmental, and behavioral and track from childhood to adulthood leading to premature CVD in adulthood. Hence, efforts for the prevention of CVD should begin right from childhood and adolescence when lifestyle habits are being formed, especially with respect to diet and physical activity, as well as during the prenatal period with respect to maternal nutrition and health.

GLOBAL TRENDS IN MAJOR DETERMINANTS OF CVD RISK EARLY IN LIFE

An understanding of the trends fueling the growing burden of childhood risk factors for chronic diseases is imperative if a reversal is to be brought about through public policy and programs. The following sections offer a brief overview of the global trends in the major determinants of CVD risk in children and youth.

Trends in Tobacco Use in Children and Adolescents

As described in Chapter 2, tobacco use is a growing worldwide epidemic (Reddy and Gupta, 2004). It is a risk factor for many chronic diseases and is the single most important preventable cause of death in the world today (WHO, 2008a). The most susceptible time for initiating tobacco use is during adolescence and early adulthood, before the age of 18 years (U.S.

Department of Health and Human Services, 1994), and the prevalence of tobacco use is increasing among children and adolescents. Due to this increasing prevalence, tobacco use is often referred to as a "pediatric disease" or a "pediatric epidemic" (Committee on Environmental Health et al., 2009; Perry et al., 1994). In India, for example, an estimated 5500 adolescents start using tobacco every day, joining the 4 million young people under the age of 15 years who already regularly use tobacco (Rudman, 2001).

The Global Youth Tobacco Survey (GYTS) provides some insight into global trends in tobacco consumption among youth. GYTS is a school-based survey of students aged 13-15 years that was undertaken at 395 sites in 131 countries. GYTS reported that, globally, about 10 percent of adolescents currently use tobacco in any form (Asma, 2009). Nearly 25 percent of them try their first cigarette before the age of 10 years, and 19 percent are susceptible to initiating smoking during the next year (Global Youth Tobacco Survey Collaborative Group, 2002).

The GYTS estimates also revealed differences within a country or a region, thereby showing how national estimates can obscure within-country differences and highlighting the need to look at subnational data. For example, India had both the highest and lowest rates of current use of any tobacco product (62.8 percent in Nagaland and 3.3 percent in Goa) (Global Youth Tobacco Survey Collaborative Group, 2002). These variations revealed by the GYTS indicate that tobacco-reduction strategies targeting youth will need to be adapted to local contexts with careful consideration paid to the unique factors influencing differential burden in each country, such as geographic regions or ethnic groups. In South Africa, for example, factors associated with race may play an important role in influencing adolescents' decision to smoke (Panday et al., 2007a, 2007b). Adolescents in different ethnic groups had different responses to the importance of information provided on the pros and cons of smoking, contextual factors, and preexisting self-efficacy (Panday et al., 2005). More research regarding the nuances of adapting approaches to local culture and context is an important priority if the global health community hopes to reduce the startlingly high rates of tobacco use among the world's youth.

Lastly, the GYTS data provide information about the exposure of children to environmental tobacco smoke. Almost half of the students (44 percent) reported that they were exposed to tobacco smoke at home and greater than 6 in 10 students (52 percent) reported being exposed to tobacco smoke in public places (Warren et al., 2006). This is of particular concern given the causal association that has been established between exposure to secondhand smoke and the prevalence of impaired vascular function, metabolic abnormalities, and chronic debilitating conditions (Peto et al., 1996).

As an example of the status of tobacco use on a national scale, the

National Youth Risk Behavior Survey, conducted with more than 10,000 school children in South Africa in 2002, revealed that 31 percent of students had smoked, and passive tobacco smoke exposure levels ranged from 56-84 percent (Reddy et al., 2003). In addition, since the study looked at a wide variety of potential risk factors, including violence-related intentional and unintentional injuries, mental health and wellness indicators, and nutrition and physical activity levels, it provided a more complete, well-rounded picture of adolescent risk behaviors, reinforcing the need to look more closely at the complex interactions that contribute to youth health status (Reddy et al., 2003). However, as it was the first study of its kind in that country, few conclusions on temporal trends can be drawn. If the study were to be repeated regularly, it could provide information on the impact of a number of national-level policy initiatives implemented in order to bring more focus onto youth and adolescent health.

Trends in Childhood Obesity

The total global prevalence of overweight in children between the ages of 5 and 17 years is 10 percent, varying from under 2 percent in Sub-Saharan Africa to more than 30 percent in the United States (Bhardwaj et al., 2008). Although still highest in high income countries, the epidemic of childhood obesity has spread from the United States and other developed countries to low and middle income countries, especially in urban areas (Prentice, 2006). Figures 6.2 and 6.3 provide an illustration—compiled by the International Association for the Study of Obesity (IASO)—of worldwide trends in the prevalence of overweight among boys and girls, respectively, over the past two decades. While the data is not age-standardized across countries or directly comparable across years, the figures suggest a trend of growing prevalence of overweight among children in an increasing number of developing countries.

For example, among school-going children and adolescents in India (rural and urban) aged 10-18 years, the prevalence of overweight was 1.7 percent in boys and 0.8 percent in girls in the year 2007 (WHO Global InfoBase, 2008). In the Middle East, Kuwait has among the highest prevalence of overweight (30 percent in boys; 31.8 percent in girls) and obesity (14.7 percent in boys; 13.1 percent in girls) among children and adolescents (10-14 years) (Al-Isa, 2004; Kelishadi, 2007). Figure 6.4 shows the prevalence of overweight and obesity among boys and girls aged 6-18 years in developing countries, demonstrating the high prevalence in the Middle East and Central and Eastern Europe. Among younger children, obesity is not a major public health issue in Asia and Sub-Saharan Africa, but in countries of Latin America, the Caribbean, the Middle East, North Africa, and Cen-

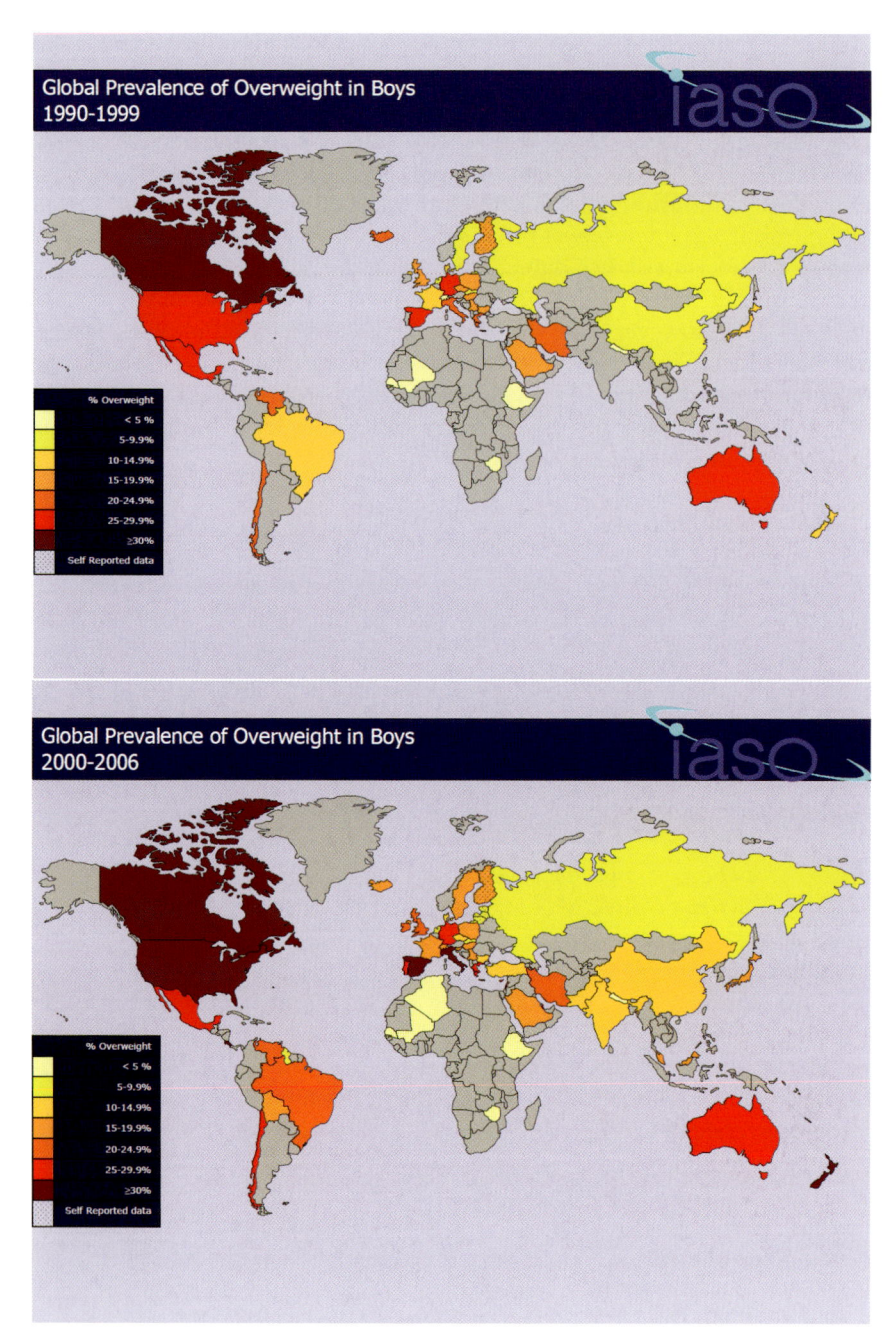

FIGURE 6.2 Illustrative prevalence of overweight in boys.
SOURCE: IASO, 2008a.

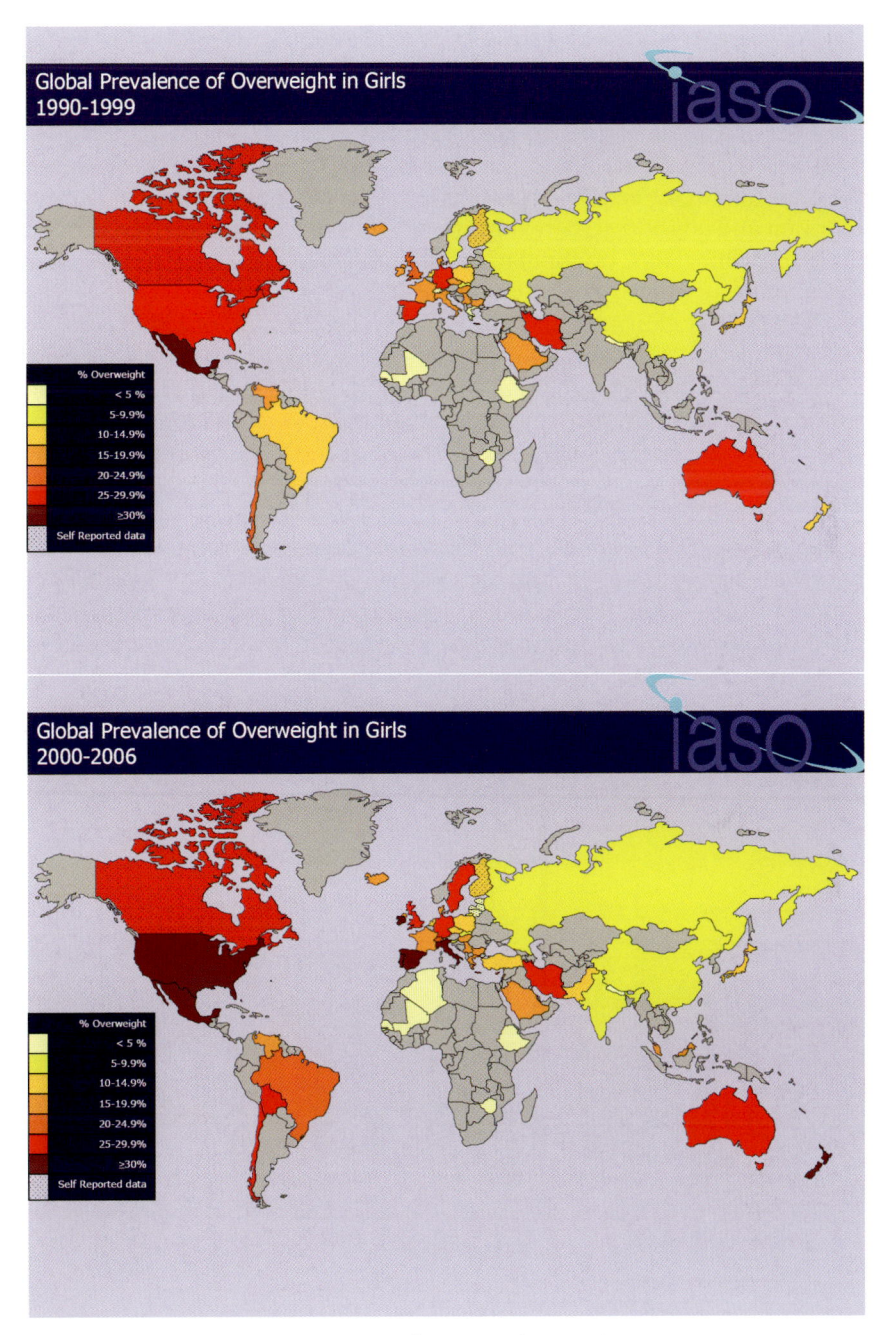

FIGURE 6.3 Illustrative prevalence of overweight in girls.
SOURCE: IASO, 2008b.

tral and Eastern Europe, its prevalence in children below 5 years of age is as high as that in the United States (Martorell et al., 2000).

Some of the most common factors to which the growing prevalence of obesity has been attributed are increasing affluence among populations and their increasing urbanization (Misra and Khurana, 2008). However, the most important determinants that have recently been widely studied are nutrition and physical activity transitions. These have direct implications on the energy imbalance of populations and are widely accepted as the cause for an increase in obesity and chronic diseases.

The present global population is in the midst of a unique phenomenon in which it is not uncommon for both undernutrition and obesity to coexist in the same populations, and indeed even in the same household. Undernutrition, with its associated communicable diseases and micronutrient deficiencies like anemia, has been the hallmark of the low and middle income countries of Africa, Latin America, and South Asia for decades. In India, for instance, between the years of 2005 and 2006, 40 percent of all children under the age of 3 years were underweight, 22 percent of newborns were born with low birth weight, and 55.3 percent of women and 69.5 percent of children were anemic (International Institute of Population Studies, 2005-2006). In one survey in South Africa, 9 percent of students were found to

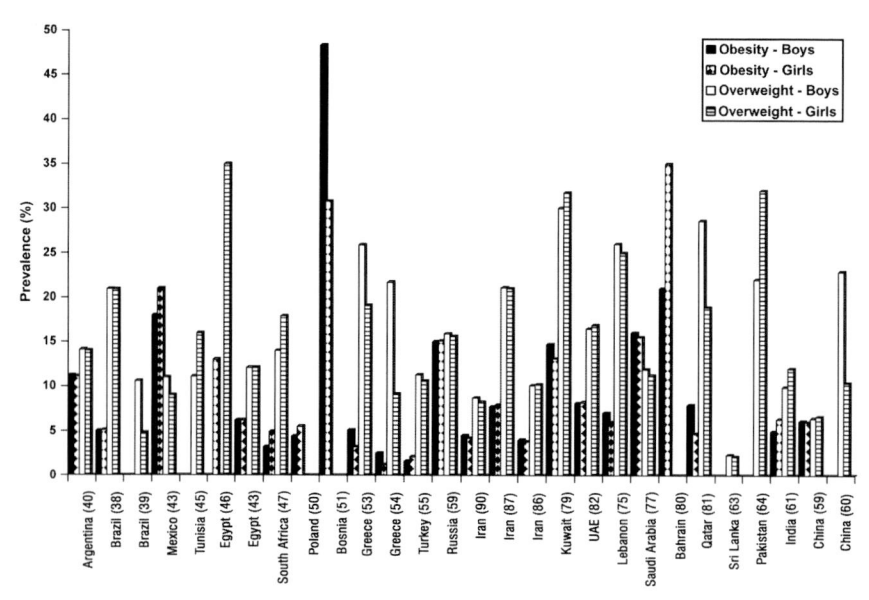

FIGURE 6.4 Prevalence of overweight and obesity among children aged 6-18 years in developing countries.
SOURCE: Kelishadi, 2007.

be either underweight or wasting, while at the same time 16.9 percent were found to be either overweight or obese (Reddy et al., 2009).

Policy makers are faced with a conundrum of sorts in addressing the dietary risks that contribute to the growing prevalence of obesity in developing countries while ensuring that the diets of children are both calorically adequate and nutritionally appropriate. As mentioned previously, there is emerging evidence that undernourishment followed by rapid weight gain in infancy is associated with increased risk of cardiovascular disease later in life. Thus it is possible that well-intentioned interventions targeting undernutrition, such as infant feeding initiatives, school meal programs, and free meals for family members may lead to an increase in adiposity among its target populations. For example, an evaluation of a school feeding program in Chile found that more than 50 percent of the children under the age of 6 years were reported to be obese (Kain et al., 1998). There is a growing need for efforts in maternal and child health and global food programs aimed at reducing malnutrition among children to take into account these potential negative impacts when developing their programmatic nutritional guidance and policies for the distribution of food products. With careful coordination, programs such as Save the Children's "Survive to 5" initiative (2010) can successfully address the challenges of reducing child hunger while not unintentionally increasing their future risk of cardiovascular disease. Such programs will thereby support not only shorter-term childhood outcomes but also promote future lifelong health.

In addition to changes in nutrition, perceived unsafe neighborhoods, limited open spaces, and inappropriate sports infrastructure can contribute to declines in physical activity, another key determinant of obesity and CVD risk. For example, the rates of participation in organized sport and physical education classes in Australia and the United Kingdom have decreased substantially in school-going children (Dollman et al., 2005). Although data on physical activity among children is generally sparse in developing countries, a 2002 national survey in South Africa found that 37.5 percent of school children in grades 8-11 were physically inactive, classified as not engaging in moderate or vigorous physical activity at least 3 or 5 days per week, respectively (Reddy et al., 2003). Sedentary leisure-time pursuits are also increasing, with more children turning to indoor entertainment. For example, in the United States, children aged 8-18 years watch an average of more than 3 hours of television daily (Roberts and Foehr, 2004). The ownership of televisions has increased dramatically in some developing countries such as China (Popkin and Gordon-Larsen, 2004), but there is limited data from developing countries on hours of television watched by children in particular. In South Africa, 25.2 percent of school-aged children were found to spend more than 3 hours per day watching television or playing computer or videogames (Reddy et al., 2003).

Trends in Marketing That Influence Tobacco Use and Nutrition

A common, although mistaken, belief about chronic diseases is that they arise out of irresponsible personal lifestyle decisions made by individuals—this is only partially true. This tendency to blame the individual for faulty lifestyle choices, and hence onset of disease, has in part led to the current situation of inadequate response from the international public health community to combat the burden. However, broader environmental and socioeconomic determinants are also at play, which lie far from the control of the individual (Yach et al., 2004). Marketing—which has the principal aim of persuasion, pushing a passive observer into becoming an active consumer of a product or service—has the potential of magnifying exposure to CVD risk factors. Marketing related to CVD risk factors is part of the broader social determinants underlying behavioral and lifestyle changes occurring among children and young adults that increase their risk for developing CVD later in life.

Children and teenagers may be disproportionately vulnerable to the effects of marketing. Children under the age of 8 years lack the level of cognitive sophistication required to understand the true persuasive motive of advertising, which has led psychologists and child development experts to view this age group as vulnerable to the effects of the marketing of potentially unhealthy products (John, 1999). While the ability to process advertisements develops by age 8 years, preadolescents (8- to 10-year-olds) do not necessarily process the information they get from ads critically (Strasburger, 2001). Moreover, adolescents, going through a physically and emotionally trying period, might be easily swayed by advertisements focusing on issues related to identity, peer culture, emotions, and sexuality (Story and French, 2004). In addition, children are targeted due to their indirect influence over household food purchases, their direct spending on food and beverages, as well as their potential as future adult consumers (Story and French, 2004). Studies have found that the amount of time spent watching TV predicts the number of times children ask for products at the grocery store, with a majority of the products being the ones advertised on TV (Arnas, 2006; Galst and White, 1976; Taras et al., 1989). One of the main aims of such advertising is to get children to convince their parents to buy their products, what marketers call "pester power" or "nag factor" (Center for Science in the Public Interest, 2003). Thus aggressive marketing of unhealthful products can be seen as a part of the larger socioeconomic environment that compels the youth to adopt lifestyles that are detrimental to their health.

One of the biggest concerns in marketing has been the impact of tobacco advertising on children and adolescents. Tobacco campaigning is often targeted at younger age groups and has tremendous potential to affect their perceptions of smoking, glossing over its harmful effects, and giving them the image of social acceptability, thereby encouraging them to try smoking early in life. Because smoking is highly addictive, any attempt to try smoking at an early age can lead to serious addictions lasting late into adulthood. Several studies have demonstrated that cigarette retail marketing increases the likelihood of youth smoking uptake (Slater et al., 2007), receptivity to tobacco promotion among adolescents increases their chances of progressing from experimentation to established smoking (Choi et al., 2002), and exposure and receptivity to tobacco advertising are highly associated with tobacco use among schoolchildren (Arora et al., 2008).

It has been argued that the role played by marketing in accelerating the tobacco epidemic has parallels in the current obesity epidemic that is affecting increasingly younger populations today (Chopra and Darnton-Hill, 2004). The food industry in the west, and now even in the developing world, relies heavily on marketing to promote global brands. In the United States, for instance, the food industry spends $30 billion on direct advertising, more than any other industry in the country (Chopra and Darnton-Hill, 2004), and the prime target population is children and adolescents. According to one of the most recent reports on food advertising on television aimed at children, published by the Henry J. Kaiser Family Foundation (2007), 2- to 7-year-olds are exposed to 4,400, 8- to 12-year-olds to 7,600, and 13- to 17-year-olds to 6,000 food ads per year. These ads are not for nutritious foods; according to the former report, 50 percent of all ad time during children's shows is for food, out of which 34 percent are for candies and snacks, 28 percent are for cereal, 10 percent are for fast food, and only 4 and 1 percent, respectively, are for dairy products and fruit juices. The report found that there were no ads for fruits and vegetables during children's television shows. With market liberalization and globalization, the effects of promotional marketing have reached all corners of the developing world. This is clearly demonstrated by global fast food and soft drink companies, which have been expanding internationally at a rapid pace. Of particular interest is a marketing strategy used by these companies, termed "glocal" marketing, the main thrust of which is to create demand by replacing traditional food consumption habits with their products, and then to increase demand by applying global marketing principles. Even in these local markets, their prime target populations are children and teenagers (Hawkes, 2002).

Several studies have shown the influence food advertising can have on children's food choices. Gorn and Goldberg (1982) experimentally manipulated the kind of ads seen by children attending a camp for a month and found that the ones that had been exposed to fruit commercials most often chose orange juice as a beverage, while the ones exposed to candy commercials picked the least amount of fruits and juice as snacks. Children and adolescents are bombarded with food advertisements and promotions from various channels. While the television is the most common mode of promotion in the United States for food products, multiple other channels are used, including in-school advertising, the Internet, product placements, kids' clubs, branded toys, and cross-promotions, (i.e., utilizing cartoon and movie characters, musicians, and athletes) (Story and French, 2004). Other indirect forms of marketing used include public-relations marketing, service-related marketing, sports sponsorship, and philanthropy (Hawkes, 2002). This multichannel targeting amplifies the effect of marketing on the food habits of children.

Conclusion 6.1: Accumulation of cardiovascular risks begins early in life, and strong evidence supports the value of starting cardiovascular health promotion during pregnancy and early childhood and continuing prevention efforts throughout the life course. Maternal and child health programs and other settings that already serve children in low and middle income countries offer an opportunity to provide care that takes into account not only shorter-term childhood outcomes but also long-term healthful behavior and reduction of chronic disease risk.

INTERVENTION APPROACHES AND OPPORTUNITIES

School-Based Programs

In places where school attendance is compulsory or attendance rates are high the school environment presents a particularly ideal location for health promotion interventions, because on school days, these children spend nearly half of their waking hours in school. However, the sizeable variations in both primary and secondary school attendance rates must be taken into account when considering the potential effectiveness and prioritization of school-based initiatives. While 80 percent of boys and 77 percent of girls reportedly attend primary schools in developing countries, in the least developed nations only 65 percent of males and 63 percent of females attend school. The lowest percentages are seen in West and Central Africa, while the highest are in Latin America and the Caribbean and the Commonwealth of Independent States. However, within each of these regions, there exists additional variation at the country level. When looking at secondary school—the ages at which youth are most susceptible to risk behavior development—those numbers drop to 48 percent male and 43 percent female, respectively, for developing and 26 percent male and 24 percent female, respectively, for least developed nations (UNICEF, 2008).

In addition, evaluations of school-based programs must be interpreted with caution. The lack of blinding of study personnel and inherent biases associated with self-reported data, selection of school sites, and even objective data collection may lead to an overestimation of treatment effects. Also, these programs have not operated or been evaluated over time and on a large scale, so the long-term benefits as well as any potential harmful effects of these interventions merit additional study. In addition, it is important to note that the data from low and middle income settings is extremely limited. Regardless of these limitations, the increasing popularity of these types of interventions makes it imperative to examine the benefits of programs that promote everything from increased physical activity and reduced tobacco use to youth empowerment.

In recognition of the importance of targeting youth for health promotion activities, WHO has recently launched the Global School Health Initiative with the goal of increasing the number of "Health-Promoting Schools" worldwide (WHO, 2010a). Of the five identified components of a health-promoting school, the focus on nutrition and food safety programs and opportunities for physical education and recreation directly address two of the key determinants of CVD in youth (WHO, 2010a). In addition to the Global School Health Initiative, the newly formed Mega Country Health Promotion Network has also included a school health component into its mission. Current priorities include the development of a "School-Based Multi-Risk Information Surveillance System," the development and implementation of pilot programs targeting youth tobacco use, and increasing collaboration effort between members (WHO Mega Country Health Promotion Network, 2001). The annual meetings of both the Global School Health Initative and the Mega Country Health Promotion Network also provide potential opportunities for the kinds of regional dissemination and partnerships that are discussed further in Chapter 8.

School-Based Tobacco Prevention Programs

School-based tobacco prevention is a frequently used mechanism to target youth. Experience in developed countries using school-level interventions for tobacco control has been mixed In recent reviews of school-based smoking prevention, Flay (2009a, 2009b) concludes that these programs can have significant long-term effects if they:

1. include 15 or more sessions over multiple years;
2. include some sessions in high school;
3. use the social influence model and interactive delivery methods;
4. include components on norms, commitment not to use, intentions not to use, and training and practice in the use of refusal and other life skills; and
5. use peer leaders in some role.

Flay estimated that this type of school-based program can reduce smoking onset by 25 to 30 percent, and school plus community programs can reduce smoking onset by 35 to 40 percent by the end of high school.

The findings were based on programs in developed countries due to lack of rigorous research on school-based smoking prevention in developing countries, although some school-based programs in middle income countries (South Africa, China, Thailand, Taiwan, India, and Pakistan) were identified in the review (Flay, 2009b). Elements of successful approaches to smoking prevention can potentially be adapted to be effective in developing countries. However, it can be challenging to adapt a successful school-based program for use with populations in different contexts, especially in other cultures and in varying levels and types of school system infrastructure. It is important to implement with fidelity, to monitor implementation, and to evaluate outcomes. Therefore, the effectiveness and implementation of such adaptation needs to be the subject of research so that the benefits of school-based smoking prevention can be evaluated objectively in low and middle income settings (Flay, 2009a).

Experience in India suggests that multicomponent intervention is effective in delaying onset and reducing tobacco use among youth. An Indo-U.S. collaborative endeavor between the University of Texas and Health Related Information Dissemination Amongst Youth (HRIDAY) is a model of collaboration between researchers in developed and developing countries in adapting and replicating the experience of U.S.-school-based smoking prevention intervention in schools in India. Project HRIDAY was a school-based cluster randomized trial in India of 30 public and private elementary schools. The study showed that an intervention that included information provision, interactive classroom activities, and roundtable discussions reduced experimentation, intentions to use tobacco, and offers of tobacco among the intervention schools (Reddy et al., 2002). Another multicomponent group randomized intervention trial designed and implemented in Indian schools was Project MYTRI (Mobilizing Youth for Tobacco Related Initiatives in India). After a rigorous 2-year tobacco use prevention intervention, students in the intervention schools were significantly less likely than controls to exhibit an increase in cigarette or bidi smoking. They were also less likely to intend to smoke or chew tobacco in the future (Perry et al., 2009). These experiences are now being applied to conduct Project ACTIVITY (Advancing Cessation of Tobacco in Vulnerable Indian Tobacco Consuming Youth), a group randomized trial to test the efficacy of a comprehensive, community-based tobacco control intervention among disadvantaged youth (10-19 years) living in low income communities of Delhi, India (Dell Center for Healthy Living, 2010).

Contrastingly, a recent attempt to "translate" existing school-based smoking prevention programs from the United States and Australia to the cultural context of South Africa was less successful. Resnicow et al. (2008) conducted a clustered randomized controlled trial of two new school-based approaches, the Life Skills Training model, shown to be effective with inner-city and urban youth in the United States, and the Harm Minimization strategy, which showed significant positive results in an experimental trial in Western Australia, and compared each to the standard tobacco use education. Following the intervention, the two new approaches did not differ significantly in their effect on preventing the initiation of tobacco use among youth. However, significant differences were seen in the approaches between boys and girls, indicating an important area for further study given the rising rates of female tobacco use in many countries (Resnicow et al., 2008). Thus, while many school-based programs currently underway in developed countries have the potential to be effective in developing-country settings, cultural, economic, and social differences may limit the transferability of these efforts. More research is needed regarding what aspects of prevention programs are sensitive to cultural variations and which adaptation strategies may be most effective when bringing an existing program to new environments.

School-Based Childhood Obesity, Physical Activity, Nutrition, and CVD Prevention Programs

In the face of the almost pandemic increase in the rates of chronic diseases over the past decade, the need to improve nutrition and increase physical activity is very apparent. In recent times, many interventions have used schools as the vehicle of change because the school culture is seen as one that fosters and supports physical activity and health. Several school-based obesity prevention and health promotion programs have been successfully implemented and evaluated in high income countries, but published efforts from low and middle income countries are scarce.

Several studies in high income countries have demonstrated some effectiveness in reducing risk among children through efforts to improve nutrition as well as to promote physical activity. These interventions have included components such as school self-assessment; nutrition education; nutrition policy for school meals; social marketing; student involvement and empowerment; curricular enhancements that focus on decreased television viewing, reduced consumption of soft drinks and foods high in total and saturated fat, increased fruit and vegetable intake, and increased moderate and vigorous physical activity; parent outreach; and home-based activities. Thus, there are models of programs that have been effective at changing behavioral risk factors and, in some cases, preventing or reducing overweight and obesity (Foster et al., 2008; Gortmaker et al., 1999; Luepker et al., 1996; Veugelers and Fitzgerald, 2005).

Programs more narrowly focused on increasing physical activity have a somewhat more robust evidence base. It is theorized that a physically active childhood would increase the likelihood of maintaining an active lifestyle throughout adult life, which in turn would enhance adult well-being and reduce the risk of chronic diseases in adulthood (Dobbins et al., 2009; Freedson, 1992). From a health perspective, therefore, it appears logical to encourage youth to engage in regular activity. Several interventions for promoting physical activity and fitness in schools have been evaluated in high income country settings using strategies such as changes in the school physical environment; changes in school curriculum to increase time spent on physical activity, particularly on vigorous physical activity during physical education classes; and provision of play equipment and activity cards (Dobbins et al., 2009).

There is convincing evidence that physical education (PE)-based strategies are effective for increasing and maintaining physical activity in school children. The strategies include increasing frequency of PE (e.g., four times per week), increasing PE duration, increasing activity levels during PE classes, and delivering PE using specialists or trained teachers (Naylor and McKay, 2009). In addition to PE, another strategy is to change the school's physical environment to be more conducive to physical activity in children. Some studies have indicated that improving playgrounds in schools, providing play equipment to schools, or incorporating activity breaks into the elementary school classroom can have positive effects on improving physical activity levels among students, but few studies have rigorously evaluated these approaches (Naylor and McKay, 2009).

In some cases, interventions have been comprised of a combination of multiple components. These approaches combine health education curricula and school environment with other approaches to improve nutrition and physical activity among children. Strategies to engage parents, as well as community-based strategies, mass media, and policy development have formed a part of some interventions. These combined interventions are typically incorporated into a broader program for obesity or chronic disease prevention. Evidence suggests that longer duration, multicomponent interventions are more effective in bringing about a positive change (Dobbins et al., 2009).

Although evidence from low and middle income countries is scarce, there have been a few studies designed to encourage physical activity in middle income countries. Liu et al. (2008) evaluated the effect of the Happy 10 program (incorporating two 10-minute activity breaks into classes) on the promotion of physical activity and obesity control in two primary schools in Beijing. This pilot study showed significantly improved physical activity levels and increased energy expenditure in the intervention group.

The prevalence of overweight and obesity was significantly reduced in the intervention group compared to the control school.

Jiang et al. (2007) conducted a 3-year multicomponent intervention program in 2,425 children (1,029 children in intervention schools and 1,396 children in control schools) in Beijing. The program involved schools and families and emphasized both nutrition and physical activity The program showed significantly reduced prevalence of overweight and obesity in intervention schools compared to the control schools.

Kain et al. (2004) assessed the impact of a 6-month multicomponent intervention on primary schoolchildren in Chile through changes in adiposity and physical fitness. The intervention included nutrition education for children and parents, "healthier" kiosks, 90 minutes of additional physical activity weekly, a behavioral physical activity program designed to teach children about the benefits of physical activity and an active lifestyle, and active recess. The study showed improved physical fitness in both boys and girls and significantly reduced adiposity only in boys.

In summary, there is sufficient evidence to support the potential effectiveness of school-based promotion programs for children in a limited number of settings that are reasonably analogous to the high income country settings in the program models described here and that have sufficient capacity and motivation for long-term sustainability. However, as described for many of the intervention approaches here and in Chapter 5, more evidence from interventions in low and middle income countries is greatly needed. Even if programs are successful on a small scale, it is not known what it will take to diffuse and implement programs on a large scale in developing countries. Demonstration programs need to be developed and evaluated in low and middle income countries before widespread implementation at scale would be justified.

Youth-Focused Policy Initiatives

Tobacco Control

There have been a number of initiatives both at the international and government levels to control the increasing use of tobacco products in both the developed and developing worlds. The World Health Organization's (WHO's) Tobacco Free Initiative was launched for tobacco control through research, policy, surveillance, capacity building, and global communications (WHO, 2010b). Events like World No Tobacco Day have become extremely popular in creating awareness about the harmful effects of tobacco. The Framework Convention for Tobacco Control (FCTC), described in Chapter 5, is a major public health treaty that was adopted by the World Health Assembly in 2003. Among its provisions is an explicit mention of banning the sale of tobacco products to legal minors, and although it has provisions that are applicable for all ages, its principles are particularly targeted to youth, the most vulnerable group to initiate tobacco use (WHO, 2003).

However, despite the adoption of the FCTC, tobacco control programs in low and middle income countries have been limited in their implementation and variable in their success. In addition, the tobacco industry has developed methods to counteract or dilute the effects of policy changes, and young adolescents may be particularly susceptible to these actions as they begin to explore the adult world (Shafey et al., 2009). This is exemplified by India's experience. The government of India adopted a comprehensive legislation for controlling tobacco use known as the Cigarette and Other Tobacco Products Act (COTPA) in 2003. This act, along with other provisions, banned the sale of all tobacco products to youth younger than 18 years and within 100 yards of educational institutions (Reddy et al., 2006). However, taxation of tobacco products was not included in COTPA, and recent taxation measures have continued the practice of exempting (or minimally taxing) bidis and chewable forms of tobacco on the grounds that these tobacco products are often consumed by the poor (Reddy and Gupta, 2004). The tobacco industry also responded to COTPA; for example, one tobacco company placed air-conditioned mobile lounges for smokers outside major attractions, such as sports stadiums and shopping malls, in four major cities in India (Reddy et al., 2006). In 2007, the government of India, in compliance with the FCTC and COTPA, launched the National Tobacco Control Program (NTCP) to build capacity of the states to effectively implement the tobacco control laws and also to bring about greater awareness about the ill effects of tobacco consumption. Under the NTCP, Tobacco Control Cells were set up in selected states in India to provide technical support to plan, coordinate, and monitor all activities related to tobacco control at the state level (Volunteer Health Association of India, 2009).

Recent progress in combating youth tobacco use has also been seen in the Philippines. The 2003 installment of the GYTS reported that current cigarette use declined significantly, from 32.6 percent (2000) to 21.8 percent (2003) for boys and from 12.9 percent (2000) to 8.8 percent (2003) in girls. The use of other forms of tobacco also experienced a precipitous decline in both adolescent boys and girls between 2000 and 2003, from 18.3 to 10.9 percent and 9.5 to 5.7 percent, respectively. Finally, the proportion of never smokers who reported being likely to initiate smoking within the next year was 13.8 percent in 2003, almost half as many who reported this likelihood in 2000 (26.5 percent). These declines both followed and coincided with a number of major changes in tobacco control policies in the Philippines. While many factors likely contributed to this decline, one significant piece of policy legislation passed in 1999 was the Philippines Clean

Air Act, which limited smoking indoors by enacting smoke-free indoor air laws. Building on this momentum, in 2003 the Youth Smoking Cessation Program led to the establishment of smoke-free campuses. In addition, the Tobacco Regulatory Act, also enacted in 2003, continues these efforts by increasing public education, banning all tobacco advertising, strengthening warning labels on tobacco products, and prohibiting the sale of tobacco to minors (Miguel-Baquilod et al., 2005).

In the face of resistance from the tobacco industry and its continued attempts to market their products, proactive steps need to be taken that can protect children and adolescents from exposure to tobacco products. A significant step in this direction has been taken with the initiation of the WHO FCTC, described previously. Antitobacco advertising, for example, can be effective in deterring children and preadolescents from taking up the habit in the first place (Penchmann, 2001; Wakefield et al., 2003). While evidence regarding the role of antitobacco advertising in encouraging young adults to quit the habit is inconclusive, antitobacco marketing, combined with other strategies to restrict tobacco use, can be an effective strategy in reducing the impact of tobacco promotion.

Restricting Food Marketing

There is a continued need for the international public health community, learning from the experience with the tobacco industry, to develop a sustained, global response to the aggressive marketing of potentially unhealthful food products, aimed pointedly at children and adolescents. Marketing restrictions, curtailing advertising of such products in children's television, and the banning of in-school marketing, accompanied by the promotion of healthful foods such as fruits and vegetables, are some examples of steps that can be and have been taken to this end. Although studies on the effectiveness of marketing restrictions is inconclusive, the Institute of Medicine examined the issue in the United States and determined that the totality of the evidence available indicates that television marketing to children under the age of 11 years does affect the dietary preferences and patterns of youth (IOM, 2006). Support for the reasonableness of marketing restrictions given the available evidence has also been articulated in other recent policy-oriented reviews (Hastings et al., 2006; IOM, 2006). This guidance must be considered with caution when addressing similar challenges in developing countries due to potential differences in advertising type and exposure levels, but it does support both measured action and additional research into effective activities to promote better nutrition.

Since 2004, a number of countries have employed a variety of strategies to limit food marketing to children. Product advertisements are largely dominated by promotion of the "big five": pre-sugared breakfast cereals, soft drinks, confectionary, savory snacks, and fast food retailers (Hastings et al., 2006). Television commercials have dominated marketing efforts in the past, but there is emerging evidence that alternative branding mechanisms, most notably for the fast food industry, are growing in importance in developing countries (Hastings et al., 2006). While statutory regulations are the most common attempt at marketing restrictions, it is in fact self-regulation by the private sector and advertising corporations that are playing the largest part in limiting advertising to children (Hawkes, 2007).

Many developed and some developing countries limit the amount or duration of advertisements permitted to air during children's television programming, from 5 minutes in Spain to 15 minutes in Venezuela. In 2006 in Brazil, the ministry of health drafted proposed legislation directly restricting and in some cases proscribing food-related advertising to children. Additionally, India has recently developed an inter-ministerial committee to review questionable television advertisements and more routinely enforce the previously established Cable Television Act Rules. Despite these promising steps, specific targeting of food products in statutory regulation remains extremely rare in both developed and developing countries (Hawkes, 2007).

Self-regulation, both by advertising agencies and individual companies, is by far the most common regulatory mechanism used in the European Union and is employed to a lesser extent in South-East Asia, New Zealand and Australia, and some African nations. The International Chamber of Commerce published a Framework for Responsible Food and Beverage Communications that focuses on reducing food and drink marketing approaches that are misleading to children, and a similar set of principles were endorsed by the Confederation of the Food and Drink Industries of the European Union (Hawkes, 2007). In addition, the International Food and Beverage Alliance's (IFBA's) Global Policy and Pledge Programs, which require participants to only market nutritionally sound products to youth, was recently expanded to Brazil, South Africa, Russia, and Thailand (International Food and Beverage Alliance, 2009). Since 2008, the IFBA reports greater than 99 percent compliance with the Pledge Programs by companies in participating countries (International Food and Beverage Alliance, 2009) Progress at monitoring and enforcing these self-regulation mechanisms in low and middle income countries has been more inconsistent and ranges from almost no action in South Africa to the very responsive Indian Advertising Standards Council (Hawkes, 2007).

There has been limited evidence demonstrating whether or not efforts to regulate food marketing will result in a positive health impact. Nonetheless, there is a strong rationale for these efforts, and the increasing prevalence of voluntary commitments by private companies and associations provides the potential for the cardiovascular disease prevention community to forge partnerships with the private sector and makes this a feasible area for further implementation, as described further in Chapter 8. Thus, while the pursuit of stronger regulation of food marketing to children may not be a nation's first priority, the presence of a growing global movement and the fact that many food and beverage companies have already taken the initiative to begin instituting self-imposed limits presents an opportunity for the global CVD community to encourage progress in this effort. In addition, enhanced efforts in policy research in this area—in collaboration with the child obesity field—would make a significant contribution to health promotion.

Youth-Focused Awareness and Advocacy

Mass Media

An important aspect of interventions for CVD prevention is health promotion through mass media campaigns. Because habits related to diet and physical activity begin to be established at an early age, and because adolescents and young adults are particularly susceptible to experimenting with alcohol and tobacco use, targeting campaigns focused on these risk factors of younger age groups is a rational strategy (IOM, 2006).

There are several examples of national-level mass media campaigns that have been successful in achieving greater awareness of the importance of healthful dietary habits and physical activity in leading a healthy life. One such example is the Australian government's two-pronged mass media strategy, with one campaign addressing the importance of healthful eating (the Go for 2&5® campaign), and the other addressing the importance of incorporating more physical activity into children's lives (the Get Moving campaign). Both campaigns targeted parents of 0- to 17-year-olds, along with children and youth aged 5-17 years. The main aims of the campaigns were to increase awareness of, improve attitudes toward, and change intentions to increase healthful eating and physical activity in the lives of the target audience. The campaigns adopted multiple elements to communicate its message, including television, radio, and print commercials; shopping center and shopping cart advertisements; media partnership activities; a campaign website; an information line; and distribution of other reading material. In an evaluation of the campaigns, Elliot and Walker (2007) found both aspects of the campaigns to be successful in generating awareness, increasing knowledge, and enhancing more positive attitudes toward healthful eating and physical activity. Although they didn't find these to translate into improved behavior to a considerable extent, they did find a trend toward the right direction, which, given a more sustained and long-term campaign, could have been more substantial. Thus, the duration for which a mass media campaign should run to bring about significant change at the population level is an important consideration when developing such campaigns.

A systematic review of mass media campaigns in the United States and Norway for prevention of smoking among youth illustrates this point (Sowden and Arblaster, 2000). Out of the six studies that met the inclusion criteria, Sowden found that only two significantly reduced smoking behavior among young people; both of these studies were of longer duration and of greater intensity than the others. In addition, both successful campaigns were based on sound theories and included extensive formative research.

Carrying out adequate formative research before developing a campaign is extremely important. The success of one campaign doesn't necessarily translate into successful implementation in all other settings. The success of mass media campaigns is greatly contingent on the characteristics and requirements of the target population, and educational levels, socioeconomic backgrounds, and cultural backdrops go a long way in determining whether such a campaign will generate results in the desired direction. Thus it is important to tailor social marketing efforts to the needs and constraints of particular contexts and peoples before anticipating a successful outcome.

Another use of the media is through direct educational programming. Sesame Workshop, for example, is a nonprofit educational organization that develops educational content delivered in a variety of ways—including television, radio, books, magazines, interactive media, and community outreach. Taking advantage of all forms of media and using those that are best suited to deliver a particular curriculum, it efficiently reaches millions of children, parents, caregivers, and educators—locally, nationally, and globally. Sesame Workshop uses a collaborative, research-intensive approach to the development of programs and activities. Its offerings strive to reflect both a deep understanding of children's developmental needs and the best ways to address those needs in order to engage children in a way that maximizes learning (Cole, 2009; Sesame Workshop, 2010).

Health and wellness is one of the key themes of Sesame Workshop, including programs to foster health habits and life skills that are active in 18 developed and developing countries. One of these programs is "Healthy Habits for Life" in Colombia, which addresses the need for nutrition and exercise learning and aims to instill healthful behaviors in children. An impact evaluation for this program is currently underway with researchers from the Children's Heart Foundation (Bogotá) and Mount Sinai Medical Center (New York); the results are expected in mid-2010 (Cole, 2009).

Youth-Driven Advocacy

Youth Advocacy for CVD Over the past decade, a number of youth-driven initiatives have targeted reduction in CVD risk factors and demonstrated the potential power in the energy and enthusiasm of young people. In the United States, for example, Kick Butts Day (KBD) is annual event for youth advocacy, leadership, and activism for tobacco control from the Campaign for Tobacco Free Kids (CTFK). This event is now in its 15th year. Youth advocacy groups can register on the KBD website. Each year, a date is decided when KBD events are organized across the United States, with resources and merchandise provided to the participating youth groups by CTFK. In addition, CTFK also facilitates media mobilization to garner media attention for the various events that are organized. This concerted youth advocacy effort organizes support for specific tobacco control policies at the national and local level, which teaches young people about the process of policy initiatives while pursuing tangible end goals (Campaign for Tobacco Free Kids, 2010).

The Global Youth Action on Tobacco (GYAT) Network was founded in 2006 during a pre-conference youth advocacy training workshop organized by Essential Action and CTFK in conjunction with the 13th World Conference on Tobacco or Health (WCTOH). The participants for this workshop included youth health advocates from 30 countries. Contact is maintained through e-connectivity, allowing members to share experiences with advocacy events focused on targeting the tobacco industry (Global Youth Action on Tobacco Network, 2009).

Another organization that can serve as a model for youth-driven advocacy in low and middle income countries is Youth For Health (Y4H). Y4H is a network comprised of nearly 220,000 youth health advocates from 45 countries across the globe. Y4H was launched during the first Global Youth Meet on Health (GYM 2006), a unique global health conclave with participation from 280 youth from 35 countries. GYM 2006 was organized by HRIDAY, a nongovernemtnal organization based in Delhi, India, engaged in awareness, advocacy, and research related to health promotion (HRIDAY–SHAN, 2006). The deliberations during GYM 2006 highlighted the need for a sustained network of global youth to take the battle forward in their respective countries while having a common platform to monitor progress and share knowledge, which led to the Y4H movement. The group aims to connect young people from around the world, forming a global alliance of national, regional, and global partnerships that can collectively promote common causes. These include advocating for tobacco control, healthful diets, regular physical activity, environmental protection, gender equality, women's health, and reduction of alcohol and drug abuse (HRIDAY–SHAN, 2006).

A dedicated forum facilitates sharing of experiences and undertaking concerted global action on health promotion by encouraging youth advocates to start in their own communities or countries and present their views to legislatures and other policy makers (Youth For Health, 2009). For example, Y4H activists from Argentina, Chile, Colombia, Mexico, and Uruguay worked together to draft an antitobacco manifesto in September 2007, and in South Africa Y4H members have called for stricter tobacco control policies. They presented their views in front of the South African Parliamentary Committee reviewing the Tobacco Act. In Georgia, a "HeartWeek" event was organized by Georgia Against Tobacco and Drugs (an organization formed by the Georgian Y4H delegates), where youth sport competitions were held to raise awareness about physical activity and its connections with heart health. More than 100 children aged 8-12 years (including 3 with diabetes and 4 with heart problems) from Georgia, Armenia, and Azerbaijan participated in these events (Youth For Health, 2009).

At the global level, an electronic signature campaign on Global Health Promotion for Youth with a focus on tobacco control, initiated by Y4H members and endorsed by more than 225,000 youth and adults worldwide, was presented by Y4H members to the Secretary General of the United Nations (UN) on October 24, 2007 (UN Day) at the UN Headquarters in New York. Y4H representatives discussed action areas of Y4H activities with the Secretary General and Special Adviser to the Secretary General on Gender Issues and Advancement of Women. In addition, in 2009, Y4H helped organize the Global Youth Meet on Tobacco Control (GYM 2009), a pre-conference to the 14th WCTOH. GYM 2009 was attended by 140 participants from 27 countries who discussed tobacco control issues (HRIDAY–SHAN, 2006).

Lessons from Youth Advocacy on HIV/AIDS Examples of youth advocacy efforts for cardiovascular disease in developing countries are limited, but lessons can be learned from some successful youth movements in the global HIV/AIDS community. For example, the Global Youth Coalition on HIV/AIDS (GYCA) was started by young people following the 2004 International AIDS Conference in Bangkok, Thailand. Now, with partnerships and support from the Joint United Nations Programme on HIV/AIDS (UNAIDS), the United Nations Population Fund (UNFPA), and other multinational NGOs, the GYCA operates programs in 150 countries through diverse initiatives ranging from the distribution of small grants to "outstanding young leaders" to participation in international summits (Global Youth Coalition on HIV/AIDS, 2010). Groups also network among themselves, allowing them to share best practices and advocacy tools. Because the entire program is led by young people, it not only provides opportunities for members to make a positive impact on their community, but also establishes connections between the next generation of HIV advocates and leaders. This is just one of the many efforts driven by the efforts of young people around the world in the fight against HIV/AIDS that can be examined for lessons learned.

In summary, the opportunity to capitalize on the momentum of youth advocacy in global health to increase awareness of the importance of cardiovascular health presents promising potential for the global CVD community. If efforts are to be successful and sustained, it will be critical to both push young people interested in heart health to think globally and to encourage young people already acting on the global health stage to recognize that cardiovascular disease is a fundamental component of youth wellness.

CHALLENGES TO IMPLEMENTING YOUTH-BASED PROGRAMS IN LOW AND MIDDLE INCOME COUNTRIES

Despite great progress in identifying increasing trends in the acquisition of risk early in life, data on the incidence and prevalence of CVD risk factors in youth remain very limited. More data is clearly needed to prioritize avenues for program implementation and intervention research, yet the best methods to pursue information specific to children and adolescents remain unclear. The Global Youth Tobacco Survey and South African Youth Risk Behavioral Survey are stand-alone efforts focused entirely on issues pertaining to children and adolescents, specifically targeting those groups through schools and other venues. Efforts such as these have the advantage of using questions, survey and interview strategies, and analytical models that are tailored to the needs of youth and produce a more comprehensive picture of the targeted risk behaviors in that age group. However, in order to accomplish surveys such as these, additional resources must be committed, and in some cases perhaps diverted away from existing surveillance efforts. Alternatively, the disaggregation of results of already established or ongoing surveillance efforts by age may also provide a relevant data picture with fewer additional resources required. The greater potential feasibility of this option in developing countries warrants further investigation into what survey methodologies might be most effective when youth are one of the many target populations. Regardless of which approach is ultimately selected, as discussed in Chapter 4, efforts must be made to ensure that local country and community capacity to conduct both the survey and analysis is strengthened. This is essential to ensuring the sustainability of such efforts, a critical need in order to reveal extended temporal trends that can identify whether youth-focused initiatives are ultimately having any impact on health status.

In addition to the need for better data on CVD risk factors in children and youth, evidence from youth-focused interventions targeted at these risk factors in low and middle countries is also quite limited. There are some promising findings, especially in the area of tobacco reduction. Other intervention approaches with some success in developed countries offer models for adaptation. However, many of these possible models did not operate over long periods of time and on a large scale. The issue of what it will take to adapt, diffuse, implement, and maintain programs on a large scale in low and middle income countries needs to be addressed. One particularly important potential barrier to adopting cardiovascular health promotion programs targeting children and youth in schools and other settings is whether there exist reasonable incentives for non-health organizations to create and maintain such programs. For schools, the advantages of implementing such programs are not often straightforward. For example, physical activity may be central in some schools, but the engagement and participation of schools are not guaranteed, especially if there is a competition for resources that would otherwise be dedicated to their primary academic mission. They may not commit limited resources to programs over the long term if the incentives for doing so are weak and the interventions are complex to implement, manage, and maintain. Thus, it is necessary to consider the long-term viability of such efforts as the programs may dissipate even if there is early enthusiasm, especially in developing countries where resources may be limited. Additionally, in order for many school-based interventions to be implemented, especially at a large scale, there may need to be interaction and cooperation between different divisions of the national government, such as the health and education sectors. The degree to which each of these independent agents work together varies in developing countries, and thus effort may be required to assist different sectors in coordinating their actions where appropriate and feasible. This coordination with the education sector is thus a critical component of the broader messages in this report supporting intersectoral and whole-of-government approaches to address CVD and related chronic diseases.

CONCLUSION

Accumulation of cardiovascular risk begins early in life, and evidence on rising rates of childhood obesity and youth smoking in low and middle income countries as well as emerging evidence on the effects of early nutrition on later cardiovascular health support the value of starting cardiovascular health promotion during pregnancy and early childhood and continuing prevention efforts throughout the life course. Maternal and child health (MCH) programs offer an opportunity to provide care that takes into account not only shorter-term childhood outcomes but also future lifelong health. In particular, emerging evidence on the effects of early nutrition on later cardiovascular health means that the CVD and MCH communities need to work together more closely to ensure that food and nutrition programs for undernourished children do not inadvertently contribute to long-term chronic disease risk. This could be accomplished through future coordination with multinational organizations that provide both service and programmatic guidance such as the United Nations World Food Program, United States Agency for International Development, Oxfam America, and Save the Children, as well as through direct consultation with local governments where possible. Increased efforts are needed to identify ways in which emergency and long-term food provision can be accomplished without unnecessarily increasing CVD risk or significantly increasing existing program costs.

The available evidence on the impact of cardiovascular health promotion and CVD prevention initiatives in childhood and adolescence is limited and of variable quality, especially in low and middle income country settings. Approaches with some success on a small scale that have emerging potential for developing countries include education initiatives targeted to children, school-based programs, and programs targeted to take advantage of the potential for adolescents and young adults to serve as powerful advocates for change. This foundation provides an opportunity to develop, evaluate, and implement child- and youth-based programs to prevent the development of CVD in later life.

REFERENCES

Aboderin, I., A. Kalache, Y. Ben-Shlomo, J. W. Lynch, C. S. Yajnik, D. Kuh, and D. Yach. 2002. *Life course perspectives on coronary heart disease, stroke and diabetes: Key issues and implications for policy and research.* Geneva: World Health Organization.

Agirbasli, M., S. Cakir, S. Ozme, and G. Ciliv. 2006. Metabolic syndrome in Turkish children and adolescents. *Metabolism: Clinical and Experimental* 55(8):1002-1006.

Al-Isa, A. N. 2004. Body mass index, overweight and obesity among Kuwaiti intermediate school adolescents aged 10-14 years. *European Journal of Clinical Nutrition* 58(9):1273-1277.

Arnas, Y. 2006. The effects of television food advertisement on children's food purchasing requests. *Pediatrics International* 48(2):138-145.

Arora, M., S. Reddy, M. H. Stigler, and C. L. Perry. 2008. Associations between tobacco marketing and use among urban youth in India. *American Journal of Health Behavior* 32(3):283-294.

Asma, S. 2009. Global tobacco surveillance system. Presentation at the Public Information Gathering Session for the Institute of Medicine Committee on Preventing the Global Epidemic of Cardiovascular Disease, Washington, DC.

Baker, J. L., L. W. Olsen, and T. I. A. Sørensen. 2007. Childhood body-mass index and the risk of coronary heart disease in adulthood. *New England Journal of Medicine* 357(23):2329-2337.

Barker, D. J. 1997. The fetal origins of coronary heart disease. *Acta Paediatrica Supplement* 422:78-82.
Barker, D. J. P. 1998. In utero programming of chronic disease. *Clinical Science* 95(2):115-128.
Barker, D. J. P. 2007. The origins of the developmental origins theory. *Journal of Internal Medicine* 261(5):412-417.
Barker, D. J. P., and S. P. Bagby. 2005. Developmental antecedents of cardiovascular disease: A historical perspective. *Journal of the American Society of Nephrology* 16(9):2537-2544.
Barker, D. J. P., C. Osmond, T. J. Forsen, E. Kajantie, and J. G. Eriksson. 2005. Trajectories of growth among children who have coronary events as adults. *New England Journal of Medicine* 353(17):1802-1809.
Berenson, G. S. 2002. Childhood risk factors predict adult risk associated with subclinical cardiovascular disease. The Bogalusa Heart Study. *American Journal of Cardiology* 90(10C):3L-7L.
Bhardwaj, S., A. Misra, L. Khurana, S. Gulati, P. Shah, and N. K. Vikram. 2008. Childhood obesity in Asian Indians: A burgeoning cause of insulin resistance, diabetes and subclinical inflammation. *Asia Pacific Journal of Clinical Nutrition* 17(Suppl 1):172-175.
Bhutta, Z. A., T. Ahmed, R. E. Black, S. Cousens, K. Dewey, E. Giugliani, B. A. Haider, B. Kirkwood, S. S. Morris, H. P. S. Sachdev, and M. Shekar. 2008. What works? Interventions for maternal and child undernutrition and survival. *Lancet* 371(9610):417-440.
Black, R. E., L. H. Allen, Z. A. Bhutta, L. E. Caulfield, M. de Onis, M. Ezzati, C. Mathers, and J. Rivera. 2008. Maternal and child undernutrition: Global and regional exposures and health consequences. *Lancet* 371(9608):243-260.
Buttross, L. S., and J. W. Kastner. 2003. A brief review of adolescents and tobacco: What we know and don't know. *American Journal of the Medical Sciences* 326(4):235-237.
Caballero, B. 2005. A nutrition paradox—underweight and obesity in developing countries. *New England Journal of Medicine* 352(15):1514-1516.
Caballero, B. 2009. Early undernutrition and risk of CVD in the adult. Presentation at Public Information Gathering Session for the Institute of Medicine Committee on Preventing the Global Epidemic of Cardiovascular Disease, Washington, DC.
Campaign for Tobacco Free Kids. 2010. *Kick butts day.* http://kickbuttsday.org (accessed February 19, 2010).
Celermajer, D. S., and J. G. Ayer. 2006. Childhood risk factors for adult cardiovascular disease and primary prevention in childhood. *Heart* 92(11):1701-1706.
Center for Science in the Public Interest. 2003. *Pestering parents: How food companies market obesity to children.* http://www.cspinet.org/pesteringparents (accessed August 23, 2009).
Choi, W. S., J. S. Ahluwalia, K. J. Harris, and K. Okuyemi. 2002. Progression to established smoking: The influence of tobacco marketing. *American Journal of Preventive Medicine* 22(4):228-233.
Chopra, M., and I. Darnton-Hill. 2004. Tobacco and obesity epidemics: Not so different after all? *British Medical Journal* 328(7455):1558-1560.
Cole, C. 2009. Plaza sésamo healthy habits for life: Colombia. Presentation at Public Information Gathering Session for the Institute of Medicine Committee on Preventing the Global Epidemic of Cardiovascular Disease, Washington, DC.
Committee on Environmental Health, Committee on Substance Abuse, Committee on Adolescence, and Committee on Native American Child Health. 2009. Tobacco use: A pediatric disease. *Pediatrics* 124:1474-1487.

Cook, S., M. Weitzman, P. Auinger, M. Nguyen, and W. H. Dietz. 2003. Prevalence of a metabolic syndrome phenotype in adolescents: Findings from the third National Health and Nutrition Examination Survey, 1988-1994. *Archives of Pediatrics and Adolescent Medicine* 157(8):821-827.

Crowther, N. J., N. Cameron, J. Trusler, and I. P. Gray. 1998. Association between poor glucose tolerance and rapid post natal weight gain in seven-year-old children. *Diabetologia* 41(10):1163-1167.

Cruz, M. L., M. J. Weigensberg, T. T. K. Huang, G. Ball, G. Q. Shaibi, and M. I. Goran. 2004. The metabolic syndrome in overweight hispanic youth and the role of insulin sensitivity. *Journal of Clinical Endocrinology and Metabolism* 89(1):108-113.

Csabi, G., K. Torok, D. Molnar, and S. Jeges. 2000. Presence of metabolic cardiovascular syndrome in obese children. *European Journal of Pediatrics* 159(1-2):91-94.

Davey Smith, G. 2007. Life-course approaches to inequalities in adult chronic disease risk: Boyd Orr lecture. *Proceedings of the Nutrition Society* 66(2):216-236.

Davey Smith, G. 2008. Assessing intrauterine influences on offspring health outcomes: Can epidemiological studies yield robust findings? *Basic and Clinical Pharmacology and Toxicology* 102(2):245-256.

Davey Smith, G., C. Steer, S. Leary, and A. Ness. 2007. Is there an intrauterine influence on obesity? Evidence from parent-child associations in the Avon Longitudinal Study of Parents and Children (ALSPAC). *Archives of Disease in Childhood* 92(10):876-880.

Dell Center for Healthy Living. 2010. Project ACTIVITY (Advancing Cessation of Tobacco In Vulnerable Indian Tobacco Consuming Youth). http://www.sph.uth.tmc.edu/Dell HealthyLiving/default.aspx?id=3995 (accessed June 4, 2010)

DiFranza, J. R., J. A. Savageau, N. A. Rigotti, K. Fletcher, J. K. Ockene, A. D. McNeill, M. Coleman, and C. Wood. 2002. Development of symptoms of tobacco dependence in youths: 30 month follow up data from the Dandy Study. *Tobacco Control* 11(3):228-235.

Dobbins, M., K. De Corby, P. Robeson, H. Husson, and D. Tirilis. 2009. School-based physical activity programs for promoting physical activity and fitness in children and adolescents aged 6-18. *Cochrane Database Syst Rev*(1):CD007651.

Dollman, J., K. Norton, and L. Norton. 2005. Evidence for secular trends in children's physical activity behaviour. *British Journal of Sports Medicine* 39(12):892-897; discussion 897.

Dong, M., W. H. Giles, V. J. Felitti, S. R. Dube, J. E. Williams, D. P. Chapman, and R. F. Anda. 2004. Insights into causal pathways for ischemic heart disease: Adverse childhood experiences study. *Circulation* 110(13):1761-1766.

Elliott, D., and D. Walker. 2007. *Evaluation of the national 'get moving' campaign*. Australian Government Department of Health and Ageing, Commonwealth of Australia, Canberra.

Eriksson, J. G., T. Forsen, J. Tuomilehto, P. D. Winter, C. Osmond, and D. J. P. Barker. 1999. Catch-up growth in childhood and death from coronary heart disease: Longitudinal study. *British Medical Journal* 318:7181.

Felitti, V. J., R. F. Anda, D. Nordenberg, D. F. Williamson, A. M. Spitz, V. Edwards, M. P. Koss, and J. S. Marks. 1998. Relationship of childhood abuse and household dysfunction to many of the leading causes of death in adults: The adverse childhood experiences (ACE) study. *American Journal of Preventive Medicine* 14(4):245-258.

Flay, B. R. 2009a. The promise of long-term effectiveness of school-based smoking prevention programs: A critical review of reviews. *Tobacco Induced Diseases* 5(1):7.

Flay, B. R. 2009b. School-based smoking prevention programs with the promise of long-term effects. *Tobacco Induced Diseases* 5(1):6.

Forsen, T., J. G. Eriksson, J. Tuomilehto, C. Osmond, and D. J. P. Barker. 1999. Growth in utero and during childhood among women who develop coronary heart disease: Longitudinal study. *British Medical Journal* 319(7222):1403-1407.

Foster, G. D., S. Sherman, K. E. Borradaile, K. M. Grundy, S. S. Vander Veur, J. Nachmani, A. Karpyn, S. Kumanyika, and J. Shults. 2008. A policy-based school intervention to prevent overweight and obesity. *Pediatrics* 121(4):e794-e802.

Freedman, D. S., W. H. Dietz, S. R. Srinivasan, and G. S. Berenson. 1999. The relation of overweight to cardiovascular risk factors among children and adolescents: The Bogalusa heart study. *Pediatrics* 103(6):1175-1182.

Freedman, D. S., L. K. Khan, W. H. Dietz, S. R. Srinivasan, and G. S. Berenson. 2001. Relationship of childhood obesity to coronary heart disease risk factors in adulthood: The Bogalusa Heart Study. *Pediatrics* 108(3):712-718.

Freedson, P. S. 1992. Physical activity among children and youth. *Canadian Journal of Sport Sciences* 17(4):280-283.

Galobardes, B., G. D. Smith, and J. W. Lynch. 2006. Systematic review of the influence of childhood socioeconomic circumstances on risk for cardiovascular disease in adulthood. *Annals of Epidemiology* 16(2):91-104.

Galst, J. P., and M. A. White. 1976. The unhealthy persuader: The reinforcing value of television and children's purchase-influencing attempts at the supermarket. *Child Development* 47(4):1089-1096.

Gillman, M. W., S. L. Rifas-Shiman, K. Kleinman, E. Oken, J. W. Rich-Edwards, and E. M. Taveras. 2008. Developmental origins of childhood overweight: Potential public health impact. *Obesity* 16(7):1651-1656.

Global Youth Action on Tobacco Network. 2009. *GYAT network*. http://www.gyatnetwork.org/ (accessed March 9, 2010).

Global Youth Coalition on HIV/AIDS. 2010. *Global youth coalition on HIV/AIDS*. http://www.youthaidscoalition.org/ (accessed February 18, 2010).

Global Youth Tobacco Survey Collaborative Group. 2002. Tobacco use among youth: A cross country comparison. *Tobacco Control* 11(3):252-270.

Glover, E. D., P. N. Glover, and T. J. Payne. 2003. Treating nicotine dependence. *American Journal of the Medical Sciences* 326(4):183-186.

Gluckman, P. D., M. A. Hanson, A. S. Beedle, and D. Raubenheimer. 2008. Fetal and neonatal pathways to obesity. In *Frontiers of hormone research*. Vol. 36. Edited by M. Korbonits. Basel: Karger. Pp. 61-72.

Gorn, G., and M. Goldberg. 1982. Behavioural evidence of the effects of televised food messages on children. *Journal of Consumer Research* 9:200-205.

Gortmaker, S. L., K. Peterson, J. Wiecha, A. M. Sobol, S. Dixit, M. K. Fox, and N. Laird. 1999. Reducing obesity via a school-based interdisciplinary intervention among youth: Planet health. *Archives of Pediatrics and Adolescent Medicine* 153(4):409-418.

Guillaume, M., L. Lapidus, F. Beckers, A. Lambert, and P. Björntorp. 1996. Cardiovascular risk factors in children from the Belgian province of Luxembourg: The Belgian Luxembourg Child Study. *American Journal of Epidemiology* 144(9):867-880.

Hastings, G. L., M. Stead, L. McDermott, A. Forsyth, A. M. MacKintosh, M. Rayner, C. Godfrey, M. Caraher, and K. Angus. 2003. *Review of research on the effects of food promotion to children*. Glasgow: Centre for Social Marketing.

Hastings, G., L. McDermott, K. Angus, M. Stead, and S. Thompson. 2006. *The extent, nature and effects of food promotion to children: A review of the evidence*. Geneva: World Health Organization.

Hawkes, C. 2002. Marketing activities of global soft drink and fast food companies in emerging markets: A review. In *Globalization, diets and noncommunicable diseases*. Geneva: World Health Organization.

Hawkes, C. 2007. *Marketing food to children: Changes in the global regulatory environment 2004-2006*. Geneva: World Health Organization.

Henry J. Kaiser Family Foundation. 2007. *Food for thought: Television food advertising to children in the United States.* Washington, DC: Henry J. Kaiser Family Foundation.

Hossain, P., B. Kawar, and M. El Nahas. 2007. Obesity and diabetes in the developing world—a growing challenge. *New England Journal of Medicine* 356(3):213-215.

HRIDAY–SHAN. 2006. HRIDAY–SHAN website. http://www.hriday-shan.org/ (accessed February 19, 2010).

IASO (International Association for the Study of Obesity). 2008a. *About: Global prevalence of overweight in boys.* http://www.iotf.org/database/documents/GlboalBoytrendsv2pdf.pdf (accessed December 9, 2009).

IASO. 2008b. *About: Global prevalence of overweight in girls.* http://www.iotf.org/database/documents/GlobalGirltrendspdf.pdf (accessed December 8, 2009).

International Food and Beverage Alliance. 2009. *IFBA update since November, 2008.* Presentation presented to the World Health Organization on August 31, 2009. Geneva, Switzerland.

International Institute of Population Studies. 2005-2006. *National family health survey 3.* Mumbai, India: International Institute of Population Studies.

IOM (Institute of Medicine). 2006. *Food marketing to children and youth: Threat or opportunity?* Washington, DC: The National Academies Press.

Jiang, J., X. Xia, T. Greiner, G. Wu, G. Lian, and U. Rosenqvist. 2007. The effects of a 3-year obesity intervention in schoolchildren in Beijing. *Child: Care, Health and Development* 33(5):641-646.

John, D. R. 1999. Consumer socialization of children: A retrospective look at twenty-five years of research. *Journal of Consumer Research* 26(3):183-213.

Johnson, M. C., L. J. Bergersen, A. Beck, G. Dick, and B. R. Cole. 1999. Diastolic function and tachycardia in hypertensive children. *American Journal of Hypertension* 12(10 I):1009-1014.

Kain, J., F. Vio, and C. Albala. 1998. Childhood nutrition in Chile: From deficit to excess. *Nutrition Research* 18(11):1825-1837.

Kain, J., R. Uauy, Albala, F. Vio, R. Cerda, and B. Leyton. 2004. School-based obesity prevention in Chilean primary school children: Methodology and evaluation of a controlled study. *International Journal of Obesity and Related Metabolic Disorders* 28(4):483-493.

Kelishadi, R. 2007. Childhood overweight, obesity, and the metabolic syndrome in developing countries. *Epidemiologic Reviews* 29:62-76.

Laird, W. P., and D. E. Fixler. 1981. Left ventricular hypertrophy in adolescents with elevated blood pressure: Assessment by chest roentgenography, electrocardiography, and echocardiography. *Pediatrics* 67(2):255-259.

Li, S., W. Chen, S. R. Srinivasan, M. G. Bond, R. Tang, E. M. Urbina, and G. S. Berenson. 2003. Childhood cardiovascular risk factors and carotid vascular changes in adulthood: The Bogalusa Heart Study. *Journal of the American Medical Association* 290(17):2271-2276.

Liu, A., X. Hu, G. Ma, Z. Cui, Y. Pan, S. Chang, W. Zhao, and C. Chen. 2008. Evaluation of a classroom-based physical activity promoting programme. *Obesity Reviews* 9(Suppl 1):130-134.

Luepker, R. V., C. L. Perry, S. M. McKinlay, P. R. Nader, G. S. Parcel, E. J. Stone, L. S. Webber, J. P. Elder, H. A. Feldman, C. C. Johnson, et al. 1996. Outcomes of a field trial to improve children's dietary patterns and physical activity. The child and Adolescent Trial for Cardiovascular Health. Catch Collaborative Group. *Journal of the American Medical Association* 275(10):768-776.

Martorell, R., L. K. Khan, M. L. Hughes, and L. M. Grummer-Strawn. 2000. Overweight and obesity in preschool children from developing countries. *International Journal of Obesity* 24(8):959-967.

Miguel-Baquilod, M., B. Fishburn, J. Santos, N. R. Jones, and C. W. Warren. 2005. Tobacco use among students age 13-15 years—Phillipines, 2000 and 2003. *Morbidity and Mortality Weekly Report* 54(4):94-97.

Misra, A., and L. Khurana. 2008. Obesity and the metabolic syndrome in developing countries. *Journal of Clinical Endocrinology and Metabolism* 93(11 Suppl 1):S9-S30.

Naylor, P. J., and H. A. McKay. 2009. Prevention in the first place: Schools a setting for action on physical inactivity. *British Journal of Sports Medicine* 43(1):10-13.

Oates, J. A., A. J. J. Wood, and N. L. Benowitz. 1988. Drug therapy: Pharmacologic aspects of cigarette smoking and nicotine addiction. *New England Journal of Medicine* 319(20):1318-1330.

Oken, E., E. B. Levitan, and M. W. Gillman. 2008. Maternal smoking during pregnancy and child overweight: Systematic review and meta-analysis. *International Journal of Obesity* 32(2):201-210.

Osmond, C., and D. J. P. Barker. 2000. Fetal, infant, and childhood growth are predictors of coronary heart disease, diabetes, and hypertension in adult men and women. *Environmental Health Perspectives* 108(Suppl 3):545-553.

Panday, S., S. P. Reddy, R. A. Ruiter, E. Bergstrom, and H. de Vries. 2005. Determinants of smoking cessation among adolescents in South Africa. *Health Education Research* 20(5):586-599.

Panday, S., S. P. Reddy, R. A. Ruiter, E. Bergstrom, and H. de Vries. 2007a. Determinants of smoking among adolescents in the Southern Cape-Karoo Region, South Africa. *Health Promotion International* 22(3):207-217.

Panday, S., S. P. Reddy, R. A. Ruiter, E. Bergstrom, and H. de Vries. 2007b. Nicotine dependence and withdrawal symptoms among occasional smokers. *Journal of Adolescent Health* 40(2):144-150.

Parliament of the Republic of India. *The cigarettes and other tobacco products (prohibition of advertisement and regulation of trade and commerce, production, supply and distribution) amendment bill, 2007. 62.* (2007).

Penchmann, C. 2001. Changing adolescent smoking prevalence. In *Smoking and tobacco control monograph no 14*. NIH Pub. No. 02-5086. Bethesda, MD: National Cancer Institute.

Perry, C. L., M. Eriksen, and G. Giovino. 1994. Tobacco use: a pediatric epidemic. *Tobacco Control* 3(2):97-98.

Perry, C. L., M. H. Stigler, M. Arora, and K. S. Reddy. 2008. Prevention in translation: Tobacco use prevention in India. *Health Promotion Practice* 9(4):378-386.

Perry, C. L., M. H. Stigler, M. Arora, and K. S. Reddy. 2009. Preventing tobacco use among young people in India: Project MYTRI. *American Journal of Public Health* 99(5):899-906.

Peto, R., A. D. Lopez, J. Boreham, M. Thun, C. Heath Jr., and R. Doll. 1996. Mortality from smoking worldwide. *British Medical Bulletin* 52(1):12-21.

Popkin, B. M., and P. Gordon-Larsen. 2004. The nutrition transition: Worldwide obesity dynamics and their determinants. *International Journal of Obesity and Related Metabolic Disorders* 28(Suppl 3):S2-S9.

Prentice, A. M. 2006. The emerging epidemic of obesity in developing countries. *International Journal of Epidemiology* 35(1):93-99.

Prentice, A. M., and S. E. Moore. 2005. Early programming of adult diseases in resource poor countries. *Archives of Disease in Childhood* 90(4):429-432.

Prokhorov, A. V., J. P. Winickoff, J. S. Ahluwalia, D. Ossip-Klein, S. Tanski, H. A. Lando, E. T. Moolchan, M. Muramoto, J. D. Klein, M. Weitzman, and K. H. Ford. 2006. Youth tobacco use: A global perspective for child health care clinicians. *Pediatrics* 118(3):e890-e903.

Raitakari, O. T., M. Juonala, M. Kahoen, L. Taittonen, T. Laitinen, N. Maki-Torkko, M. J. Jarvisalo, M. Uhari, E. Jokinen, T. Ronnemaa, H. K. Akerblom, J. S. A. Viikari. 2003. Cardiovascular risk factors in childhood and carotid artery intima-media thickness in adulthood: The Cardiovascular Risk in Young Finns Study. *Journal of the American Medical Association* 290(17):2277-2291.

Reddy, K. S., and P. C. Gupta. 2004. *Report on tobacco control in India.* New Delhi, India: Ministry of Health & Family Welfare, Government of India, CDC, and WHO.

Reddy, K. S., M. Arora, C. L. Perry, B. Nair, A. Kohli, L. A. Lytle, M. Stigler, and D. Prabhakaran. 2002. Tobacco and alcohol use outcomes of a school-based intervention in New Delhi. *American Journal of Health Behavior* 26(3):173-181.

Reddy, K. S., C. L. Perry, M. H. Stigler, and M. Arora. 2006. Differences in tobacco use among young people in urban India by sex, socioeconomic status, age, and school grade: Assessment of baseline survey data. *Lancet* 367(9510):589-594.

Reddy, S. P., S. Panday, D. Swart, C. C. Jinabhai, S. L. Amosun, S. James, K. D. Monyeki, G. Stevens, N. Morejele, N. S. Kambaran, R. G. Omardien, and H. W. Van den Borne. 2003. *Umthenthe uhlaba usamila: The South African Youth Risk Behavior Survey 2002.* Cape Town: South African Medical Research Council.

Reddy, S. P., K. Resnicow, S. James, N. Kambaran, R. Omardien, and A. D. Mbewu. 2009. Underweight, overweight and obesity among South African adolescents: Results of the 2002 national youth risk behaviour survey. *Public Health and Nutrition* 12(2):203-207.

Resnicow, K., S. P. Reddy, S. James, R. Gabebodeen Omardien, N. S. Kambaran, H. G. Langner, R. D. Vaughan, D. Cross, G. Hamilton, and T. Nichols. 2008. Comparison of two school-based smoking prevention programs among South African high school students: Results of a randomized trial. *Annals of Behavioral Medicine* 36(3):231-243.

Richter, L., S. Norris, J. Pettifor, D. Yach, and N. Cameron. 2007. Cohort profile: Mandela's children: The 1990 birth to twenty study in South Africa. *International Journal of Epidemiology* 36(3):504-511.

Roberts, D. F. and U. G. Foehr. 2004. *Kids and media in America.* Cambridge: Cambridge University Press.

Rocchini, A. P. 2002. Childhood obesity and a diabetes epidemic. *New England Journal of Medicine* 346(11):854-855.

Rosner, B., R. Prineas, S. R. Daniels, and J. Loggie. 2000. Blood pressure differences between blacks and whites in relation to body size among US children and adolescents. *American Journal of Epidemiology* 151(10):1007-1019.

Rudman, A. 2001. *India inhales.* USA: Bullfrog Films.

Save the Children. 2010. *Survive to 5.* http://www.savethechildren.org/programs/health/child-survival/survive-to-5 (accessed March 9, 2010).

Sesame Workshop. 2010. Inside the Workshop. http://www.sesameworkshop.org/insidetheworkshop (accessed June 4, 2010).

Sinaiko, A. R., D. R. Jacobs Jr., J. Steinberger, A. Moran, R. Luepker, A. P. Rocchini, and R. J. Prineas. 2001. Insulin resistance syndrome in childhood: Associations of the euglycemic insulin clamp and fasting insulin with fatness and other risk factors. *Journal of Pediatrics* 139(5):700-707.

Singh, R., A. Bhansali, R. Sialy, and A. Aggarwal. 2007. Prevalence of metabolic syndrome in adolescents from a north Indian population. *Diabetic Medicine* 24(2):195-199.

Singhal, A., M. Fewtrell, T. J. Cole, and A. Lucas. 2003. Low nutrient intake and early growth for later insulin resistance in adolescents born preterm. *Lancet* 361(9363):1089-1097.

Singhal, A., T. J. Cole, M. Fewtrell, J. Deanfield, A. Lucas, A. Singhal, T. J. Cole, M. Fewtrell, J. Deanfield, and A. Lucas. 2004. Is slower early growth beneficial for long-term cardiovascular health? *Circulation* 109(9):1108-1113.

Sinha, R., G. Fisch, B. Teague, W. V. Tamborlane, B. Banyas, K. Allen, M. Savoye, V. Rieger, S. Taksali, G. Barbetta, R. S. Sherwin, and S. Caprio. 2002. Prevalence of impaired glucose tolerance among children and adolescents with marked obesity. *New England Journal of Medicine* 346(11):802-810.

Slater, S. J., F. J. Chaloupka, M. Wakefield, L. D. Johnston, and P. M. O'Malley. 2007. The impact of retail cigarette marketing practices on youth smoking uptake. *Archives of Pediatrics and Adolescent Medicine* 161(5):440-445.

Sorof, J., and S. Daniels. 2002. Obesity hypertension in children: A problem of epidemic proportions. *Hypertension* 40(4):441-447.

Sorof, J. M., A. V. Alexandrov, G. Cardwell, and R. J. Portman. 2003. Carotid artery intimal-medial thickness and left ventricular hypertrophy in children with elevated blood pressure. *Pediatrics* 111(1):61-66.

Sowden, A. J., and L. Arblaster. 2000. Mass media interventions for preventing smoking in young people. *Cochrane Database of Systematic Reviews* (2):CD001006.

Stein, A. D., A. M. Thompson, A. Waters, A. D. Stein, A. M. Thompson, and A. Waters. 2005. Childhood growth and chronic disease: Evidence from countries undergoing the nutrition transition. *Maternal and Child Nutrition* 1(3):177-184.

Stein, C. E., C. H. D. Fall, K. Kumaran, C. Osmond, V. Cox, and D. J. P. Barker. 1996. Fetal growth and coronary heart disease in south India. *Lancet* 348(9037):1269-1273.

Story, M., and S. French. 2004. Food advertising and marketing directed at children and adolescents in the U.S. *International Journal of Behavioral Nutrition and Physical Activity* 1(1):3.

Strasburger, V. C. 2001. Children and TV advertising: Nowhere to run, nowhere to hide. *Journal of Developmental and Behavioral Pediatrics* 22(3):185-187.

Strong, J. P., G. T. Malcom, C. A. McMahan, R. E. Tracy, W. P. Newman, 3rd, E. E. Herderick, and J. F. Cornhill. 1999. Prevalence and extent of atherosclerosis in adolescents and young adults: Implications for prevention from the Pathobiological Determinants of Atherosclerosis in Youth Study. *Journal of the American Medical Association* 281(8):727-735.

Swart, D., S. Panday, S. P. Reddy, E. Bergstrom, and H. de Vries. 2006. Access point analysis: What do adolescents in South Africa say about tobacco control programmes? *Health Education Research* 21(3):393-406.

Taras, H. L., J. F. Sallis, T. L. Patterson, P. R. Nader, and J. A. Nelson. 1989. Television's influence on children's diet and physical activity. *Journal of Developmental and Behavioral Pediatrics* 10(4):176-180.

Tyas, S. L., and L. L. Pederson. 1998. Psychosocial factors related to adolescent smoking: A critical review of the literature. *Tobacco Control* 7:409-420.

UNICEF (United Nations Children's Fund). 2009. *State of the world's children 2009: Maternal and newborn health*. New York: UNICEF.

U.S. Department of Health and Human Services. 1994. *Preventing tobacco use among young people: A report of the surgeon general*. Atlanta, GA: Centers for Disease Control and Prevention, National Center for Chronic Disease Prevention and Health Promotion, Office on Smoking and Health, U.S. Department of Health and Human Services, Public Health Service.

van Sluijs, E. M. F., A. M. McMinn, and S. J. Griffin. 2007. Effectiveness of interventions to promote physical activity in children and adolescents: Systematic review of controlled trials. *British Medical Journal* 335(7622):703.

Verma, M., J. Chhatwal, and S. M. George. 1994. Obesity and hypertension in children. In *Indian Pediatrics* 31(9):1065-1069.

Veugelers, P. J., and A. L. Fitzgerald. 2005. Effectiveness of school programs in preventing childhood obesity: A multilevel comparison. *American Journal of Public Health* 95(3):432-435.

Victora, C. G., L. Adair, C. Fall, P. C. Hallal, R. Martorell, L. Richter, and H. S. Sachdev. 2008. Maternal and child undernutrition: Consequences for adult health and human capital. *Lancet* 371(9609):340-357.

Volunteer Health Association of India. 2009. *Tobacco control in India: What have we achieved till date?* New Delhi: Volunteer Health Association of India.

Wakefield, M., B. Flay, M. Nichter, and G. Giovino. 2003. Effects of anti-smoking advertising on youth smoking: A review. *Journal of Health Communication* 8(3):229-247.

Walker, S., and S. George. 2007. *Young@heart.* USA: Fox Searchlight Pictures.

Warren, C. W., N. R. Jones, M. P. Eriksen, and S. Asma. 2006. Patterns of global tobacco use in young people and implications for future chronic disease burden in adults. *Lancet* 367(9512):749-753.

Whitaker, R. C. 2004. Predicting preschooler obesity at birth: The role of maternal obesity in early pregnancy. *Pediatrics* 114(1):e29-e36.

WHO (World Health Organization). 2003. *WHO Framework Convention on Tobacco Control.* Geneva: World Health Organization.

WHO. 2008a. *WHO report on the global tobacco epidemic, 2008: The mpower package.* Geneva: World Health Organization.

WHO. 2008b. *Childhood overweight and obesity.* http://www.who.int/dietphysicalactivity/childhood/en/ (accessed December 12, 2008).

WHO. 2009. *Aging and life course.* Geneva: World Health Oranization.

WHO. 2010a. *Global school health initiative.* http://www.who.int/school_youth_health/gshi/en/ (accessed March 9, 2010).

WHO. 2010b. *Tobacco free initiative.* http://www.who.int/tobacco/en/index.html (accessed March 9, 2010).

WHO Global InfoBase. 2008. Overweight & obesity (BMI) country data. Geneva: World Health Organization.

WHO Mega Country Health Promotion Network. 2001. *Recommendations from the fourth annual meeting of the school health component of the WHO mega country health promotion network.* Paris: World Health Organization.

Yach, D., C. Hawkes, C. L. Gould, and K. J. Hofman. 2004. The global burden of chronic diseases: Overcoming impediments to prevention and control. *Journal of the American Medical Association* 291(21):2616-2622.

Yajnik, P. C., and C. S. Yajnik. 2009. Predictive equations for body fat in Asian Indians. *Obesity* 17(5):935-936.

Youth For Health. 2009. *Y4H.* http://www.y4h.hriday-shan.org (accessed February 19, 2010).

7

Making Choices to Reduce the Burden of Cardiovascular Disease

It is clear from preceding chapters that the health and economic burden of cardiovascular disease (CVD) is high. This burden is likely to rise and remain unacceptably high in developing countries unless bold moves are made to implement policies and programs to contain the growth in prevalence of CVD and other chronic diseases, to develop and implement affordable and accessible health services and technology, and to reduce the financial risks to individuals and economies.

Aggressively reducing population and individual CVD risks would not only help low and middle income countries avert a potential crisis by reducing their chronic disease burden, it could also be viewed as an opportunity to improve both their economies and their public health. However, many developing countries face a difficult challenge: to make further headway against infectious diseases and other health concerns where they remain rampant while transforming health systems to accomplish chronic disease prevention and care. Very limited resources are available for health in developing countries, and there are great gaps in meeting needs. Therefore, the strategy in developing countries should be to seek low-cost approaches with a high potential return on investment to achieve structural and behavioral changes to reduce risk, and low-cost technology and health delivery to effectively treat and manage CVD.

There is a particular urgency to the need to identify and implement those interventions that can reap the biggest CVD reduction benefits in low and middle income countries while at the same time offering good "value for money." Many of these countries are confronting a mounting gap between the dual disease burden they experience and the ability of their health systems to deliver adequate care. Other countries are making headway as they and/or donors increase resource allocations to health. In both instances, informed choices about what the available resources will buy can better align needed and realized health improvements.

ECONOMIC INFORMATION TO HELP ALLOCATE RESOURCES

Economic measurements and analysis are critically important to inform decisions both about allocating resources and choosing among alternative solutions to the problem within and beyond the health sector. The health economics literature relies almost exclusively on cost-effectiveness measures to assess value for money. Cost-effectiveness analysis of interventions can be an important tool for choosing among interventions targeted to the same outcomes, and the first section of this chapter summarizes the available cost-effectiveness evidence for CVD interventions in low and middle income countries. However, cost-effectiveness provides little information about the affordability of given interventions or the actual value to the beneficiaries, and it does not allow for ready comparisons of interventions across different sectors and different health and development priorities. The potential return on investment needs to be assessed within a broad socioeconomic context, and guidance derived from cost-effectiveness analysis may be superseded by broader policy choices for allocating resources across competing priorities within the parameters that society sets for achieving better health and well-being. Economic benefit–cost analysis can be used to balance tradeoffs in choosing among alternatives, such as new technologies or investments in structural and policy changes. However, the analytical and data demands are much higher, and there are almost no cost–benefit studies available from developing countries on CVD interventions. Ultimately, decisions about how to prioritize investments will necessitate carefully defining feasible options for change and determining the willingness of stakeholders to shift resources to implement those changes.

Summary of Cost-Effectiveness Evidence[1]

The preceding chapters have provided a thorough summary of the relevant CVD interventions under consideration in low and middle income countries. This section discusses the available evidence on their cost-effectiveness, drawing primarily on two rapid reviews commissioned for this report, which built on and updated major recent efforts such as the Disease Control Priorities Project (DCP2) (Musgrove and Fox-Rushby, 2006) and the WHO initia-

---

[1] This section is based in part on papers written for the committee by Marc Suhrcke et al. and by Stephen Jan and Alison Hayes.

tive on Choosing Interventions That are Cost-effective (CHOICE) (WHO, 2010).[2] While there is a large body of evidence on the cost-effectiveness of CVD-related interventions in developed countries, this chapter considers only evidence with an explicit focus on low and middle income countries.

Most of the available studies identified in the commissioned reviews were focused on clinical prevention strategies and case management for individuals, with far fewer studies on population-based prevention approaches. Overall, most studies in both of these categories focused on risk-factor reduction.

About half the economic studies relied on modeling analysis using estimated cost assumptions and secondary data for intervention effectiveness and epidemiological conditions rather than on primary empirical data on costs and effectiveness from observational trials or randomized controlled trials in the setting of interest. In these models, developing-country data was the source for most of the epidemiological data, but developed countries were the source of data for intervention effectiveness. The advantages and limitations of these secondary versus primary analyses will be discussed further in the final section of this chapter on future research needs.

It is also important to note that cost-effectiveness studies are difficult to compare because the threshold of what is considered cost-effective varies (the standard is 3× the per capita gross domestic product [GDP] for the country, but 1× GDP is sometimes used). In addition, the outcome measures and comparator are often not the same across studies (the standard comparator is either no intervention or current standard care in the country). Different approaches for economic evaluation are also used, as well as different measures to express cost-effectiveness (the standard is an incremental cost-effectiveness ratio [ICER] reporting the cost per averted disability-adjusted life year [DALY] or quality-adjusted life year [QALY], but an average cost-effectiveness ratio [CER] is also used).

Cost-Effectiveness of Population-Based and Other Lifestyle Interventions

Population-based and other public health interventions typically target nutrition, physical activity, and tobacco risk-factor reduction. There has been remarkably little research on non-clinical, population-based approaches, such as legislative actions, education campaigns, or health promotion through social marketing, as a way to tackle CVD in developing

---

[2] Searches were conducted using the PubMed and EconLit databases. In addition, the references of retrieved articles and the relevant publications of the DCP2 and the WHO CHOICE program were hand-searched for relevant articles. The search strategy consisted of freetext and MeSH terms related to economic evaluation and CVD disease or risk factors endpoints, filtered for the occurrence of the term "developing countries" or any country name defined as middle or low income country according to the World Bank definition. Only published full economic evaluations were included.

countries. Changes in health policy are beginning to be observed in developed countries such as the United Kingdom, Finland, and the United States. New strategies are being implemented, such as legislation for salt reduction and labeling of food (Karppanen and Mervaala, 2006), and some analysis has been done about the potential revenue and dietary benefits of taxes on sugared drinks and junk food (Brownell and Frieden, 2009) as well as the potential cost-effectiveness of community-based physical activity programs in the United States (Roux et al., 2008).

However, most of these strategies have yet to be implemented with a rigorous economic evaluation component. In addition, since interventions targeted to change health behaviors are highly dependent on political, cultural, infrastructural, and other system-related aspects, it is deemed less feasible to assume effectiveness results from studies in developed regions can be applied to developing regions than is commonly accepted for clinical effectiveness evidence (Jamison et al., 2006). In pharmaceutical research, for example, a common assumption is that a drug affecting biomedical processes would have approximately identical effects, irrespective of the context in which it is applied. This is less likely to be the case for a health communication campaign or for legislative or regulatory approaches.

Nonetheless, evidence from both modeling and some primary economic analysis is building that population-level interventions targeted to reduce CVD are likely to be cost-effective in low and middle income countries. Table 7.5a at the end of this chapter summarizes the cost-effectiveness results for population-based CVD interventions in a developing-country setting.

The antitobacco regulatory interventions, such as taxation, smoke-free public places, restrictions on marketing, and youth cessation are strongly supported. In particular, taxation and legislation options have been relatively well evaluated, certainly for developed regions and countries but also for developing-country settings (Chisholm et al., 2006). Those include reviews such as an article by Shibuya et al. (2003) and the *Disease Control Priorities in Developing Countries* publication (Jha et al., 2006), both of which describe an increase in tobacco tax as the most cost-effective strategy to reduce smoking prevalence, followed by comprehensive advertisement campaigns and bans on smoking in public places. Tobacco taxes combined with smoking and advertising bans is also cost-effective (Gaziano, 2008; Lai et al., 2007). A modeling study also showed cost savings from a community-based pharmacist-driven education and counseling program for prevention of CVD risk from smoking among high-risk groups of men and women in Thailand (Thavorn and Chaiyakunapruk, 2008).

A number of studies have found food regulation (including regulation of salt or substitution of transfats) to be highly cost-effective, even cost-saving. These studies included cooperation among government, industry, and consumer organizations to reduce the salt content in bread in Argentina

(Rubinstein et al., 2009) and salt reduction in processed foods through industry agreements or legislation in South-East Asia, Latin America, and Sub-Saharan Africa (Gaziano, 2008; Murray et al., 2003). However, the few studies of this type that exist have not conducted a thorough examination of the true costs of achieving policy or regulatory change, which can be high during the policy advocacy phase and then generally diminish.

Promoting physical activity is a CVD prevention intervention that has been largely overlooked by economic evaluation. The Agita São Paulo program, described in Chapter 5, is known globally as an effective intervention to promote physical activity in Brazil. It was evaluated by the World Bank and also found to be cost-effective (Matsudo et al., 2006). In a more narrow approach, a randomized controlled trial of home-based physical activity education for rehabilitation of post-MI coronary patients in Brazil showed significant improvements in all domains at a low cost (Salvetti et al., 2008).

Educational campaigns for outcomes beyond tobacco use are also shown as highly cost-effective in the few studies of this type (mainly addressing high blood pressure, high cholesterol, and lowering body mass index [BMI]), and some are even cost-saving. Cost-effectiveness modeling of health education programs for multi-risk reduction in multiple regions demonstrated positive results (Murray et al., 2003). Salt reduction through communication and mass media programs were deemed likely to be cost-effective, as well as similar programs for tobacco control, in a range of low and middle income countries at about $0.40 per person per day (Asaria et al., 2007). A population-based social marketing study with experimental and control groups in Thailand shows effective hypertension risk reduction at very low cost when village health workers were mobilized with trained health workers (Getpreechaswas et al., 2007). Bi-weekly home counseling visits by a trained health professional in Mexico were also very cost-effective in reducing hypertension (García-Peña et al., 2002). A community-based primary prevention program in Beijing to alter food intake also showed cost savings (Huang et al., 2001). However, the reported ICERs for health education interventions were quite variable. This suggests a degree of variation and uncertainty in the parameters used for such studies. It is also difficult to judge the effects of mass education programs due to difficulties in assessing numbers of persons reached.

In summary, legislated reductions in salt and transfats in foods, tobacco taxation and restrictions, and health education campaigns all show some promising cost-effectiveness across a range of countries. However, except for antitobacco measures in developed countries, the cost-effectiveness of population-based interventions has been measured almost entirely through modeling techniques. These few studies are generally supportive of one another, but need confirmation from a broad range of empirical examples using primary data.

Cost-Effectiveness of Pharmaceutical and Other Clinical Interventions

Cost-effectiveness results for pharmaceutical and other clinical interventions for CVD in a developing-country setting are summarized in Table 7.5b at the end of this chapter. These strategies have been the predominant focus of economic analysis to date. In summary, the cost-effectiveness of pharmaceutical interventions to reduce CVD depends heavily on the risk group targeted. Prevention with pharmacological treatment for high-risk individuals is likely to be cost-effective across a range of country settings. Prevention with pharmacological treatment is not generally likely to be cost-effective for reducing risk factors in individuals without high absolute risk.

In conclusion, just as with the available intervention effectiveness reviewed in Chapter 5, there are limitations on the available economic analyses. These limitations guide future needs, which will be discussed later in this chapter. However, they do not preclude intervening now, and some determinations can be made about priorities for investment in intervention approaches. Indeed, both intervention and economic evidence support selected population-based interventions and pharmacological interventions for high-risk target groups to reduce CVD and hypertension. Although there are interventions that are likely to be cost-effective, it remains difficult to make comparisons to draw definitive conclusions about which interventions are the most cost-effective. This is both due to the challenges of making comparisons across the available studies and due to gaps in the economic evaluation literature in some important areas of intervention that have promise for effective impact on health outcomes.

Economic Information to Compare Prevention and Treatment Strategies

When comparing interventions to reduce the burden of CVD, it is tempting to try to look to the economic analysis to make a determination about whether it would be more advisable to invest in prevention strategies or treatment strategies. To many, prevention seems like the most promising investment because of its potential for avoidance of costly treatment interventions (technology, hospitalization, etc.). On the other hand, many see potential for a high return on investment in terms of health outcomes from advances in technology and health services if made more available in the developing world.

The evidence does not provide a definitive choice between prevention and treatment on economic grounds. There is economic evidence to support the cost-effectiveness of implementation on a wider scale of certain pharmaceutical strategies in developing countries (Gaziano et al., 2007). However, the issue of how best to approach implementation remains unresolved (Gaziano, 2007), which was also a central message of Chapter 5. There is also an unresolved discussion between those who advocate for the targeting of patients with a single but high-risk factor (e.g., high blood pressure) and those arguing for an overall absolute risk approach (e.g., on the basis of 10-year risk of CVD), independent from the particular risk factor. These are debates on medical effectiveness, but they also spill over into the economic evaluation literature, as evidenced by the differences in therapeutic combinations and assessments of patient risks across the cost-effectiveness studies summarized in Table 7.5b at the end of this chapter. In addition, there has been limited economic evaluation of screening strategies, a necessary component of scaling up interventions to target individuals at high risk that is certainly not without cost. Therefore, considering the potential costs of scaling up and screening for risk factors as well as for delivering adequate supplies of drugs for persons identified through screening, there is still room for debate about whether pharmaceutical interventions are the right priority. In addition, factors such as the risk of adverse events in such a large untreated population, inequalities in access to care, and limited patient and system compliance need to be addressed.

Despite a general endorsement of scaling up pharmaceutical support from the economic perspective, it is also important to be mindful of the limitations of a strategy focused narrowly on pharmaceutical support. Clinically managed chronic care can be expensive and is often necessary for the remaining lifetime of an individual. In addition, clincial approaches targeted at segments of the population with higher risk (e.g., based on blood pressure) miss the typically large number of people below the threshold but nevertheless with risk factor-related ailments (Blackburn, 1983; Kottke et al., 1985; Puska et al., 1985; Schooler et al., 1997). A population-based approach, like one aiming for a reduction in salt intake, would at least in principle effect change in the entire population and not only those in the population at the highest risk, and in principle over the long term this could reduce the ultimate need for costly clinical interventions. This may render such population-based approaches attractive because of the rationale for a likelihood of cost-effectiveness over time, although the population risk reduction with these approaches can be limited (Neal et al., 2007).

In reality, the issue of prevention versus treatment is probably not the most useful question. The epidemic of CVD is not going to be addressed through the eradication of the disease in an entire population, the way one might hope to eradicate a disease with an acute infectious etiology. Instead, the goals for reducing the population burden of disease are that a greater proportion of the population can avoid developing the disease, that the average age of onset can be delayed, and that morbidity, mortality, and financial consequences due to CVD can be reduced. Indeed, the totality of the available epidemiological, intervention, and economic evidence support a balanced approach in which health promotion and prevention is emphasized but which also recognizes the need for effective, appropriate, quality delivery of medical interventions for risk reduction and treatment. The distribution of investment in health promotion, prevention, and treatment approaches within that balance is something that will need to be determined based on the specific needs, capacity, and political and societal will of the stakeholder making the investment. The potential for improving the information available to inform this decision making is described in the final section of this chapter.

Costs to Address Gaps in CVD Needs[3]

One of the key questions asked by policy makers wishing to make investments to address an unmet health need is, "What will it cost?" The total cost to reduce the burden of disease is determined not only by the costs of interventions but also by the number of affected people in need of them. The difference between the proportion of the population that could benefit from intervention and that currently receiving such intervention is commonly called the "treatment gap." This treatment gap can be defined in terms of any intervention approach, including population-based approaches and individual prevention or treatment. Determining the treatment gap depends on knowing four key parameters: prevalence in the population of a health condition; proportion of people with the condition that are treated and, conversely, the proportion that are not; proportion with the condition under control and, conversely the proportion not controlled; and cost of treatment. It is generally recognized that, particularly in developing countries, there are significant numbers of individuals who are in need but have not benefited from potentially effective and cost-effective interventions to treat or reduce risk for CVD and related chronic diseases. However, this treatment gap would need to be more specifically defined and linked to accurate cost information in order to more precisely determine the investment that would be required. This section of the chapter offers a discussion of illustrative evidence to demonstrate the analytic approaches available to determine what it will cost to reduce the burden of CVD in developing countries.

A short review was commissioned for this report of the treatment gaps in the developing world for CVD and related risk factors (Jan and Hayes, 2009).[4] The objective of the review was to assess the feasibility of an approach to investment appraisal that brings together two sources of data:

---

[3] This section is based in part on papers written for the committee by Stephen Jan and Alison Hayes and by Thomas Gaziano and Grace Kim.

[4] The authors conducted a non-systematic search of the published and grey literature using PubMed and Google Scholar databases as well as hand-searches and snowballing. Search terms included "treatment gap and chronic diseases" and "treatment gap and cardiovascular disease."

the nature and the scale of treatment gaps in CVD in developing countries and the costs and cost-effectiveness of a range of interventions. The review extracted evidence on treatment gaps from systematic reviews of treatment gaps for hypertension, comparative studies of risk reduction in individuals with CVD, and numerous studies of treatment gaps for specific diseases and risk factors in individual countries. A fair degree of standardization in the approaches taken to measuring treatment gaps enables some comparisons to be made across studies, but the appropriateness of generalizations about average overall rates is limited because the studies are derived from multiple sources across different settings and involve varying methodologies. In addition, although the available evidence establishes the treatment gap for some risk factors related to CVD, there remain methodological problems that make it difficult to reliably link the current evidence on treatment gaps with the current evidence on costs and cost-effectiveness in order to determine the total investment required to fill the treatment gap.

The studies extracted in this review provided sufficient information to assess treatment gaps in some countries for some risk factors for CVD, including hypertension, high cholesterol, and diabetes as well as ongoing risk reduction in individuals with CVD. The results show large treatment gaps. For other risk factors, such as obesity, lack of physical activity, and tobacco use, there is sufficient data to derive population estimates that indicate the potential numbers of individuals who could benefit from added intervention but not sufficient data on the numbers receiving interventions to determine a treatment gap.

For hypertension, a number of recent studies indicate that hypertension prevalence is on average around 30 percent of the adult population in developing countries, with a wide variation across settings, from 5 percent in rural India to 70 percent in Poland (Kearney et al., 2004). The available evidence indicates that around 30 percent of individuals with reported hypertension across developing countries are receiving treatment—thus a 70 percent treatment gap (Pereira et al., 2009). This gap varies not only across countries but also over time. For example, evidence from China indicates treatment levels at 17 percent in urban populations and 5 percent in rural populations in 1991 (Whelton et al., 2004), but levels were more recently observed at 28.2 percent overall in 2000-2001 (Gu et al., 2002). These variations demonstrate the difficulties with generalizing over time and across countries that are at differing stages of epidemiological and economic transition.

An interesting finding from the studies reviewed is that even in countries with relatively high proportions of patients getting treatment, the percent of hypertension under control is sometimes low. Across countries, around 30 percent of those receiving treatment in developing countries have their hypertension under control, which is similar to the rate of around 35 percent that has been observed in developed countries (Pereira et al., 2009).

Although most studies review gaps in treatment using pharmaceutical interventions to reduce hypertension, recent evidence from China through the InterASIA study sheds some light on treatment coverage for nonpharmacotherapies. This study found that 47.2 percent of people with hypertension were using at least one of five nonpharmacological approaches, including salt reduction, weight loss or weight control therapies, exercise, alcohol reduction, and potassium supplementation at the time of the survey (Gu et al., 2002).

For cholesterol and diabetes, data is much less available than for hypertension. Evidence for both derives mainly from recent systematic reviews in China. The prevalence of moderate hypercholesterolemia (defined as ≥ 200 mg/dl total cholesterol) was 32.8 percent and the prevalence of high hypercholesterolemia (defined as ≥ 240 mg/dl total cholesterol or taking cholesterol lowering medications) was 9.0 percent. For those with moderately high cholesterol levels, 3.5 percent of men and 3.4 percent of women were receiving treatment, while 14 percent of men and 11.6 percent of women with very high cholesterol levels were receiving treatment. This suggests significant treatment gaps as high as 96 percent or 86 percent, depending on the criteria used for treatment (He et al., 2004). The prevalence of diabetes in China is around 5 percent, but only 20.3 percent are currently on treatment and 8.3 percent report being able to achieve control (Hu et al., 2008).

A study based on the WHO Study on Prevention of Recurrences of Myocardial Infarction and Stroke (PREMISE) project examined the level at which patients already diagnosed with coronary heart disease or cerebrovascular disease are being treated for ongoing risk-factor reduction. This study was conducted across 10 countries (Brazil, Egypt, India, Indonesia, Iran, Pakistan, Russia, Sri Lanka, Tunisia, and Turkey) and assessed patients' awareness and uptake of lifestyle and pharmacological interventions (Mendis et al., 2005). Table 7.1a shows the percentage of patients with coronary heart disease and cerbrovascular disease on pharmaceutical interventions for risk reduction. For both conditions, the levels of medication use are highest for aspirin and lowest for statins. Also, although there was a high level of awareness of the benefits of various lifestyle interventions, uptake of these interventions was variable (Table 7.1b). Looking at a country-specific analysis, India was quite similar to the overall findings in terms of pharmaceutical interventions (Table 7.1c). However, another study in rural India showed much lower levels of patients on medication antiplatelet therapy, blood pressure-lowering drugs, and statins (Joshi et al., 2009) (Table 7.1d).

Estimated Costs to Fill the Hypertension Treatment Gap in 10 Countries

In addition to the review of the available literature described earlier, a modeling analysis of treatment gaps for hypertension and costs to achieve

TABLE 7.1a Patients on Medications in 10 Low and Middle Income Countries

	Coronary Heart Disease	Cerebrovascular Disease
Aspirin	81.2%	70.5%
Beta-Blocker	48.1%	22.1%
ACE-Inhibitor	39.8%	38.1%
Statin	29.8%	12.2%

NOTE: WHO PREMISE data from Brazil, Egypt, India, Indonesia, Iran, Pakistan, Russia, Sri Lanka, Tunisia, and Turkey.
SOURCE: Mendis et al., 2005.

TABLE 7.1b Awareness and Uptake of Lifestyle Interventions in Patients in 10 Low and Middle Income Countries

	Awareness of Benefits	Behavior
Smoking Cessation	82%	12% tobacco users
Healthful Diet	89%	35% did not follow healthful diet
Physical Activity	77%	52.5% less than 30 mins exercise/day

NOTE: WHO PREMISE data from Brazil, Egypt, India, Indonesia, Iran, Pakistan, Russia, Sri Lanka, Tunisia, and Turkey.
SOURCE: Mendis et al., 2005.

TABLE 7.1c Patients on Medications in India

	Coronary Heart Disease	Cerebrovascular Disease
Aspirin	94.5%	90.1%
Beta-Blocker	46.2%	28.4%
ACE-Inhibitor	41.3%	23.5%
Statin	38.4%	37.0%

NOTE: WHO PREMISE data from India.
SOURCE: Mendis et al., 2005.

TABLE 7.1d Patients on Medications in Rural India

	Coronary Heart Disease	Stroke
Antiplatelet (aspirin, copidogrel)	19.4%	11.8%
Blood Pressure-Lowering (beta-blocker, ACE-Inhibitor, diuretic, and others)	41.1%	53.9%
Statin	6.0%	1.0%

SOURCE: Joshi et al., 2009.

reductions in blood pressure in select countries representing the different World Bank regions was commissioned for this report (Gaziano and Kim, 2009). This analysis was not focused on aggregated findings to determine global treatment gap and costs, but rather on country-specific analyses of the kind that might be most useful for decisions about funding and implementing country-specific policies and programs.

Based on a meta-analysis of published articles on nationally representative health surveys, Table 7.2 shows the prevalence, awareness, treatment, and control rates for hypertension in adult populations across 9 developing countries, including at least 1 country in each of the World Health Organization Developing World Regions, as well as in the United States as a comparison. Overall, control of hypertension is poor, with most countries having control rates of less than 15 percent. In the 10 countries examined in the commissioned analysis there were nearly 400 million individuals with hypertension, and it was currently controlled in fewer than 50 million (Gaziano and Kim, 2009).

The goal of the analysis was to provide, for each of the countries examined, an estimate of the likely total costs to address this "treatment gap" by achieving reduction of hypertension using one of two strategies. The first

TABLE 7.2 Global Prevalence, Awareness, and Control Rates for Hypertension

Country	Year	Age	Population (1000s)	% Prevalence	% Aware	% Treated	% Controlled
USA	1999-2004	≥18	187709	28.90	71.80	61.40	35.10
China	2000	35-74	476057	27.20	44.70	28.20	8.10
Czech Republic	2000-2001	25-64	5684	36.59	67.52	51.40	20.31
Mexico	2000	25-64	41695	33.30	25.20	12.90	3.70
Chile	2003	>17	11539	33.70	59.80	36.30	11.80
Iran	2005	25-64	28345	25.20	33.90	24.80	6.00
Egypt	1991-1993	≥25	36236	26.30	37.50	23.90	8.00
South Africa	1998	>15	28592	21.00	41.03	30.00	14.80
Pakistan	1990-1994	45-64	13634	30.82	17.61	9.40	3.04
India	2004	20-69	593906	28.00	51.50	50.00	7.00

NOTES: Hypertension is high blood pressure defined as systolic blood pressure/diastolic blood pressure over 140/90 mmHg and/or use of antihypertensive medication.

Awareness rate is the percentage of hypertensive individuals who were aware of their elevated blood pressure or had been told by a physician.

Control rate is the percentage of hypertensive individuals who successfully controlled their high blood pressure to below 140/90 mmHg.

Treatment rate is the percentage of hypertensive individuals were currently taking medications for their elevated blood pressure.
SOURCE: Gaziano and Kim, 2009.

is a treatment program, where all individuals with hypertension would be treated and given medications to successfully control their high blood pressure. The second is a lifestyle change strategy aimed at reducing the mean blood pressure across the population. This analysis estimates only the cost of additional control and treatment programs; it does not report or evaluate current expenditures on efforts already implemented for drug treatment and population strategies to decrease blood pressure (Gaziano and Kim, 2009).

Table 7.3 shows the estimated total cost per country for the first approach, to treat and control all those with a blood pressure greater than 140 mmHg to a level below 140 mmHg, where the benefits of reducing risk are most robust. The estimate of costs reflects the overall population; the prevalence of hypertension; the blood pressure distribution in the country; and country-specific costs of care, including lab costs, health worker wages, use of facilities, and the costs of medication regimens administered according to current treatment guidelines and tailored to the starting blood pressure. It is important to note that this estimate only includes costs to achieve control once diagnosed and does not include the costs of screening, which would add necessary expenditures to identify those in need of treatment (Gaziano and Kim, 2009).

The total estimated cost that would be accrued to meet treatment needs is also shown in Table 7.3 as a percentage of the nation's gross domestic product (GDP) in 2008 and as a percentage of the nation's total health expenditures in 2006. The estimated costs relative to both GDP and total health expenditures show considerable variability across countries, with India and Chile standing out at the high end of the range.

TABLE 7.3 Estimated Annual Cost to Control Hypertension with Medication

Country	Total Population Cost of Controlling Hypertension (Intl $ millions)	% of GDP (2008, Intl $ millions)	% of Total Health Expenditures
USA	14,404	0.10	0.66
China	4,346	0.05	1.22
Czech Republic	200	0.08	1.14
Mexico	1,662	0.11	1.74
Chile	411	0.17	3.20
Iran	469	0.06	0.72
Egypt	254	0.06	0.91
South Africa	230	0.05	0.54
Pakistan	150	0.03	1.71
India	4,821	0.14	2.90

SOURCE: Gaziano and Kim, 2009.

In summary, the available evidence from a sample of developing countries shows relatively low treatment coverage of the estimated at-risk population, with an even lower proportion of cases of hypertension under control. The costs that would need to be added to current health expenditures in order to address this unmet need are variable across countries. In some countries it may seem like a manageable shift in expenditures, whereas in others it is much higher. India is a particularly alarming case. The current estimate is that 28 percent of the population is hypertensive, but only half of those individuals are aware of their condition and half of that number receive treatment. Most alarmingly, only 7 percent of those treated have their blood pressure under control. Using current costs, it is estimated that India would need to add on additional spending of almost 3 percent of health care expenditures to control hypertension. This suggests that addressing the unmet needs for screening and effective treatment would require a much more effective health system to reduce those costs.

Hypertension can also be successfully averted through lifestyle and dietary changes, and implementing nation-wide strategies to promote lifestyle changes would possibly reduce mean blood pressure in a population. A population-wide strategy, by reducing the incidence of hypertension, could also produce cost reductions in the long term due to fewer patients requiring the treatment costs estimated above. The most reliable cost estimates currently available for population-based lifestyle changes to reduce hypertension are for salt-reduction strategies (Asaria et al., 2007). For the analysis commissioned for this report, a population-wide salt-reduction strategy assumed to result in a 3 mmHg reduction in mean population blood pressure was used to estimate the costs that would be accrued to achieve this in each country, as shown in Table 7.4 (Gaziano and Kim, 2009).

Combining population-based strategies with treatment approaches theoretically should produce some cost efficiencies, as one outcome of the population-based approaches would be to reduce the number in need of treatment. Successfully filling the treatment gap for hypertension could also potentially produce cost savings in the longer term by reducing not only the burden of CVD but also the burden of complications of other chronic diseases, such as diabetes and kidney failure.

This analysis provided an example of country-specific analyses of one risk factor for CVD. Further analyses using country-specific costs and treatment needs, taking into account other risk factors and other disease endpoints, would serve to inform the investment priorities of national governments and other stakeholders.

TABLE 7.4 Estimated Total Cost to Achieve Mean Systolic Blood Pressure Reduction via Population Salt-Reduction Strategies (Intl $ millions)

Country	Total Population (2009, 1000s)[a]	3 mmHg Reduction[b]
USA	307,212	307.21
China	1,338,613	535.45
Czech Republic	10,212	4.08
Mexico	111,212	44.48
Chile	16,602	6.64
Iran	66,429	26.57
Egypt	78,867	31.55
South Africa	49,052	19.62
Pakistan	174,579	69.83
India	1,156,898	462.76

[a] U.S. Census International Database.
[b] Salt reduction: cost per individual is $1 for the United States, $0.4 for all other countries.
SOURCE: Gaziano and Kim, 2009.

FUTURE NEEDS IN ECONOMIC ANALYSIS OF INTERVENTIONS[5]

As the previous sections demonstrate, economic analysis is a critical tool for evaluating different interventions to address CVD in developing countries, but there has been relatively little carried out in those settings, and what exists is not easily comparable (Behrman et al., 2009). Given the growing importance of CVD and other chronic diseases in developing countries, and the potential to seriously thwart or delay economic development—further research will be critical to determine, for specific countries, which investments are needed to address CVD and which investments are likely to produce the highest returns.

***Conclusion 7.1**: Governments need better health-sector and intersectoral economic analysis to guide decision making about resource allocations among health conditions and interventions.*

This section details several high-priority areas for economic research on CVD.

---

[5] This section is based in part on papers written for the committee by Stephen Jan and Alison Hayes, by Marc Suhrcke et al., and by Thomas Gaziano and Grace Kim.

Costs, Cost-Effectiveness, and Potential for Return on Investment in Public Health and Health Systems

The available evidence for low and middle income countries on cost-effectiveness of CVD interventions is informative and valuable, but scarce when compared to developed countries (Schwappach et al., 2007). Although the number of published economic evaluations of interventions for CVD in developing countries has increased substantially in recent years, beyond antitobacco strategies, the gaps in the evidence base limit the ability to conclude with confidence general recommendations that would apply to CVD in developing countries across countries and across all available intervention approaches. This is because there is a lack of primary economic analyses in developing countries, variation in costs and population health across countries, and reason to question whether and how the evidence-based strategies to prevent and manage CVD that have been shown to be cost-effective in developed countries are applicable in a developing-country context where resources are more limited and health care systems are less strong and more variable.

The available research studies are biased toward individual interventions, mostly pharmaceutical, targeted at persons with already established risk factors. Approaches using a population-based, public health intervention strategy, such as communications strategies or legislative actions, have not undergone cost-effectiveness analysis as extensively in developing-country contexts, especially using primary effectiveness data. However, the available studies do show promise for the likely cost-effectiveness of these approaches. There are even fewer cost-effectiveness studies from developing countries on multi-level and multi-valent CVD interventions.

Therefore, as described in the following section, there is a pressing need for research efforts to improve methodologies to evaluate the transferability of cost-effectiveness evidence from developed to developing settings and to increase the primary evidence base for cost-effectiveness evaluations in developing-country settings. There is also a need to expand economic analyses to be more inclusive of countries and regions that have a high burden of disease but are not well represented in the available economic literature, such as former Soviet Republics and the Middle East. Increasing the research in these and other neglected regions should be part of an international global health strategy to address CVD.

Improving the Use of Modeling to Transfer Cost-Effectiveness Evidence from Developed to Developing Countries

It is not realistic to expect primary economic evaluations to be conducted for every intervention in every developing country. The use of modeling methodologies to transfer results from developed to developing countries and between developing countries, as well as to estimate long-term effects, remains a necessary alternative that has and will continue to be highly informative, as described earlier in this chapter. However, there are several major challenges to using this approach to guide implementation choices at the national level in low and middle income countries. These include differences in health care costs across countries, differential effectiveness of interventions in different settings, differential disease prevalence, differential valuation of outcomes, and differential efficiency in implementing interventions. As a result, the applicability of economic modeling results is highly dependent on the methods applied and the assumptions that are incorporated in the model.

Broadly speaking, there is a need to improve modeling methods to take into account the potential effects, including regional/country-level variations, of demographics, epidemiological transition, emerging changes in availability of technology, and financial conditions. In particular, there are two key areas that emerge as a priority to improve models used to evaluate interventions to address CVD.

First, the available modeling analyses almost exclusively calculate effectiveness based on studies conducted in developed countries. Therefore, there is a great need to perform effectiveness studies in developing-country settings and for these results to inform economic models. This is especially important for interventions targeted to changing health behaviors and those that use methods such as communications, which are highly dependent on cultural and infrastructural characteristics. In addition, for interventions to target high-risk individuals, the effectiveness of strategies for screening/identification must be taken into account. The predominance of the use of developed-country effectiveness data in these models is due primarily to the lack of effectiveness data for CVD interventions in developing countries, as has been described in Chapters 5 and 6. Efforts to fill this knowledge gap will also serve to improve the quality of economic analyses by making more relevant secondary data available.

Second, and similarly, many models calculate resource utilization based on implemented data from developed countries. Therefore, there is also a great need for modeling that instead calculates resource utilization based on implemented data from developing-country settings. This is true for all types of interventions. Even interventions for which effectiveness data is arguably more readily transferred across populations and stage of development (such as pharmaceutical interventions), developing-country settings will have vastly different implementation resources and infrastructure. Addressing this gap will require greater research efforts to project, or ideally measure, the actual costs of implementing interventions in at least a representative sample of developing countries. This includes realistic assessments of the costs of implementing non-clinical primary prevention and population-based strategies in these settings, the true costs of which can be very difficult to determine. As above for effectiveness, this also means that to conduct realistic assessments of the costs of interventions to target high-risk individuals, costs of screening/identification must be taken into account.

Although the challenges of transferring evidence using modeling methodologies is acknowledged by both the Disease Control Priorities Project (Musgrove and Fox-Rushby, 2006) and the WHO CHOICE project (Evans and Ulasevich, 2005), there are currently no validated methodologies or consensus guidelines within the scientific community on how to handle this uncertainty in modeling interventions for developing countries. Consensus standards for conducting and reviewing evaluations among researchers and journals in the field could elevate the quality of evidence and allow for greater comparability across studies. A potential model for such standards could come from the task force on research practices in modeling studies of the International Society for Pharmacoeconomics and Outcomes Research (ISPOR) (Weinstein et al., 2003). At a minimum, the capacity for this kind of data to be useful for policy decisions would be greatly improved if information about the assumptions influencing the model and the sources of secondary data were more clearly stated in the published literature. In both reviews commissioned by this committee, for example, the authors found that there was a lack of full information in many modeling studies.

Increasing the Evidence Base of Primary Economic Analyses of Interventions Conducted in Developing-Country Settings

Modeling methodologies to transfer results from developed to developing countries and between developing countries will continue to be an important approach to assessing the most cost-effective ways to address CVD. However, it is also a crucial goal to increase the evidence base of primary economic analyses from developing countries. Once again, this relates directly to the need for more primary intervention evidence from developing countries. Therefore, it is important that steps taken to increase effectiveness and implementation research in these countries be accompanied by an emphasis on conducting economic analyses as part of the evaluation, especially for population-based and public health approaches such as community-based interventions, communications strategies, or legislative actions. These are areas where economic evidence is lacking and the specificity of the setting potentially has the largest impact on effectiveness. This should be an achievable goal if made a priority by global health funders (see Chapter 8).

Making the Evidence More Useful for Policy Makers

Few of the currently available economic analyses adopted a comprehensive perspective in their analysis. In general, the more comprehensive a study is, the easier it is for decision makers to compare the intervention to other alternatives available for funding. In developing countries, budgets are highly constrained, and not only is CVD competing with other health priorities, but also all investments in health care are in crucial competition with other budgetary sectors, such as education or public infrastructure. A greater focus on comprehensive evaluations would facilitate policy decisions.

One way to address this is through the expression of health benefits in comprehensive units (such as "life-years gained" or the surrogate measure of QALYs or DALYs) rather than CVD-specific measures that may be easier to measure but are difficult to compare to other interventions within or outside the health care sector. In addition, the utility to policy makers can be improved through the use of methods such as benefit–cost analysis, which offers the capability of expressing all benefits of an intervention, occurring in the health care sector or not, in monetary units. With respect to affordability and adherence to treatment, the use of willingness to pay approaches could also be informative, especially in health care systems in which patients are required to contribute some or all of the costs. For example, in a rare willingness-to-pay analysis from a developing country, patients in China were not willing to pay the annual cost of $73 for antihypertensive medicine until their 5-year absolute risk for CVD exceeded 35 percent (Tang et al., 2009).

This also applies to the economic perspective applied in the analysis, which relates to the question of who will incur the costs of an intervention and who will receive the benefits. Key perspectives that are relevant to policy makers include, for example, the health care provider, the patient, the government, third-party payers, and the societal perspective, which has not yet been explicitly applied to the evaluation of interventions for CVD in the developing world.

Defining Resource Needs

As described in this chapter, there has not been sufficient analysis to determine what it will cost to reduce the burden of CVD in developing countries. Ideally, this type of analysis—linking evidence of prevention and disease management needs (the "treatment gap") with evidence of costs and cost-effectiveness—would be carried out at a country level to inform the implementation of interventions to address high-priority health conditions. If provided within a specific macroeconomic and epidemiological context, it would give decision makers an indication of not only what options represent the "best buys" but also how investment in such buys is anticipated to contribute to a reduction in the overall burden of disease. For instance it would indicate that, for a defined population, $X invested in treatment Y would be needed to eliminate a particular treatment gap. Health and finance policy makers would then have clear guidance on where to shift resources to achieve the maximum health benefit. There is very limited available evidence for this type of health investment appraisal. Therefore, there needs to be an ongoing program of research in this area, especially given the rapid changes over time in risk-factor prevalence, treatment levels (and gaps), technology, and costs of treatment.

Recommendation: Define Resource Needs

The Global Alliance for Chronic Disease should commission and coordinate case studies of the CVD financing needs for five to seven countries representing different geographical regions, stages of the CVD epidemic, and stages of development. These studies should require a comprehensive assessment of the future financial needs within the health, public health, and agricultural systems to prevent and reduce the burden of CVD and related chronic diseases. Several scenarios for different prevention and treatment efforts, technology choices, and demographic trends should be evaluated. These assessments should explicitly establish the gap between current investments and future investment needs, focusing on how to maximize population health gains. These initial case studies should establish an analytical framework with the goal of expanding beyond the initial pilot countries.

A number of considerations should be taken into account for these studies and other future research to accurately project costs to address untreated CVD. First, as mentioned earlier, if estimates of treatment gaps are to offer specific guidance to decision makers they must be contextualized based on local circumstances—including demographics, epidemiological transition, and financial conditions—and must be provided in conjunction with cost and cost-effectiveness analysis. The reasons for treatment gaps are likely to be varied and differ according to context and intervention. Factors such as cost, geographical access, availability of treatment technologies, and provider incentives are likely to be significant determinants. At present the treatment gap literature focuses mainly on patient awareness. Further work should be conducted into investigating the broader determinants of treatment gaps because they are crucial in establishing any policy response.

Second, existing evidence of treatment gaps generally focuses on a single risk factor. However, ideally this assessment would take into account multiple risk factors based on an absolute risk approach. This includes reorienting risk-factor prevalence studies so that they are based on absolute risk rather than on the prevalence of a single risk factor. This would also allow such studies to be better linked with most of the available cost-effectiveness evidence. However, it is important to consider that risk-factor measures required by models such as the risk assessment tool based on the Framingham Study may not always be available or may be cost-prohibitive in a low income setting (e.g., if they include lab tests). These measures also may not be readily applicable to different populations in developing countries. A priority for future research is the development of specific risk-prediction screening tools appropriate for low income settings and for such forms of risk stratification to then be reflected in cost-effectiveness and treatment gap analysis.

In addition, the role of system constraints in determining treatment gaps needs to be assessed (e.g., geographical and financial constraints on access to health care; human resource constraints such as lack of staff, misaligned incentives for providers, lack of infrastructure, and inadequate regulatory systems), as well as the effectiveness and cost-effectiveness of addressing these constraints. Better information is also needed on the extrapolation of cost-effectiveness estimates in relation to the scaling up of interventions to meet the treatment gap. Assumptions made in economic modeling of constant returns to scale and of continued and constant treatment effect are currently not well supported by evidence. Finally, studies on costs and cost-effectiveness of interventions to address CVD are generally health sector-specific. Further research is required to investigate intersectoral approaches that work beyond conventional health-sector boundaries as potential innovations in interventions to address the treatment gap.

CONCLUSION

Given limited resources and political energy to allocate to CVD programming, many countries will want to focus their efforts on goals that are economically feasible, have the highest likelihood of intervention success, and have the largest morbidity impact. The limitations on the available evidence do not preclude intervening now as initial priorities can be ascertained. Indeed, the totality of intervention and economic analysis suggests that substantial progress in reducing CVD can be made in the near term through a prioritized subset of intervention approaches—if they can be successfully and efficiently adapted and implemented. These include staretgies for tobacco control, reduction of salt in the food supply and in consumption, and improved delivery of clinical prevention using pharmaceutical interventions in high-risk patients, especially if linked to existing health systems strengthening efforts. The evidence for lowered CVD morbidity associated with achieving these priority goals is credible, there are examples of successful implementation of programs in each of these focus areas with the potential to be adapted for low and middle income countries, and economic analyses have shown that they are likely to be cost-effective.

TABLE 7.5a Summary of Economic Analyses for Population-Based and Other Lifestyle CVD Intervention Approaches for Low and Middle Income Countries

Intervention Type	Reference	Country/ Setting	Intervention	Comparator
Tobacco Control[b]				
	Lai et al., 2007	Estonia	Increase taxes from 49% to 60%	Current situation
		Estonia	Taxes and advertising bans on smoking	Taxes only
		Estonia	Taxes, ad ban, and clean indoor air	Taxes and ad ban
	Gaziano, 2008	Sub-Saharan Africa	Tobacco taxation—price increase 33%	Null
		Sub-Saharan Africa	Tobacco regulation (non-price intervention such as labeling, advertising bans)	Null
	Thavorn and Chaiyakunapruk, 2008	Thailand	Individual health education for tobacco cessation	Usual care: screening and brief advice and support

---

[a] Sources of data on intervention effectiveness and costs for modeling assumptions vary widely across studies and in some cases are drawn from high income country information.
[b] For tobacco control, see also reviews by Chisholm et al., 2006; Jha et al., 2006; and Shibuya et al., 2003.

Method[a]	Outcome or Assumed Outcome[a]	Economic Analysis Result[a]	Cost Effective?
WHO CHOICE Modeling	Assumed 3.4% decline in tobacco consumption	ICER: 218 EEK/DALY averted	Y <per capita GDP (90454 EEK)
WHO CHOICE Modeling	Assumed 3.4% decline in tobacco consumption PLUS 5% decline in new smokers	ICER: 304 EEK/DALY	Y
WHO CHOICE Modeling	Assumed 3.4% decline in tobacco consumption PLUS 5% decline in new smokers PLUS 5% decline in the incidence of smoking among male smokers, and 2.4% decline among female smokers	ICER: 453 EEK/DALY	Y
Modeling	Assumed a reduction in future tobacco deaths of 5.4%-15.9%	ICER: US$2-26/DALY	Not reported
Modeling	Assumed a reduction in future tobacco deaths of 1.6%-7.9%	ICER: US$33-417/DALY	Not reported
Modeling	Assumed a 14.3% smoking cessation rate (with no relapse) with a corresponding assumed reduction in events and mortality due to COPD, AMI, CHF, angina, and stroke	Cost savings of 17503 baht (£250; €325; US$500) to the health system and life year gains of 0.18 years for men Cost savings of 21 499.75 baht (£307; €399; $614) and life year gains of 0.24 years for women	Y

continued

TABLE 7.5a Continued

Intervention Type	Reference	Country/Setting	Intervention	Comparator
Food Regulation				
	Rubinstein et al., 2009	Argentina (Buenos Aires)	Regulation of salt content of bread	Null
	Murray et al., 2003	Latin America	Salt reduction—industry agreements	Null
		Latin America	Salt reduction—legislation	Null
		South-East Asia	Salt reduction—industry agreements	Null
		South-East Asia	Salt reduction—legislation	Null
	Gaziano, 2008	Sub-Saharan Africa	Substitution of polyunsaturated fats for 2% of dietary transfats	Null
Physical Activity				
	Matsudo et al., 2006	Brazil	Population-based physical activity promotion	

Method[a]	Outcome or Assumed Outcome[a]	Economic Analysis Result[a]	Cost Effective?
Modeling Popmod (WHO)	Assumed that a 1g of salt reduction per 100g of bread led to a reduction of 1.33mmHg in systolic blood pressure per person and 1% of the population-attributable risk of CHD and stroke	ICER: 151 ARG$/DALY	Y Based on <3× per capita GNI
Popmod multi-state modeling	Assumed blood pressure changes specific for region, age, and sex associated with a 15% reduction in total dietary salt intake	Average CER: US$24/DALY	Y based on < per capita GDP
Popmod multi-state modeling	Assumed blood pressure changes specific for region, age, and sex associated with a 30% reduction in total dietary salt intake	Average CER: US$13/DALY	Y
Popmod multi-state modeling	Assumed blood pressure changes specific for region, age, and sex associated with a 15% reduction in total dietary salt intake	Average CER: US$37/DALY	Y
Popmod multi-state modeling	Assumed blood pressure changes specific for region, age, and sex associated with a 30% reduction in total dietary salt intake	Average CER: US$19/DALY	Y
Popmod multi-state modeling	Assumed reduction in CAD of 7% to 40%	ICER: US$53-1344/DALY at 7% Cost saving US$ −184 at 40%	Y
Modeling	Assumptions for model unknown	Cost Utility Analysis: Cost saving	Y

continued

TABLE 7.5a Continued

Intervention Type	Reference	Country/Setting	Intervention	Comparator
Physical Activity (cont.)	Salvetti et al., 2008	Brazil	Home-based training for physical post-MI	Standard care
Health Education	Murray et al., 2003	South-East Asia	Health education focusing on lowering BMI and cholesterol	Null
		Latin America	Health education focusing on lowering BMI and cholesterol	Null
	Getpreechaswas et al., 2007	Thailand	Social marketing through trained health personnel, village health volunteers, and family health leaders	Interview only
	García-Peña et al., 2002	Mexico	Health education in home visits by nurse to elderly people with hypertension	No intervention

Method[a]	Outcome or Assumed Outcome[a]	Economic Analysis Result[a]	Cost Effective?
RCT	Overall biomedical measures of cardiovascular function and self-reported measures of quality of life improved in the intervention group and remained constant or worsened in the control group	Protocol cost $502.71 (BHCMP) per patient for 3 months	Not reported
Popmod multi-state modeling	Assumed a 2% reduction in total blood cholesterol concentrations	Average CER: US$14/DALY	Y based on < per capita GDP
Popmod multi-state modeling	Assumed a 2% reduction in total blood cholesterol concentrations	Average CER: US$14/DALY	Y
Observational trial	The intervention group showed a significant improvement in dietary patters, physical activity, and stress reduction and a significant decrease in tobacco and alcohol use compared to the control group	Costs: 74.89 baht per head of population	Not reported
RCT	A reduction of 3.31 mm Hg in SBP and 3.67 mm Hg in DBP in the intervention group compared to the control group. In the intervention group, 12.9% of participants reported an increase in brisk walking, compared with 5.2% in the control group. The proportion of people on anti-hypertensive medication decreased from 28.4% to 15.9%, compared to a decrease from 32.2% to 26.9% in the control group	CER: 10.46 pesos (US$1.14) per mmHg reduced for SBP 9.43 (US$1.03) per mmHg reduced for DBP	Not possible to conclude

continued

TABLE 7.5a Continued

Intervention Type	Reference	Country/Setting	Intervention	Comparator
Health Education (cont.)	Huang et al., 2000, and Chen et al., 2008	Beijing China	Community-based CVD program including education and risk-targeted high blood pressure medication (Beijing Fangshan CVD Prevention Program)	Null
	Rubinstein et al., 2009	Argentina (Buenos Aires)	Health education through mass media	Null
	Rossouw et al., 1993	South Africa	Social Marketing (CORIS)	No intervention

Method[a]	Outcome or Assumed Outcome[a]	Economic Analysis Result[a]	Cost Effective?
Observational cohort	Observed a net reduction in SBP/DBP in the intervention group compared to the control group of −1.4/.05 mmHg in men and −3.4/−1.0 in women. Observed a reduction in morbidity and mortality of stroke of 18.7% in the intervention group compared to 17.7% in the control group. Observed a reduction in morbidity and mortality of CHD of 4.9% in the intervention group compared to 4.3% in the control group.	ICER: 1992 1586 yuan/DALY 1993 1380 yuan/DALY ICER: Cost saving from 1994-1997	Cost saving
Modelling Popmod (WHO)	Assume a reduction of 1.83mmHg in systolic blood pressure and 0.02mm/l in cholesterol (t), leading to a reduction of 2% of the population attributable risk of CHD and stroke	ICER: 547 ARG$/DALY	Y Based on <3× per capita GNI
Observational trial	For men there was a reduction in risk score of 1.3% in the control group, 3.7% in the low-intensity intervention group, and 3.7% in the high-intensity intervention group For women there was a reduction in risk score of 1.6% in the control group, 4.7% in the low-intensity intervention group, and 4.4% in the high-intensity intervention group	$5 per capita cost for low intensity; $22 per capita cost for high intensity	Not reported

continued

TABLE 7.5a Continued

Intervention Type	Reference	Country/Setting	Intervention	Comparator
Multiple Strategies	Asaria et al., 2007	Multi-national	Population-based strategies to reduce salt consumption by 15% and a 43.2% increase in the price of tobacco combined with non-price interventions	No treatment

NOTE: AMI = Acute Myocardial Infarction; CAD = Coronary Artery Disease; CER = Cost-Effectiveness Ratio; CHD = Coronary Heart Disease; CHF = Congestive Heart Failure; COPD = Chronic Obstructive Pulmonary Disease; CVD = Cardiovascular Disease; DALY = Disability-Adjusted Life Year; GDP = Gross Domestic Product; GNI = Gross National Income; ICER = Incremental Cost-Effectiveness Ratio; RCT = Randomized Controlled Trial; WHO = World Health Organization.

Method[a]	Outcome or Assumed Outcome[a]	Economic Analysis Result[a]	Cost Effective?
Modeling	Salt Reduction Assumed the reduction in salt intake lead to an age-stratified decrease in mmHg of SPB of 1.24 (30-44), 1.7 (45-59), 2.34 (60-69), 2.83 (70-79), 3.46 (80-100) Tobacco prices Assumed the non-price interventions lead to a 12% decrease in smoking prevalence Assumed the increase in price of tobacco lead to a 20.8% decrease in smoking prevalence	Costs range from US$0.14-1.04 per person per year to avert approximately 13.8 million deaths from CVD, respiratory disease, and cancer over 10 years	Not reported

TABLE 7.5b Summary of Cost Effectiveness Evidence for Pharmaceutical Intervention Approaches Against Cardiovascular Disease for Low and Middle Income Countries

Intervention Type	Reference	Country/ Setting	Intervention	Comparator
Pharmaceutical				
	Lim et al., 2007	Multi-national	Secondary prevention (aspirin, ACE-inhibitor, β-blocker, statin) Primary prevention targeted to high risk (aspirin, ACE-inhibitor, thiazide, statin)	No treatment
	Gaziano et al., 2006	East Asia and the Pacific	Secondary prevention (aspirin, β-blockers, ACE-inhibitor, statins)	Null
		East Europe and Central Asia	Secondary prevention (aspirin, β-blockers, ACE-inhibitor, statins)	Null
		Latin America and Caribbean	Secondary prevention (aspirin, β-blockers, ACE-inhibitor, statins)	Null
		Middle East and North Africa	Secondary prevention (aspirin, β-blockers, ACE-inhibitor, statins)	Null
		South Asia	Secondary prevention (aspirin, β-blockers, ACE-inhibitor, statins)	Null

[a] Sources of data on intervention effectiveness and costs for modeling assumptions vary widely across studies and in some cases are drawn from high income country information.

Methodology[a]	Outcome or Assumed Outcome[a]	Economic Analysis Result[a]	Cost-Effective?
Modeling	Assumed achievement of a 50% drug coverage rate in the more constrained countries Assumed achievement of an 80% coverage rate in the less constrained countries Assumed between 40% and 60% drug adherence	Financial resources needed to scale up average $5 billion per year, or $1.08 per head per year	Not reported
Markov model	Assumed a 7% reduction in lifetime risk for CVD	ICER: US$336/QALY	Y based on <3× per capita GNI
Markov model	Assumed a 15% reduction in lifetime risk for CVD	ICER: US$362/QALY	Y
Markov model	Assumed a 12% reduction in lifetime risk for CVD	ICER: US$388/QALY	Y
Markov model	Assumed a 15% reduction in lifetime risk for CVD	ICER: US$341/QALY	Y
Markov model	Assumed a 13% reduction in lifetime risk for CVD	ICER: US$306/QALY	Y

continued

TABLE 7.5b Continued

Intervention Type	Reference	Country/ Setting	Intervention	Comparator
Pharmaceutical (cont.)	Gaziano et al., 2006 (cont.)	Sub-Saharan Africa	Secondary prevention (aspirin, β-blockers, ACE-inhibitor, statins)	Null
		East Asia and the Pacific	Primary prevention absolute risk 5% and 25% (aspirin, calcium channel blocker, ACE-inhibitor, statin)	Null
		East Europe and Central Asia	Primary prevention absolute risk 5% and 25% (aspirin, calcium channel blocker, ACE-inhibito, statin)	Null
		Latin America and Caribbean	Primary prevention absolute risk 5% and 25% (aspirin, calcium channel blocker, ACE-inhibitor, statin)	Null
		Middle East and North Africa	Primary prevention absolute risk 5% and 25% (aspirin, calcium channel blocker, ACE-inhibitor, statin)	Null
		South Asia	Primary prevention absolute risk 5% and 25% (aspirin, calcium channel blocker, ACE-inhibitor, statin)	Null
		Sub-Saharan Africa	Primary prevention absolute risk 5% and 25% (aspirin, calcium channel blocker, ACE-inhibitor, statin)	Null
	Amira and Okubadejo, 2006	Nigeria	Pharmaceutical treatment of hypertension; Targeted to high risk	Respective drug

Methodology[a]	Outcome or Assumed Outcome[a]	Economic Analysis Result[a]	Cost-Effective?
Markov model	Assumed a 9% reduction in lifetime risk for CVD	ICER: US$312/QALY	Y
Markov model	Assumed a 54% and 40% reduction in lifetime risk for CVD	ICER: US$1214/QALY US$890/QALY	Y
Markov model	Assumed a 43% and 30% reduction in lifetime risk for CVD	ICER: US$1207/QALY US$858/QALY	Y
Markov model	Assumed a 53% and 32% reduction in lifetime risk for CVD	ICER: US$1219/QALY US$881/QALY	Y
Markov model	Assumed a 50% and 29% reduction in lifetime risk for CVD	ICER: US$1221/QALY US$872/QALY	Y
Markov model	Assumed a 50% and 27% reduction in lifetime risk for CVD	ICER: US$1039/QALY US$746/QALY	Y
Markov model	Assumed a 59% and 32% reduction in lifetime risk for CVD	ICER: US$1145/QALY US$771/QALY	Y
Other	Blood pressure control was achieved in 39.6% of the target population	Most cost-effective was coamiloride with CER 42.9, least was combination CCB with ACEI, CER 3145.2	See comparison result

continued

TABLE 7.5b Continued

Intervention Type	Reference	Country/ Setting	Intervention	Comparator
Pharmaceutical (cont.)	Rubinstein et al., 2009	Argentina (Buenos Aires)	Treatment of hypertension (lifestyle change promotion and hydrochlorothiazide, atenol, enalapril); Not risk targeted	Null
		Argentina (Buenos Aires)	Treatment of high cholesterol (low cholesterol diet plus statin) Not risk targeted	Null
		Argentina (Buenos Aires)	Polypill based on three different target populations (risk determined with Framingham equations) 20% CVD risk	Null
		Argentina (Buenos Aires)	As above—10% CVD risk	Null
		Argentina (Buenos Aires)	As above—5% CVD risk	Null
	Robberstad et al., 2007	Tanzania	Diuretic hydrochlorothiazide; Not risk targeted	Null

Methodology[a]	Outcome or Assumed Outcome[a]	Economic Analysis Result[a]	Cost-Effective?
Modeling Popmod (WHO)	Assumed that 40% of the population would take one drug, 40% at least two drugs, and 20% three or more drugs Assumed a 50% rate of disease detection and drug compliance leading to a reduction in the population-attributable risk of CVD and stroke by 8%	ICER: 7716 ARG$/DALY	N
Modeling Popmod (WHO)	Assumed reduction of cholesterol to less than 240mg/dl, (6.2mm/l) leading to a reduction of 8% of the population-attributable risk of CHD and stroke Assumed a 50% detection and drug compliance rate	ICER: 70994 ARG$/DALY	N
Modeling Popmod (WHO)	Assumed a reduction of population-attributable risk of CHD and stroke of 60% Assumed an 80% detection and drug compliance rate	ICER: 3599 ARG$/DALY	Y Based on <3× per capita GNI
Modeling Popmod (WHO)	Assumed a reduction of population-attributable risk of CHD and stroke of 40% Assumed a 50% detection and drug compliance rate	ICER: 4113 ARG$/DALY	Y Based on <3× per capita GNI
Modeling Popmod (WHO)	Assumed a reduction of population-attributable risk of CHD and stroke of 15% Assumed a 50% detection and drug compliance rate	ICER: 4533 ARG$/DALY	N
Life cycle Markov model	Assumed 1.6 life years saved and a very high risk population	ICER: US$85/DALY	Y based on < per capita GDP of $300

continued

TABLE 7.5b Continued

Intervention Type	Reference	Country/ Setting	Intervention	Comparator
Pharmaceutical (cont.)	Robberstad et al., 2007 (cont.)	Tanzania	Aspirin + diuretic hydrochlorothiazide; Not risk targeted	Null
		Tanzania	Aspirin, diuretic, β-blocker; Not risk targeted	Null
		Tanzania	Aspirin, diuretic, β-blocker, statin; Not risk targeted	Null
		Tanzania	Hypothetical polypill; Not risk targeted	Null
	Moreira et al., 2009	Brazil	Treatment of hypertension with diuretics	Null
		Brazil	Treatment of hypertension with β-blockers	Null
		Brazil	Treatment of hypertension with ACEI	Null
	Gaziano, 2005	South Africa	Targeted drug treatment based on blood pressure 160/95mmHg	No treatment
		South Africa	Targeted drug treatment based on blood pressure 140/90mmHg	No treatment

Methodology[a]	Outcome or Assumed Outcome[a]	Economic Analysis Result[a]	Cost-Effective?
Life cycle Markov model	Assumed 3.1 life years saved and a very high risk population	ICER US$143/DALY	Y based on < per capita GDP of $300
Life cycle Markov model	Assumed 3.6 life years saved and a very high risk population	ICER US$317/DALY	N
Life cycle Markov model	Assumed 5.4 life years saved and a very high risk population	ICER US$999/DALY	N
Life cycle Markov model	Assumed 6.3 life years saved and a very high risk population	ICER US$1476/DALY	N
Observational cohort >40 years	Observed a 56.6% blood pressure control rate	Average CER: US$15.5 (total monthly cost/controlled patients)	Not reported
Observational cohort >40 years	Observed a 66.4% blood pressure control rate	Average CER: US$34.7	Not reported
Observational cohort >40 years	Observed a 44.8% blood pressure control rate	Average CER: US$176.7	Not reported
Markov CVD model	Treatment was assumed to lead to a 10mmHg reduction in SDP, which was assumed to lead to a 40% relative risk reduction for stroke and a 14% relative risk reduction for CHD	Dominated	N
Markov CVD model	Treatment was assumed to lead to a 10mmHg reduction in SDP, which was assumed to lead to a 40% relative risk reduction for stroke and a 14% relative risk reduction for CHD	Dominated	N

continued

TABLE 7.5b Continued

Intervention Type	Reference	Country/ Setting	Intervention	Comparator
Pharmaceutical (cont.)	Gaziano, 2005 (cont.)	South Africa	Targeted drug treatment based on 10-year absolute CVD risk >40%	No treatment
		South Africa	Targeted drug treatment based on 10-year absolute CVD risk >30%	Treatment at 40% risk
		South Africa	Targeted drug treatment based on 10-year absolute CVD risk >20%	Treatment at 30% risk
		South Africa	Targeted drug treatment based on 10-year absolute CVD risk >15%	Treatment at 20% risk
	Shafiq et al., 2006	India	Low molecular weight heparin in patients with unstable angina	No treatment
	Murray et al., 2003	Latin America	Hypertension treatment (β-blocker, diuretic) and education; Not risk targeted	No treatment

Methodology[a]	Outcome or Assumed Outcome[a]	Economic Analysis Result[a]	Cost-Effective?
Markov CVD model	Treatment was assumed to lead to a 10mmHg reduction in SDP, which was assumed to lead to a 40% relative risk reduction for stroke and a 14% relative risk reduction for CHD	ICER: US$700/QALY	Y Based on <US$9000/QALY (3× per capita GDP)
Markov CVD model	Treatment was assumed to lead to a 10mmHg reduction in SDP, which was assumed to lead to a 40% relative risk reduction for stroke and a 14% relative risk reduction for CHD	ICER: US$1600/QALY	Y
Markov CVD model	Treatment was assumed to lead to a 10mmHg reduction in SDP, which was assumed to lead to a 40% relative risk reduction for stroke and a 14% relative risk reduction for CHD	ICER: US$4900/QALY	Y
Markov CVD model	Treatment was assumed to lead to a 10mmHg reduction in SDP, which was assumed to lead to a 40% relative risk reduction for stroke and a 14% relative risk reduction for CHD	ICER: US$11000/QALY	N
Prospective RCT	Primary endpoints of death, MI, or angina occurred in 24% to 30% of patients	ICER: US$54.72 to US$119.91/composite endpoint	See comparison result
Popmod multi-state modeling	Assumed a 33% reduction in difference between the actual SBP and 115mm Hg	Average CER: US$81/DALY	N Based on < per capita GDP

continued

TABLE 7.5b Continued

Intervention Type	Reference	Country/Setting	Intervention	Comparator
Pharmaceutical (cont.)	Murray et al., 2003 (cont.)	Latin America	High cholesterol treatment (statins) and education; Not risk targeted	No treatment
		Latin America	Blood pressure and cholesterol treatment and education; Not risk targeted	No treatment
		Latin America	Treatment based on absolute risk (>35% risk in 10 years)	No treatment
		South-East Asia	Hypertension treatment (β-blocker, diuretic) and education; Not risk targeted	No treatment
		South-East Asia	High cholesterol treatment (statins) and education; Not risk targeted	No treatment
		South-East Asia	Blood pressure and cholesterol treatment and education; Not risk targeted	No treatment
		South-East Asia	Treatment based on absolute risk (>35% risk in 10 years)	No treatment
	Ker et al., 2008	South Africa	Pharmaceutical interventions with tobacco cessation	No treatment

Methodology[a]	Outcome or Assumed Outcome[a]	Economic Analysis Result[a]	Cost-Effective?
Popmod multi-state modeling	Assumed a 20% reduction in total blood cholesterol	Average CER: US$87/DALY	N
Popmod multi-state modeling	Assumed a 33% reduction in difference between the actual SBP and 115mmHg and a 20% reduction in total blood cholesterol	Average CER: US$183/DALY	N
Popmod multi-state modeling	Assumed a 33% reduction in difference between the actual SBP and 115mmHg, a 20% reduction in total blood cholesterol, and an additional 20% reduction of absolute risk for antiplatelet therapy	Average CER: US$37/DALY	Y
Popmod multi-state modeling	Assumed a 33% reduction in difference between the actual SBP and 115mmHg	Average CER: US$36/DALY	N
Popmod multi-state modeling	Assumed a 20% reduction in total blood cholesterol	Average CER: US$47/DALY	N
Popmod multi-state modeling	Assumed a 33% reduction in difference between the actual SBP and 115mmHg and a 20% reduction in total blood cholesterol	Average CER: US$84/DALY	N
Popmod multi-state modeling	Assumed a 33% reduction in difference between the actual SBP and 115mmHg, a 20% reduction in total blood cholesterol, and an additional 20% reduction of absolute risk for antiplatelet therapy	Average CER: US$33/DALY	Y
Modeling	Assumed an absolute risk reduction of 7% to 22%	Costs per % of risk reduction ranges from R12.7 to R23.84	Not reported

continued

TABLE 7.5b Continued

Intervention Type	Reference	Country/ Setting	Intervention	Comparator
Pharmaceutical (cont.)	Rubinstein et al., 2009	Argentina (Buenos Aires)	Tobacco cessation therapy (bupropion)	Null
	Redekop et al., 2008	Poland	Prevention of CVD endpoints with perindopril in CHD patients	Placebo
	Wessels, 2007	South Africa	Prevention of cardiovascular or cerebrovascular events with eprosartan in stroke patients	Use of amlodipine and perindopril
	Dias da Costa et al., 2002	Brazil	Treatment of hypertension with diuretics, β-blockers, calcium channel blockers, and ACE-inhibitors	Alternative drugs
	Anderson et al., 2000	South Africa	Treatment with angiotensin II type 1 receptor blockers in patients with mild to moderate hypertension	Alternative drugs

Methodology[a]	Outcome or Assumed Outcome[a]	Economic Analysis Result[a]	Cost-Effective?
Modeling Popmod (WHO)	Assumed a reduction of 4% of the population-attributable risk of CHD and stroke	ICER: 33563 ARG$/DALY	N
Combined Trial-modeling	Observed a 1.88% decrease in risk of primary endpoints. Increase of .182 years life expectancy	ICER of PLN10896 per life year gained	Highly likely to be Y (<PLN60000)
Modeling	Assumed prevention of 23 CVD events per 1000 patients and 29.1 CBV events per 1000 patients	Cost-utility analysis of eprosartan estimated cost saving of ZAR 53132/QALY compared with amlodipine, and a cost saving of ZAR 72888 compared with perindopril	Y based on < per capita GDP
Population survey	Percent of patients using a drug category whose hypertension was controlled (<160mmHg SBP) Diuretics: 54.9% β-blockers: 71% ACE-inhibitors: 52% Calcium channel blockers: 80%	Cost-effectiveness relationship (ratio of annual mean cost to proportion of patients using drug/drug combination whose hypertension was controlled) Diuretics: 116.3 β-blockers: 228.5 ACEI: 608.5 Calcium channel blockers: 762	See comparison result
Modeling	Assumed reduction in SDBP for each drug of candesartan 10.57mmHg irbesartan 9.07mmHg losartan 8.89mmHg valsartan 7.11mmHg	Reduction in SDBP per R100 spent: candesartan was most cost-effective at 4.48 mmHg/R1OO; losartan was 3.77; irbesartan was 3.37; valsartan was 3.04mmHg Cost to achieve 1mmHg reduction in SDBP: candesartan (R22.34/mmHg); losartan (R26.54/mmHg); irbesartan (R29.65/mmHg); valsartan (R32.86/mmHg)	See comparison result

continued

TABLE 7.5b Continued

Intervention Type	Reference	Country/Setting	Intervention	Comparator
Pharmaceutical (cont.)	Edwards et al., 1998	South Africa	Reducing availability for routine prescribing of less cost-effective antihypertensive drugs or drug combinations	Current drug treatment
	Oyewo, 1989	Nigeria	Treatment of hypertension with antihypertensives	Respective alternative drug
Treatment and Prevention of Cardiac Events	Biccard et al., 2006	South Africa	Use of β-blocker or statin following surgery to avoid cardiovascular complications in patients with >10% risk	Placebo
	Orlewska et al., 2003	Poland	Treatment with enoxaparin in acute coronary syndrome	

Methodology[a]	Outcome or Assumed Outcome[a]	Economic Analysis Result[a]	Cost-Effective?
Observational trial	Observed blood pressure control did not change	Monthly cost per patient decreased 24.2% due to decrease in prescriptions of less cost-effective drugs for more cost-effective drugs	Not applicable
Cross-sectional	Efficacy coded based on systolic blood pressure reduction observed Mean values of coding Thiazide 2.94 Thiazide and methyldopa 4.05 Thiazide, methyldopa, and hydralazine 4.95 Propranolol 3.10 Propranolol and thiazide 2.53 Brinerdine 3.20 Minizide 1.30	Effectiveness score/average monthly cost Thiazide 0.49 Thiazide and methyldopa 0.27 Thiazide, mMethyldopa, and hydralazine 0.18 Propranolol 0.26 Propranolol and thiazide 0.14 Brinerdine 0.21 Minizide 0.06	See comparison result
Modeling	Assumed the use of β-blockers reduced the risk of non-fatal CVD events from 7.7% to 4% and risk of death from 8.2% to 4.2% but increased the risk of adverse events from 33.8% to 49.2% Assumed the use of statins reduced the risk of non-fatal CVD events from 11.3% to 6.5% and risk of death from 4% to 2.2%	Peri-operative β-blocker therapy may potentially save R869 per patient, statin treatment R1,822 per patient	Not reported
Modeling	Assumed a 19.8% 30-day event (MI, recurrent angina, or death) rate for those using enoxaparin and a 23.3% 30-day event rate for those using UFH	Cost/patient of enoxaparin = Z1085; cost/patient of UFH = Z1097	See comparison result

continued

TABLE 7.5b Continued

Intervention Type	Reference	Country/ Setting	Intervention	Comparator
Treatment and Prevention of Cardiac Events (cont.)	Araujo et al., 2008	Brazil	Pre-hospital thrombolysis in acute MI	In-hospital
	Rodriguez et al., 1993	Argentina	Percutaneous transluminal coronary angioplasty (PTCA)	Coronary artery bypass graft (CABG) surgery
	Grines et al., 1998	Multi-national: (developed and developing nations)	Early discharge after primary angioplasty in low-risk patients after acute MI	Traditional Care
Health Care Delivery				
	Diaz et al., 2006	Chile	Stroke unit	Regular hospital care

Methodology[a]	Outcome or Assumed Outcome[a]	Economic Analysis Result[a]	Cost-Effective?
Modeling	Assumed a gain of .1585 life years over 20 years with use of pre-hospital thrombolysis versus in-hospital thrombolysis	Dominated Pre-hospital thrombolysis cost R$176 less per .1585 life year gained (over 20 years)	See comparison result
RCT	In-hospital complication rate for PTCA was death 1.5%, AMI 6.3%, emergency CABG 1.5%, and stroke 1.5% In-hospital complication rate for CABG was death 4.6%, AMI 6.2%, emergency PTCA 1.5%, stroke 3.1%	Cumulative (group) costs at 1-year: PTCA (US$438,000), CABG (US$828,000)	Not reported
RCT	Rates of readmission in early discharge patients were 4.2% for recurrent unstable ischemia or MI, target vessel revascularization 9.8%, death 0.8%, reinfarction 0.8%, unstable ischemia 10.1%, stoke 0.4%, CHF 4.6%, and any event 15.2% Rates of readmission in traditional care patients were 3.9% for recurrent unstable ischemia or MI, target vessel revascularization 8.6%, death 0.4%, reinfarction 0.4%, unstable ischemia 12.0%, stroke 2.6%, CHF 4.3%, and any event 17.5%	Early discharge patients had significantly lower hospital costs (US$9,658 +/−5,287) compared to traditional care (US$11,604 +/−6,125)	Not reported
Observational trial	Stroke unit: Mean length of stay: 6.6 days Hospital: Mean length of stay: 9.9 days	Stroke unit: Mean cost per patient: US$5.550; Hospital: Mean cost per patient US$4.815	Not reported

continued

TABLE 7.5b Continued

Intervention Type	Reference	Country/ Setting	Intervention	Comparator
Health Care Delivery (cont.)	Pannarunothai et al., 2001	Thailand	Health care delivery by urban health center for hypertension and diabetes	Healthcare delivery by home visit program at the regional hospital and no home visit program
	Hauswald and Yeoh, 1997	Malaysia	EMS system to treat acute MI	Current care (performed by police/ private vehicle)

NOTE: ACE-inhibitor = Angiotensin converting enzyme inhibitor; AMI = Acute Myocardial Infarction; CABG = Coronary Artery Bypass Graft; CBV = Cerebrovascular; CER = Cost-Effectiveness Ratio; CHD = Coronary Heart Disease; CHF = Congestive Heart Failure; CVD = Cardiovascular Disease; DALY = Disability-Adjusted Life Year; GDP = Gross Domestic Product; GNI = Gross National Income; ICER = Incremental Cost-Effectiveness Ratio; MI = Myocardial Infarction; PTCA = Percutaneous Transluminal Coronary Angioplasty; QALY = Quality-Adjusted Life Year; RCT = Randomized Controlled Trial; SBP = Systolic Blood Pressure; SDBP = Sitting Diastolic Blood Pressure; UFH = Unfractionated Heparin; WHO = World Health Organization.

Methodology[a]	Outcome or Assumed Outcome[a]	Economic Analysis Result[a]	Cost-Effective?
Retrospective analysis	Identified the % of patients with controlled hypertension (SBP <160mmHg) was 79.4% at the urban health center, 72.8% at the Maharaj Hospital, and 79.8% of people receiving no home visit care	Total costs per % of patients with controlled disease Hypertension: Urban health center 5729 baht Maharaj Hospital home visit 7137 baht No home visit 7195 baht	See comparison result
	Identified the % of patients with controlled diabetes (fasting blood sugar 80-140mg/dl) was 50% at the urban health center, 49% at the Maharaj Hospital, and 33% of people receiving no home visit care	Diabetes: Urban health center 7468 baht Maharaj Hospital home visit 12313 baht No home visit 17861baht	
Modeling	Assumed delivery of a defibrillator to 85% of patients in less than 6 minutes and a 6% increase in survival rate from pre-hospital defibrillation with 50% having significant neurologic injury	Pre-hospital system for Kuala Lumpur would cost approximately US$357,000 per life saved with approximately 40% having significant neurological damage	Not reported

REFERENCES

Amira, O., and N. Okubadejo. 2007. Frequency of complementary and alternative medicine utilization in hypertensive patients attending an urban tertiary care centre in Nigeria. *BMC Complementary and Alternative Medicine* 7(1):30.

Anderson, A. N., F. Wessels, I. Moodley, and K. Kropman. 2000. At1 receptor blockers—cost-effectiveness within the South African context. *South African Medical Journal* 90(5):494-498.

Araujo, D. V., B. R. Tura, A. L. Brasileiro, H. Luz Neto, A. L. Pavao, and V. Teich. 2008. Cost-effectiveness of prehospital versus inhospital thrombolysis in acute myocardial infarction. *Arquivos Brasileiros de Cardiologia* 90(2):91-98.

Asaria, P., D. Chisholm, C. Mathers, M. Ezzati, and R. Beaglehole. 2007. Chronic disease prevention: Health effects and financial costs of strategies to reduce salt intake and control tobacco use. *Lancet* 370(9604):2044-2053.

Behrman, J. R., J. A. Behrman, and N. M. Perez. 2009. On what diseases and health conditions should new economic research on health and development focus? *Health Economics* 18(S1):S109-S128.

Biccard, B. M., J. W. Sear, and P. Foex. 2006. The pharmaco-economics of peri-operative beta-blocker and statin therapy in South Africa. *South African Medical Journal* 96(11):1199-1202.

Blackburn, H. 1983. Research and demonstration projects in community cardiovascular disease prevention. *Journal of Public Health Policy* 4(4):398-421.

Brownell, K. D., and T. R. Frieden. 2009. Ounces of prevention: The public policy case for taxes on sugared beverages. *New England Journal of Medicine* 360(18):1805-1808.

Chisholm, D., C. Doran, K. Shibuya, and J. R. Rehm. 2006. Comparative cost-effectiveness of policy instruments for reducing the global burden of alcohol, tobacco and illicit drug use. *Drug and Alcohol Review* 25(6):553-565.

Dias da Costa, J. S., S. C. Fuchs, M. T. Olinto, D. P. Gigante, A. M. Menezes, S. Macedo, and S. Gehrke. 2002. Cost-effectiveness of hypertension treatment: A population-based study. *São Paulo Medical Journal* 120(4):100-104.

Diaz, T. V., D. S. Illanes, M. A. Reccius, V. J. Manterola, C. P. Cerda, L. C. Recabarren, and V. R. Gonzalez. 2006. Evaluation of a stroke unit at a university hospital in Chile. *Revista Médica de Chilé* 134(11):1402-1408.

Edwards, P. R., D. W. Lunt, G. S. Fehrsen, C. J. Lombard, and K. Steyn. 1998. Improving cost-effectiveness of hypertension management at a community health centre. *South African Medical Journal* 88(5):549-554.

Evans, W. D., and A. Ulasevich. 2005. News media tracking of tobacco control: A review of sampling methodologies. *Journal of Health Communication* 10(5):403-417.

Ford, E. S., and S. Capewell. 2007. Coronary heart disease mortality among young adults in the U.S. from 1980 through 2002: Concealed leveling of mortality rates. *Journal of the American College of Cardiology* 50(22):2128-2132.

García-Peña, C., M. Thorogood, D. Wonderling, and S. Reyes-Frausto. 2002. Economic analysis of a pragmatic randomised trial of home visits by a nurse to elderly people with hypertension in Mexico. *Salud Publica de Mexico* 44:14-20.

Gaziano, T. A. 2005. Cardiovascular disease in the developing world and its cost-effective management. *Circulation* 112(23):3547-3553.

Gaziano, T. A. 2007. Reducing the growing burden of cardiovascular disease in the developing world. *Health Affairs* 26(1):13-24.

Gaziano, T. A. 2008. Economic burden and the cost-effectiveness of treatment of cardiovascular diseases in Africa. *Heart* 94(2):140-144.

Gaziano, T., and G. I. Kim. 2009. *Cost of treating non-optimal blood pressure in select low and middle income countries in comparison to the United States.* Boston, MA: Background Paper Commissioned by the Committee on Preventing the Global Epidemic of Cardiovascular Disease.

Gaziano, T.A., L. H. Opie, and M. C. Weinstein. 2006. Cardiovascular disease prevention with a multidrug regimen in the developing world: A cost-effectiveness analysis. *Lancet* 368(9536):679-86.

Gaziano, T. A., G. Galea, and K. S. Reddy. 2007. Chronic diseases II: Scaling up interventions for chronic disease prevention: The evidence. *Lancet* 370(9603):1939-1946.

Gaziano, T. A., A. Bitton, S. Anand, M. C. Weinstein. 2009. The global cost of nonoptimal blood pressure. *Journal of Hypertension* 27(7):1472-1477.

Getpreechaswas, J., N. Boontorterm, and P. Yospol. 2007. A model of health services for hypertension in primary care unit in Patumthani province. *Journal of the Medical Association of Thailand* 90(1):129-136.

Grines, C. L., D. L. Marsalese, B. Brodie, J. Griffin, B. Donohue, C. R. Costantini, C. Balestrini, G. Stone, T. Wharton, P. Esente, M. Spain, J. Moses, M. Nobuyoshi, M. Ayres, D. Jones, D. Mason, D. Sachs, L. L. Grines, and W. O'Neill. 1998. Safety and cost-effectiveness of early discharge after primary angioplasty in low risk patients with acute myocardial infarction. PAMI-II investigators. Primary angioplasty in myocardial infarction. *Journal of the American College of Cardiology* 31(5):967-972.

Gu, D., K. Reynolds, X. Wu, J. Chen, X. Duan, P. Muntner, G. Huang, R. F. Reynolds, S. Su, P. K. Whelton, and J. He. 2002. Prevalence, awareness, treatment, and control of hypertension in China. *Hypertension* 40(6):920-927.

Hauswald, M., and E. Yeoh. 1997. Designing a prehospital system for a developing country: Estimated cost and benefits. *American Journal of Emergency Medicine* 15(6):600-603.

He, J., D. Gu, K. Reynolds, X. Wu, P. Muntner, J. Zhao, J. Chen, D. Liu, J. Mo, and P. K. Whelton. 2004. Serum total and lipoprotein cholesterol levels and awareness, treatment, and control of hypercholesterolemia in China. *Circulation* 110(4):405-411.

Hu, D., P. Fu, J. Xie, C. S. Chen, D. Yu, P. K. Whelton, et al. 2008. Increasing prevalence and low awareness, treatment and control of diabetes mellitus among Chinese adults: The InterASIA study. *Diabetes Research and Clinical Practice* 81(2):250-257.

Huang, G. Y., D. F. Gu, X. F. Duan, X. S. Xu, W. Q. Gan, J. C. Chen, B. Y. Xie, and X. G. Wu. 2000. [effects of 8 years community intervention on risk factors of cardiovascular diseases in Fangshan Beijing]. *Zhongguo Yi Xue Ke Xue Yuan Xue Bao* 23(1):15-18.

Jamison, D. T., J. G. Breman, A. R. Measham, G. Alleyne, M. Claeson, D. B. Evans, P. Jha, A. Mills, and P. Musgrove, eds. 2006. *Disease control priorities in developing countries.* 2nd ed. New York: Oxford University Press.

Jan, S., and A. Hayes. 2009 (unpublished). *A review of the evidence on treatment gaps, costs and cost-effectiveness of interventions for the prevention of cardiovascular disease in developing countries.*

Jha, P., F. J. Chaloupka, J. Moore, V. Gajalakshmi, P. C. Gupta, R. Peck, S. Asma, and W. Zatonski. 2006. Tobacco addiction. In *Disease control priorities in developing countries.* 2nd ed. Edited by D. T. Jamison, J. G. Breman, A. R. Measham, G. Alleyne, M. Claeson, D. B. Evans, P. Jha, A. Mills and P. Musgrove. New York: Oxford University Press. Pp. 869-886.

Joshi, R., C. K. Chow, P. K. Raju, R. Raju, K. S. Reddy, S. Macmahon, et al. 2009. Fatal and nonfatal cardiovascular disease and the use of therapies for secondary prevention in a rural region of India. *Circulation* 119(14):1950-1955.

Karppanen, H., and E. Mervaala. 2006. Sodium intake and hypertension. *Progress in Cardiovascular Diseases* 49(2):59-75.

Kearney, P. M., M. Whelton, K. Reynolds, P. K. Whelton, and J. He. 2004. Worldwide prevalence of hypertension: A systematic review. *Journal of Hypertension* 22(1):11-19.

Ker, J. A., H. Oosthuizen, and P. Rheeder. 2008. Decision-making using absolute cardiovascular risk reduction and incremental cost-effectiveness ratios: A case study. *Cardiovascular Journal of Africa* 19(2):97-101.

Kottke, T., P. Puska, J. T. Salonen, J. Tuomilehto, and A. Nissinen. 1985. Projected effects of high-risk versus population-based prevention strategies in coronary heart disease. *American Journal of Epidemiology* 121(5):697-704.

Lai, T., J. Habicht, M. Reinap, D. Chisholm, and R. Baltussen. 2007. Costs, health effects and cost-effectiveness of alcohol and tobacco control strategies in Estonia. *Health Policy* 84(1):75-88.

Lim, S. S., T. A. Gaziano, E. Gakidou, K. S. Reddy, F. Farzadfar, R. Lozano, and A. Rodgers. 2007. Prevention of cardiovascular disease in high-risk individuals in low-income and middle-income countries: Health effects and costs. *Lancet* 370(9604):2054-2062.

Manuel, D. G., J. Lim, P. Tanuseputro, G. M. Anderson, D. A. Alter, A. Laupacis, and C. A. Mustard. 2006. Revisiting rose: Strategies for reducing coronary heart disease. *British Medical Journal* 332(7542):659-662.

Matsudo, S. M., V. K. R. Matsudo, D. R. Andrade, T. L. Araújo, and M. Pratt. 2006. Evaluation of a physical activity promotion program: The example of Agita São Paulo. *Evaluation and Program Planning* 29(3):301-311.

Mendis, S., D. Abegunde, S. Yusuf, S. Ebrahim, G. Shaper, H. Ghannem, et al. 2005. WHO study on Prevention of REcurrences of Myocardial Infarction and StrokE (WHO-PREMISE). *Bulletin of the World Health Organization* 83(11):820-829.

Moreira, G. C., J. P. Cipullo, J. F. Martin, L. A. Ciorlia, M. R. Godoy, C. B. Cesarino, et al. 2009. Evaluation of the awareness, control and cost-effectiveness of hypertension treatment in a Brazilian city: Populational study. *Journal of Hypertension* 27(9):1900-1907.

Murray, C. J., J. A. Lauer, R. C. Hutubessy, L. Niessen, N. Tomijima, A. Rodgers, C. M. Lawes, and D. B. Evans. 2003. Effectiveness and costs of interventions to lower systolic blood pressure and cholesterol: A global and regional analysis on reduction of cardiovascular-disease risk. *Lancet* 361(9359):717-725.

Musgrove, P., and J. Fox-Rushby. 2006. Cost-effectiveness analysis for priority setting. In *Disease Control Priorities in Developing Countries*. 2nd ed, edited by D. T. Jamison, J. G. Breman, A. R. Measham, G. Alleyne, M. Claeson, D. B. Evans, P. Jha, A. Mills and P. Musgrove. New York: Oxford University Press. Pp. 271-286.

Neal, B., W. Yangfeng, and N. Li. 2007. *The effectiveness and costs of population interventions to reduce salt consumption*. Geneva: World Health Organization.

Orlewska, E., A. Budaj, and D. Tereszkowski-Kaminski. 2003. Cost-effectiveness analysis of enoxaparin versus unfractionated heparin in patients with acute coronary syndrome in Poland: Modelling study from the hospital perspective. *Pharmacoeconomics* 21(10):737-748.

Oyewo, E. A., A. A. Ajayi, and G. O. Ladipo. 1989. A therapeutic audit in the management of hypertension in Nigerians. *East African Medical Journal* 66(7):458-467.

Pannarunothai, S., M. Kongpan, and R. Mangklasiri. 2001. Costs-effectiveness of the urban health center in Nakhon Ratchasima: A case study on diabetes and hypertension. *Journal of the Medical Association of Thailand* 84(8):1204-1211.

Pereira, M., N. Lunet, A. Azevedo, and H. Barros. 2009. Differences in prevalence, awareness, treatment and control of hypertension between developing and developed countries. *Journal of Hypertension* 27(5):963-975.

Puska, P., A. Nissinen, J. Tuomilehto, J. T. Salonen, K. Koskela, A. McAlister, T. E. Kottke, N. Maccoby, and J. W. Farquhar. 1985. The community-based strategy to prevent coronary heart disease: conclusions from the ten years of the North Karelia project. *Annual Review of Public Health* 6:147-193.

Ravishankar, N., P. Gubbins, R. J. Cooley, K. Leach-Kemon, C. M. Michaud, D. T. Jamison, and C. J. Murray. 2009. Financing of global health: tracking development assistance for health from 1990 to 2007. *Lancet* 373(9681):2113-2124.

Redekop, W. K., E. Orlewska, P. Maciejewski, F. F. Rutten, and L. W. Niessen. 2008. Costs and effects of secondary prevention with perindopril in stable coronary heart disease in Poland: An analysis of the Europa Study including 1251 Polish patients. *Pharmacoeconomics* 26(10):861-877.

Robberstad, B., Y. Hemed, O. F. Norheim. 2007. Cost-effectiveness of medical interventions to prevent cardiovascular disease in a Sub-Saharan African country—the case of Tanzania. *Cost Effectiveness and Resource Allocation* 5:3.

Rodriguez, A., F. Boullon, N. Perez-Balino, C. Paviotti, M. I. Liprandi, and I. F. Palacios. 1993. Argentine randomized trial of percutaneous transluminal coronary angioplasty versus coronary artery bypass surgery in multivessel disease (ERACI): In-hospital results and 1-year follow-up. Eraci group. *Journal of the American College of Cardiology* 22(4):1060-1067.

Rossouw, J. E., P. L. Jooste, D. O. Chalton, E. R. Jordaan, M. L. Langenhoven, P. C. Jordaan, M. Steyn, A. S. Swanepoel, and L. J. Rossouw. 1993. Community-based intervention: The coronary risk factor study (CORIS). *International Journal of Epidemiology* 22(3):428-438.

Roux, L., M. Pratt, T. O. Tengs, M. M. Yore, T. L. Yanagawa, J. Van Den Bos, C. Rutt, R. C. Brownson, K. E. Powell, G. Heath, H. W. Kohl, 3rd, S. Teutsch, J. Cawley, I. M. Lee, L. West, and D. M. Buchner. 2008. Cost-effectiveness of community-based physical activity interventions. *American Journal of Preventive Medicine* 35(6):578-588.

Rubinstein, A., S. Garcia Marti, A. Souto, D. Ferrante, and F. Augustovski. 2009. Generalized cost-effectiveness analysis of a package of interventions to reduce cardiovascular disease in Buenos Aires, Argentina. *Cost Effectiveness and Resource Allocation* 7(1):10.

Salvetti, X. M., J. A. Oliveira, D. M. Servantes, and A. A. Vincenzo de Paola. 2008. How much do the benefits cost? Effects of a home-based training programme on cardiovascular fitness, quality of life, programme cost and adherence for patients with coronary disease. *Clinical Rehabilitation* 22(10-11):987-996.

Schooler, C., J. W. Farquhar, S. P. Fortmann, and J. A. Flora. 1997. Synthesis of findings and issues from community prevention trials. *Annals of Epidemiology* 7(Suppl 1):S54-S68.

Schwappach, D., T. Boluarte, and M. Suhrcke. 2007. The economics of primary prevention of cardiovascular disease—a systematic review of economic evaluations. *Cost-Effectiveness and Resource Allocation* 5(1):5.

Shafiq, N., S. Malhotra, P. Pandhi, N. Sharma, A. Bhalla, and A. Grover. 2006. A randomized controlled clinical trial to evaluate the efficacy, safety, cost-effectiveness and effect on PAI-1 levels of the three low-molecular-weight heparins—enoxaparin, nadroparin and dalteparin. The ESCAPe-END study. *Pharmacology* 78(3):136-143.

Shibuya, K., C. Ciecierski, E. Guindon, D. W. Bettcher, D. B. Evans, and C. J. L. Murray. 2003. WHO Framework Convention on Tobacco Control: Development of an evidence based global public health treaty. *British Medical Journal* 327(7407):154-157.

Tang, J.-L., W.-Z. Wang, J.-G. An, Y.-H. Hu, S.-H. Cheng, and S. Griffiths. 2009. How willing are the public to pay for anti-hypertensive drugs for primary prevention of cardiovascular disease: A survey in a Chinese city. *International Journal of Epidemiology* 39(1):244-254.

Thavorn, K., and N. Chaiyakunapruk. 2008. A cost-effectiveness analysis of a community pharmacist-based smoking cessation programme in Thailand. *Tobacco Control* 17(3): 177-182.

Weinstein, M. C., B. O'Brien, J. Hornberger, J. Jackson, M. Johannesson, C. McCabe, and B. R. Luce. 2003. Principles of good practice for decision analytic modeling in health-care evaluation: Report of the ISPOR task force on good research practices modeling studies. *Value in Health* 6(1):9-17.

Wessels, F. 2007. Eprosartan in secondary prevention of stroke: The economic evidence. *Cardiovascular Journal of Africa* 18(2):95-96.

Whelton, P. K., J. He, and P. Muntner. 2004. Prevalence, awareness, treatment and control of hypertension in North America, North Africa and Asia. *Journal of Human Hypertension* 18(8):545-551.

WHO (World Health Organization). 2006. *WHO country health information.* http://www.who.int/nha/country/en/ (accessed February 5, 2010).

WHO. 2010. *Choosing Interventions that are Cost-Effective (WHO-CHOICE).* http://www.who.int/choice/en/ (accessed March 15, 2010).

8

Framework for Action

The actions needed to prevent and treat cardiovascular disease (CVD) in individuals are at first glance beguilingly simple. People should follow healthful balanced diets, remain active throughout their lives, never smoke, and seek health care regularly. Declarations have called on governments to invest more in CVD, to develop laws and policies to protect the health of people, and to provide health services that respond to the CVD needs of people. International conference recommendations have demanded that companies restrict the marketing of certain products such as tobacco and unhealthful foods and beverages to children; eliminate transfats, reduce salt, and introduce healthful oils in their products; and make healthful foods more affordable and available to communities.

The reality is much more complex. Each action is subject to a cascade of breakdowns. Behavior change is difficult, and individual choices are influenced by broader environmental factors. Governments need to juggle many competing priorities, and some countries have limited infrastructure and capacity to address the problem. Companies need to meet the needs of their shareholders. These realities are often not fully considered in the understandable call for needed action. This call has been driven by good intentions, but there has been less success than in other areas of global health in attracting international attention and action, despite overwhelming evidence of the need. The failure to have the scaled impact needed has been due to concern that attention to CVD would detract from other health needs; uncertainty about the effectiveness and feasibility of policies, programs, and services in the contexts in which they need to be implemented; fragmentation of efforts among stakeholders and a need for focused leadership and collaboration centered on clearly defined goals and outcomes; a lack of financial, individual, and institutional resources; and insufficient capacity to meet CVD needs in low and middle income countries, including health workforce and infrastructure capacity as well as implementation and enforcement capacity for policies and regulatory approaches.

Deeper reflection suggests that to prevent and control CVD in the developing world, a number of essential functions are needed to develop and implement effective approaches. Successfully carrying out these functions will require the combined efforts of many players over long periods of time. This chapter first describes these essential functions. This is followed by a discussion of the relative strengths and responsibilities for key players, proposing new or expanded accountabilities and responsibilities where needed and highlighting the need for more effective coordination of efforts to address CVD. Taken together, these functions and key stakeholders form a framework for implementing the actions needed to address the global epidemic of cardiovascular disease.

ESSENTIAL FUNCTIONS REQUIRED FOR IMPLEMENTATION

The effective implementation of efforts to address global CVD requires that certain actions be executed. The functions required to do this include advocacy and leadership at global and national levels, developing policy, program implementation, capacity building, research focusing on evaluating approaches in developing countries that are context specific and culturally relevant, ongoing monitoring and evaluation, and funding. All of these also require resources—financial, technical, and human. These functions and resource needs are described below, with examples of their role in CVD and indications of how they are tied to messages from previous chapters.

Advocacy and Leadership

Advocacy for policy change and for individuals to take actions in their everyday lives are not the same. Both approaches are critical and need to be led by recognized leaders who might be drawn from the community, academia, industry, or government. The first targets governments at local, national, and international levels to encourage policies that will support prevention and control efforts, which is discussed in more detail here. The second focuses on influencing and supporting individuals within their homes and communities to follow healthful lifestyles throughout their lives. National governments, nongovernmental organizations (NGOs), local media, and local governments can each be well placed to do this; these approaches were discussed in Chapter 5.

International advocacy efforts to raise awareness of the growing CVD epidemic in low and middle income countries have continued to grow with increasing intensity over the past several decades. Professional organizations (national and international) as well as CVD and chronic disease advocacy organizations initially spearheaded this push, organizing a steady stream of declarations, campaigns, and conferences to raise awareness (see Chapter 1 for a more detailed description of these efforts). These succeeded in catching the attention of the international community, which, over the course of the 1990s and early 2000s, has begun to embrace the cause.

Since the mid-1990s, the World Health Organization (WHO) has joined in these advocacy efforts, sponsoring a series of white papers, declarations, and events aimed at convincing donor agencies and national ministries of health of the importance of addressing CVD as well as preparing a toolkit for chronic disease advocacy efforts (WHO Department of Chronic Diseases and Health Promotion, 2006). These efforts have yet to result in significant investment; however, they do appear to have had some success in starting to convince some in the international development assistance and global health donor community that chronic diseases should be a part of the global health agenda. Part of the reason for this lack of success in stimulating investment in chronic disease prevention is that, although there are many advocacy groups working on chronic disease issues, there is little coordination and communication among them, and thus efforts can be fragmented and lack unified messages. More recently this has begun to change, most notably through a partnership for chronic disease advocacy among the World Heart Federation, International Diabetes Federation, and International Union Against Cancer (International Diabetes Federation et al., 2009).

The challenge for advocacy efforts, moving forward, will be to convince ministries of health in low and middle income countries, development assistance agencies, and other donors that investment in CVD prevention and control is critical despite their highly constrained health budgets and many competing health and development priorities. A key challenge in this effort will be to target advocacy efforts at infectious disease, maternal and child health, health systems strengthening, and other global health programs to better communicate the reasons and opportunities to promote the integration of basic chronic disease prevention and management into their existing programs.

In addition to the direct advocacy efforts of CVD and related chronic disease stakeholders, strategies using mass media, media advocacy, social marketing, and social mobilization can serve as conduits of information and mechanisms for advocacy to build support among the various other stakeholders in the global health arena: governments, multinational agencies, scientists and academic institutions, civil society organizations, public health and health care practitioners, and the general public.

The media can interpret and convey scientific information and government policies to the public, and at the same time they can represent the concerns of the general public to policy makers and global health leaders (WHO, 2002). For example, the United Nations has advocated a strategic use of mass media in the effort to control the global HIV/AIDS epidemic, recognizing mass media's role in influencing public attitudes, behavior, and policy making (UNAIDS, 2005). A similar strategic use of mass media can be used in the global CVD effort in countries where media coverage is reliable and operates within a system that guarantees freedom of the press and thus contributes to a robust and balanced public discourse.

Policy

Policies include national and international norms and standards, regulation, fiscal and trade policies, and professional and clinical guidelines. They indirectly affect individual choices and behavior by changing the available default options. In countries that have adequate regulatory and enforcement capacity, policy makers have a range of policy solutions that are related to CVD, which were discussed in detail in Chapter 5. They include, for example, clinical guidelines, tobacco taxes, restrictions on marketing of certain foods to children, school physical education policies, and subsidies or import duties on certain foods. This is not an exhaustive list but does show the diversity of approaches available.

Because the determinants of CVD extend beyond the realm of the health sector, coordinated approaches are needed so that policies in non-health sectors of government, such as agriculture, urban planning, transportation, and education, can be developed synergistically with health policies to reduce, or at least not adversely affect, risk for CVD. In addition to coordinating among different sectors of government, policies in each of these domains can be developed with input from civil society and the private sector. This coordinated, intersectoral approach can help determine the balance of regulatory measures, incentives, and voluntary measures that is likely to be most effective and realistic in the local political and governmental context, especially when the feasibility of policy changes is challenged by economic aims that may be in conflict with goals for improving health outcomes.

Some approaches work best when initiated globally, like the WHO Framework Convention on Tobacco Control (FCTC). Other approaches do well when initiated locally. Still others, such as clinical guidelines, are best developed and implemented by national agencies or professional societies. There are numerous sets of standards and guidelines in existence that articulate the best practices for CVD care. Most of these are produced by national health and nutrition agencies, national and international professional organizations, and organizations focusing on individual risk factors or related diseases (such as tobacco, obesity, and diabetes). Unfortunately, as described in Chapter 5, a significant barrier can be that guidelines are not sufficiently disseminated or followed up with training, making it difficult to ensure provider adherence.

Program Implementation

A broad-based set of programmatic initiatives will need to be implemented in a sustained fashion in order to control global CVD and promote cardiovascular health. These programs need to include a range of approaches such as the provision of health services to patients, including clinical prevention as well as diagnosis and treatment; health communications and education in communities; and policy initiatives in a range of sectors. Depending on the available infrastructure, national and subnational authorities are responsible for implementing public health and health programs as well as policy initiatives in other sectors. Other program implementers include universities, NGOs and other organizations in civil society, and, in some low and middle income countries, development agencies and their subcontractors. For all implementers, leveraging existing infrastructure and engaging the local workforce to implement programs and deliver services is crucial for successful solutions in the short term, while building the skills and capacity locally to develop, manage, and maintain programs is a crucial goal for longer-term, sustainable approaches to address the burden of CVD and related chronic disease programs.

Ideally, programs conducted by implementing agencies will be evidence-based. As described earlier in this report, at this time the strength of evidence is variable with limited knowledge about direct applicability to low and middle income settings. However, implementation of initiatives need not wait for full evidence to be generated. It is clear that there is potential for substantial impact on global CVD with adaptations of current knowledge and available tools. The practical solution both to begin to intervene and to build the knowledge base is to conduct research on effectiveness and impact alongside the implementation of programs. This can be achieved through partnerships between research funders and implementation agencies, with the development of pilot programs that are designed from the beginning with the ultimate goal of feasible scale-up in mind.

Capacity Building

Among the most enduring investments in public health over the past century have been those that established institutions that trained leaders in public health, health care, and health research and supported their career development over decades. Nonetheless, there remains an absolute shortage of public health and clinical workers to mount and sustain public health or health care delivery programs in low and middle income countries (Crisp et al., 2008; World Health Organization, 2006). The focus of investments in global health capacity has to date mainly addressed infectious diseases and maternal and child health. However, to truly meet the health needs of the developing world, strategies to address the workforce shortage need to broaden their scope to include better preparation for CVD and related chronic diseases in training programs for clinical health care, public health, epidemiology, health research, health communications, economics, health systems and program management, and behavioral disciplines. To meet gaps in chronic disease capacity needs in low and middle income countries will require years of sustained support to have a meaningful impact, including building the necessary academic, NGO, and government institutions, as well as training government health officials in the effective use of relevant policies. A health and public health workforce that is well equipped to address CVD and related chronic disease also needs to include training beyond technical competencies to understand the broader systemic and social determinants of health and to be prepared to participate in the policy process as well as in partnerships across disciplines and sectors.

The WHO Global Health Workforce Alliance, a partnership of national governments, civil society, international agencies, finance institutions, researchers, educators and professional associations dedicated to working toward solutions for the global health care workforce shortage issue, needs to explicitly include chronic disease needs as part of its efforts in order to truly address global health workforce needs. This will encourage other major efforts to build the health workforce in low and middle income countries to ensure that, even if funded through disease-specific funding streams, they are supporting appropriately comprehensive health and public health training and not inadvertently creating educational programs and curricula that are narrowly focused on specific diseases to the exclusion of training in basic health promotion and chronic disease competencies.

University and academic global health centers have also assumed an increasingly important role in building leadership and research capacity. In addition to training the next generation of global health leaders, these centers also support and collaborate with training and research centers in low and middle income countries, thereby building workforce and expertise locally. Because the majority of these centers are interdisciplinary, they also provide an opportunity for the collaboration of experts from seemingly disparate specialties. In general, these global health centers in high income countries and the training programs in low and middle income countries tend to lack any strong emphasis on chronic disease. Gathering more information about the current status and gaps in the chronic disease curricula of medical schools, schools of nursing, and schools of public health in both global health programs in high income countries and institutions in low and middle income countries could inform systematic plans to develop future public health and health care leaders and workforce who are better prepared with chronic disease competencies.

Another critical component of capacity building is the dissemination of knowledge. Recently, CVD professional organizations, major global health organizations, and academic global health centers have convened international and regional meetings to share the latest developments in CVD treatment and prevention. While the global meetings provide an opportunity to gather stakeholders and focus on international issues, the regional meetings (especially those in low and middle income countries) are key opportunities to provide local providers with training and information that they might otherwise not have access to. In addition to convening meetings, a number of professional organizations publish journals that highlight the latest advances in research. Most of these journals, however, focus on clinical and technological advances and place little emphasis on global CVD prevention research. ProCor is a wide-reaching global network that serves as a model in its innovative use of low-cost communication technologies to provide people in clinical, community, advocacy, and policy-making settings in developing countries and other low-resource environments with the information they need to promote heart health through access to cost-effective preventive strategies and noninvasive medical management of cardiac conditions.

Research

Research should underpin all actions and is a critical element of the overall package of global CVD efforts. Although the health and economic burden of global CVD have been elucidated as described in Chapters 2 and 3, further research will be required to develop initiatives to control global CVD. While there exists greater awareness about which risk factors require the most attention, less is known about what intervention approaches will be most effective and feasible in the resource-constrained settings of low and middle income countries. This lack of knowledge about program and policy effectiveness within local realities not only constrains program implementers, but also prevents national governments, NGOs, and multilateral organizations from effectively making and implementing decisions to address the cardiovascular disease epidemic.

Some broad-based priorities for chronic diseases have recently been defined at the global level (Daar et al., 2007), and illustrative examples of the research needs described throughout this report are summarized in Box 8.1. An agenda for CVD research priorities needs to address the diversity of actions required for successful impact. In general, research funds

BOX 8.1
Summary of Research Needs

Chapter 2: Epidemiology and Cardiovascular Disease

- Future prospective epidemiological studies (including birth cohort studies) to determine the role of specific factors in causing CVD in low and middle income countries, including their interaction with infectious and environmental factors as well as factors in pregnancy, infancy, and childhood such as early nutrition.
- Better data from large-scale community-based intervention studies in developing countries that address multiple individual and environmental risk factors to confirm causal relationships of the determinants of CVD.
- Improvement of national and regional statistics on CVD prevalence, mortality, and risk factors to improve both surveillance and global burden of disease data.
- Investigation of the effects of nutrition transitions, changes in physical activity, and changes in dietary patterns—including types of oils and the amount of sugar—on CVD risk in low and middle income countries, including overweight and obesity.
- Investigation into the relationship between food production, food distribution, food trade patterns, and food consumption in different parts of the world, including comparative studies of whole diets.
- Further research on psychosocial determinants of CVD risk in low and middle income countries (e.g., depression, income inequality).
- Additional research on genetics of CVD, including the interactions between genetic susceptibility and environmental risk factors in the development of CVD in low and middle income countries.
- Further exploration of gender differences in CVD risk in low and middle income countries, including unique CVD risk factors in women.
- Investigation of the burden and determinants of both infectious causes of CVD and disease-specific cardiovascular manifestations among individuals with HIV, TB, and other infectious diseases.

Chapter 3: Development and Cardiovascular Disease

- Future research with greater uniformity in definitions and methods to allow comparative assessments across countries and regions of both the economic impact of CVD and the impact of development on CVD.
- Additional use of panel datasets of CVD and social and health inequalities in developing countries in order to develop explicit approaches to reduce such inequalities.
- Measures of microeconomic impacts that focus on impacts on employment and earnings, disaggregated by sex and across the life cycle, based on labor market studies.
- Research in collaboration with employers and insurance companies to explore the workplace impacts of CVD and how they relate to household consequences of CVD.

Chapter 4: Measurement and Evaluation

- Costs of measurement including national surveillance, surveys, and ongoing program evaluation with the goal of better informing budgeting decisions.
- Improved long-term program evaluation tools for CVD interventions in low and middle income countries that can also inform local and national level information gathering and decision making.
- Improved tools for identifying the transferable and scalable components of existing interventions.
- Improved tools for measuring clinical practice and quality of care for CVD in low and middle income countries.
- Development of standardized proxy metrics for behavioral risk factors.
- Refinement of risk stratification tools that are relevant to developing country settings.
- Research on the impact of measurement and data on policy and programmatic decision making in developing countries and on the best ways to report and present data for greatest influence.

Chapter 5: Reducing the Burden of Cardiovascular Disease: Intervention Approaches

- Identification of interventions that will be low-cost, effective, and feasible in low and middle income countries with constraints on resources and capacity.
- Adaptation and evaluation of CVD interventions that have proven effective in high income countries.
- Setting-specific and culturally relevant programs: formative research, tailoring, adaptation.
- Partnerships between research funders and implementation agencies to develop pilot programs for interventions that are designed from the beginning with the ultimate goal of feasible scale-up in mind.
- Health services research to develop models for improving health care delivery.
- Implementation research to evaluate methods to implement large-scale interventions and manage complex evolving large-scale programs.
- Research on how to disseminate successful programs.
- Research on different social and private insurance models and their ability to reach different population segments, especially the poor.
- Policy effectiveness studies for intersectoral policies, with assessment of unintended negative consequences across sectors as well as cost analyses. This should include examples of public–private sector collaborations intended to change investor and market choices.
- Research on financing models to determine how best to pay for approaches implemented across multiple sectors.

Chapter 6: Cardiovascular Health Promotion Early in Life

- Estimating the incidence and prevalence of CVD risk factors among youth in low and middle income countries through appropriate epidemiological designs, including long-term cohort studies, ideally starting in pregnancy. These studies should

continued

> **BOX 8.1 Continued**
>
> emphasize the developmental origins of CVD, including prenatal, infancy, and early childhood risk factors.
> - Gathering qualitative data for identifying beliefs, attitudes, and social norms influencing risk behaviors in young people as well as the barriers to change.
> - Identifying risk behavior surveillance systems that can be easily and inexpensively integrated into the routine health care and educational systems of low and middle income countries.
> - Studying the geographic, socioeconomic, gender, and cultural correlates of CVD risk factors in different youth populations.
> - Identifying effective interventions that can influence the early life determinants of adult CVD.

should be invested primarily in projects that generate knowledge about how to translate what is already known into action and implementation—in other words, to close the knowledge–action gap. This research agenda will need to be multidisciplinary, spanning basic sciences, behavioral and social sciences, media and communication analysis, information technology and engineering, epidemiology, health policy and economics, clinical trials, and service delivery and implementation science. CVD research should also extend beyond traditional basic, clinical, and community-based research into areas of agriculture, economics, health systems, and intersectoral actions.

As described in Chapters 5, 6, and 7, to date research has been extensively carried out in developed countries, and going forward it is critical that the research agenda be refined to meet the needs of specific countries. The priority needs to be research aimed explicitly at adapting what works in developed countries for developing-country realities, as well as work to develop novel solutions that draw on developing-country opportunities and innovation.

The Institute of Medicine (IOM) has recently stated that the U.S. research community, in collaboration with global partners, should leverage its traditional strength and area of competitive advantage—the creation of knowledge through research—to further the global health agenda (IOM, 2009). Part of the research endeavor should include capacity building to foster and develop high-quality research infrastructure and trained researchers in the field of global chronic disease, both in high income and low and middle income countries.

> **Chapter 7: Making Choices to Reduce the Burden of Cardiovascular Disease**
> - Primary cost-effectiveness studies in low and middle income countries.
> - Integrating treatment gap analysis with cost-effectiveness studies to provide better epidemiological and macroeconomic context to evaluate potential investment options.
> - Economic evaluation of innovative intersectoral interventions, including valuation of social, environmental, and health benefits and consequences.
> - Modeling of policy changes in multiple sectors, such as trade and agriculture, to define potential winners and losers as a result of policy changes to promote cardiovascular health, including possible compensation schemes.
> - Analysis of system constraints to close treatment gaps in CVD.

Recommendation: Research to Assess What Works in Different Settings

The National Heart, Lung, and Blood Institute (NHLBI) and its partners in the newly created Global Alliance for Chronic Disease, along with other research funders and bilateral public health agencies, should prioritize research to determine what intervention approaches will be most effective and feasible to implement in low and middle income countries, including adaptations based on demonstrated success in high income countries. Using appropriate rigorous evaluation methodologies, this research should be conducted in partnership with local governments, academic and public health researchers, nongovernmental organizations, and communities. This will serve to promote appropriate intervention approaches for local cultural contexts and resource constraints and to strengthen local research capacity.

A. Implementation research should be a priority in research funding for global chronic disease.
B. Research support for intervention and implementation research should include explicit funding for economic evaluation.
C. Research should include assessments of and approaches to improve clinical, public health, and research training programs in both developed and developing countries to ultimately improve the status of global chronic disease training.
D. Research should involve multiple disciplines, such as agriculture, environment, urban planning, and behavioral and social sciences, through integrated funding sources with research funders in these

disciplines. A goal of this multidisciplinary research should be to advance intersectoral evaluation methodologies.
E. In the interests of developing better models for prevention and care in the United States, U.S. agencies that support research and program implementation should coordinate to evaluate the potential for interventions funded through their global health activities to be adapted and applied in the United States.

Monitoring and Evaluation

Monitoring and evaluation will be a critical part of any successful effort to reduce the burden of CVD in developing countries. As described in full in Chapter 4, measuring population health status and evaluation interventions, policies, and programs is critical to inform investments in CVD and ensure that strategies and programs are being implemented as intended and have their desired impact. Efforts to improve monitoring and evaluation at program, country, and global levels and to disseminate the knowledge gained will collectively contribute to an ongoing cycle of evaluation and feedback at the level of global action. Stakeholders of all kinds, from national governments to development agencies and other donors, who have committed to addressing chronic diseases will need to carefully assess the needs of the target population, the state of current efforts, the available capacity and infrastructure, and the political will to support the different available opportunities for action. This assessment will inform priorities and should lead to specific and realistic goals for the implementation of intervention strategies that are both adapted to local baseline capacity and burden of disease and designed to improve that baseline over time.

As highlighted in Chapter 4, while basic epidemiologic knowledge has been expanding, many low and middle income countries still lack sufficient local data to inform their decisions about how to prioritize actions to target CVD. In general, monitoring of chronic disease risk factors and evaluation of interventions, health services, and policies targeted to CVD are underemphasized and underfunded. These efforts are hampered by the lack of monitoring and surveillance programs and evaluation expertise in many low and middle income countries. However, there has been substantial progress in many areas of monitoring and evaluation in global health that can offer important lessons and models to meet chronic disease measurement needs. For example, there are well-established models for evaluation and data collection in developing countries, such as models for national surveillance, behavioral surveys, electronic medical records, and tools for program evaluation, that can be adapted to include or be applied to CVD-related measures. Although there will also be a need for some CVD-specific measurement approaches, it is important, when feasible, to build upon current approaches used in monitoring and evaluation both locally and globally in order to take advantage of existing infrastructure, to build capacity in measurement and monitoring, and to avoid the inefficiencies of duplicate systems.

Funding

Adequate funding is a critical requirement to execute each of the actions needed at local and national levels. A recent analysis of current trends in global funding showed that chronic diseases are the least funded area in global health. Chronic diseases received less than 3 percent of all official development assistance for health from 2001 through 2007 (Nugent and Feigl, 2010). This is consistent with several earlier analyses showing that donor assistance for health is heavily skewed toward infectious diseases, especially HIV/AIDS (Sridhar and Batniji, 2008; Stuckler et al., 2008; Yach and Hawkes, 2004). However, the trend is rising for chronic disease funding. Considering the full range of global health donor sources, including not only bilateral development assistance for health but also sources such as multilateral organizations, private organizations, disease membership associations, and research institutions, external funding for CVD and other chronic diseases increased from $236 million in 2004 to more than $618 million in 2008 in real terms. Much of this growth has come from private non-profit organizations and multilateral organizations. Of this amount, about $10 million (in 2007) was directly identifiable as CVD funding.

Despite some recent growth, this is still a very small proportion of total external donor funding, which is even more apparent when viewed in the context of the disease burden. Table 8.1 shows that in 2007, $0.78 cents/disability-adjusted life year (DALY) of external donor health funding was spent on noncommunicable diseases in low and middle income countries, compared to $12.5/DALY on infectious diseases (HIV/AIDS, TB, and malaria combined). Overall external donor health funding was $16.4/DALY for all conditions combined (Nugent and Feigl, 2010).

Given the alarming trends in disease burden, it is critical that funders take chronic disease into account to truly improve health globally. This investment could occur as an expansion of their primary global health mission and also as part of existing programs where objectives overlap and minimal new investment would be needed, such as early prevention in maternal and child health; chronic care models for infectious and noninfectious disease; health systems strengthening; and health and economic development. In order to marshal the resources needed to implement actions that are aligned with the priorities outlined in this report, CVD stakeholders need to build a case for investment in CVD by more effectively communicating with existing and potential new funders.

TABLE 8.1 External Chronic Disease Funding and Disease Burden

	2004 DALYs, Low and Middle Income Countries (million)[a]	Health Development Assistance 2007 (million US$)	Funding per DALY (US$)
Infectious diseases	518	6,516[b]	12.5
Noncommunicable chronic diseases	646	503[c]	0.78
All conditions	1,338	21,790[b]	16.4

[a] SOURCE: WHO, 2008b.
[b] SOURCE: Ravishankar et al., 2009.
[c] SOURCE: Nugent and Feigl, 2010.

Going forward, support for CVD and related chronic diseases will be needed from national governments (health and nonhealth sectors), bilateral and multilateral international agreements, private foundations, international NGOs, civic groups, community-based organizations, and public–private partnerships. The proportion of funds originating from these various sources will be specific to each country, program, and community. Over the long term, new sources of funding may emerge as a result of CVD prevention efforts. For example, there are expenditures in current disease management of CVD that could be reallocated to prevention efforts. In addition, some proposed approaches generate revenue that could be applied to prevention efforts, such as tobacco taxes. Although this revenue is rarely dedicated to additional tobacco reduction or other health promotion programs, in some cases this has been an earmarked funding stream to support health promotion, including examples such as Thailand's Health Promotion Foundation (WHO Western Pacific Regional Office, 2004).

Foreign assistance, in the form of bilateral or multilateral agreements, can include financial, technical, research, and trade inputs. The World Bank and International Monetary Fund (IMF) have historically provided financial and technical assistance to many low income countries. WHO has served as a resource for policy recommendations, data repositories, technical advice, and international treaties. The U.S. President's Emergency Plan for AIDS Relief (PEPFAR) is one example of a high income country substantially increasing the funding available for treatment of a worldwide health problem, HIV/AIDS (PEPFAR, 2009). NHLBI's recent initiatives in the area of global health are yet another example of a high income country financially supporting the development of clinical, research, and training excellence in the field of cardiovascular and pulmonary health (NHLBI Global Health Initiative, 2009).

Private foundations are another important source of funding for global health; in 2005, nearly $4 billion was given for international projects, nearly half of which were health-related (Foundation Center, 2006). There are several large private foundations that fund global health, such as the William J. Clinton Foundation and the Bill & Melinda Gates Foundation, among others. The Gates Foundation dwarfs most other private sources of funding with respect to the absolute amount of the outlay; its global health grants are nearly equal to the annual budget of WHO (McCoy et al., 2009). The Gates Foundation funds tobacco control and has recently launched a new initiative to support anti-smoking programs in Africa, but otherwise does not include chronic diseases as one of its "priority areas"(Bill & Melinda Gates Foundation, no date), despite the large and growing burden of such diseases in low income countries. It has also worked extensively in agricultural development through its efforts to help farmers improve productivity and to link farmers in developing countries to markets, and through its support of research to create crops with greater nutritional value (Bill & Melinda Gates Foundation, 2008). These agricultural programs provide the potential for integration of key chronic disease prevention goals, such as improving the accessibility of healthful foods to people in low and middle income countries. The Gates Foundation has also provided substantially more funding toward implementation and service delivery than the U.S. National Institutes of Health (NIH) (Black et al., 2009); this avenue of research and inquiry is predicted to assume increasing prominence in the field of global health (Madon et al., 2007) and is another area that has significant overlap with the needs of chronic diseases.

Philanthropy and development aid can play a leveraging role in starting essential programs and in supporting the development of academic centers by governments. However, for true success the responsibility for maintaining financial resources over the long term will ultimately fall to governments. Leadership by national governments can take the form of financing and coordinating agenda setting, policy formulation, facilitation among various stakeholders, and advocacy. In the Philippines, for example, the national government financed and coordinated the inputs of several local governments and NGOs and took a lead role in advocacy for promoting the prevention of noncommunicable diseases (Epping-Jordan et al., 2005).

In terms of research funding, as described above there is a relative lack of support for research into the effectiveness and scalability of CVD interventions in low and middle income countries. National health research funding agencies have invested heavily in the advancement of acute coronary and cerebrovascular care, but their funding of prevention research that is transferrable to low income settings has been limited. Initial progress in this area has already been initiated. A number of multilateral organizations, foreign aid agencies, international health NGOs, and academic global health centers have helped fund chronic disease centers in low and middle income countries, although to date these investments are generally localized and small in scale. In addition, in June 2009, six of the world's largest national health research agencies (Australia's National Health Medical Research Council, Canada's Institutes for Health Research, The Chinese Academy of Medical Sciences, The United Kingdom's Medical Research Council, and the National Heart, Lung, and Blood Institute and the Fogarty International Center of the U.S. NIH) announced the formation of the Global Alliance for Chronic Disease (Daar et al., 2009). The Alliance's mission is to coordinate key elements of global research in chronic disease prevention, develop the evidence base to guide public policy on global chronic disease prevention, and identify the most effective interventions. It appears poised to take the lead in promoting global investments in CVD research as well as low and middle income country CVD capacity building.

> ***Conclusion 8.1:*** *National and subnational governments as well as international stakeholders will be critical to the success of global CVD control efforts, and it will be important to use the relative and specific strengths of different levels and institutions of government and international agencies.*

> ***Conclusion 8.2:*** *Most agencies that provide development assistance do not include chronic diseases as an area of emphasis. Given the compelling health and economic burden, these agencies will not truly meet their goals of improving health and well-being worldwide without committing to address chronic diseases in alignment with their evolving global health priorities. Eliminating this gap at these agencies is a critical first step to encourage a greater emphasis on chronic diseases among all stakeholders and policy makers from the global to national and local levels.*

> **Recommendation: Recognize Chronic Diseases as a Development Assistance Priority**
>
> Multilateral and bilateral development agencies that do not already do so should explicitly include CVD and related chronic diseases as an area of focus for technical assistance, capacity building, program implementation, impact assessment of development projects, funding, and other areas of activity.

> ***Conclusion 8.3:*** *Organizations investing resources in global health currently focus efforts toward acute health needs, chronic infectious diseases, and maternal and child health. Global donor funding and other forms of assistance are heavily weighted toward such disease entities, but there is a much higher burden of disease that is attributable*

to CVD and related chronic diseases. To truly improve health globally, funders need to take chronic disease into account, both as an expansion of their primary global health mission and as part of existing programs where objectives overlap, such as early prevention in maternal and child health, chronic care models in infectious disease, health systems strengthening, and health and economic development.

Recommendation: Advocate for Chronic Diseases as a Funding Priority

Leading international and national NGOs and professional societies related to CVD and other chronic diseases should work together to advocate to private foundations, charities, governmental agencies, and private donors to prioritize funding and other resources for specific initiatives to control the global epidemic of CVD and related chronic diseases. To advocate successfully, these organizations should consider (1) raising awareness about the population health and economic impact and the potential for improved outcomes with health promotion and chronic disease prevention and treatment initiatives, (2) advocating for health promotion and chronic disease prevention policies at national and subnational levels of government, (3) engaging the media about policy priorities related to chronic disease control, and (4) highlighting the importance of translating research into effective individual- and population-level interventions.

ORGANIZING FOR ACTION

For the functions described above to become actions, they need to be owned by stakeholders with the capabilities and commitment to take leadership. That is easier said than done. The process of translating goals into action is a complex, difficult, and long-term effort that succeeds when groups work together. Such partnerships have proven highly effective at mobilizing commitments toward the prevention and treatment of infectious diseases such as AIDS, tuberculosis, malaria, measles, and polio. Current global efforts toward CVD prevention and control, however, are still relatively nascent and lack widespread, coordinated, and well-financed action.

This section first outlines some of the broad principles the committee proposes as guidance for stakeholders to take action for CVD control. This section then more fully describes current and emerging accountabilities and responsibilities of key players for each of the essential functions in tackling CVD, including proposals for new or expanded responsibilities where needed. The section also highlights the need for bold action and more effective coordination of efforts, ending with a discussion of the conditions needed to achieve successful partnerships, including clear articulation of the roles of partners, agreement on priorities and outcomes, and transparent monitoring.

Principles for Organizing Action

The effort to elevate CVD within the global health agenda and effectively organize the many committed stakeholders to implement action requires a broad shared vision for collaboration and partnership. The key principles for this shared vision are summarized in Box 8.2. First and foremost is a recognition of the realities of tight global health budgets with multiple competing priorities. Second, there needs to be a balance between disease-specific approaches and integrated approaches that place the CVD epidemic within the context of chronic diseases worldwide by emphasizing shared-risk-factor reduction. This builds on the reality that tobacco use, physical inactivity, and poor diet are the primary underlying causes of the chronic diseases responsible for 60 percent of the world's deaths (WHO, 2005). In addition, the determinants of CVD, including those shared with other chronic diseases, extend beyond the realm of the health sector, and coordinated approaches are needed to maximize the capacity to build partnerships across sectors such as agriculture, development, and the private sector. Most chronic diseases—and indeed many communicable diseases—also share the same social determinants. Thus, an integrated and intersectoral approach to health promotion is also appropriate and should

---

BOX 8.2
Key Principles for Organizing for Action Around a Shared Vision

- Recognize and respect the realities of multiple competing priorities
- Recognize the realities of resource constraints
- Integrate health promotion and prevention efforts with other diseases that share common risk factors and common social, structural, economic, and development-related determinants
- Build partnerships across sectors such as agriculture, finance, education, transportation, and the private sector
- Integrate health care delivery and capacity building efforts with ongoing health systems strengthening initiatives
- Balance integrated approaches with disease-specific approaches where appropriate for research, training, and clinical care

be encouraged. Organizations focused on CVD and other chronic diseases can maximize their efforts by jointly developing approaches to health promotion and primary prevention for reduction of shared risk factors, while at the same time retaining disease-specific programs, especially in the areas of research and technical expertise required to develop and implement secondary prevention and treatment.

Focusing on health promotion, shared-risk-factor reduction and framing the CVD epidemic within the broader context of other chronic diseases creates a common goal around which CVD and non-CVD organizations can concentrate their efforts and maximize the impact of their resources. This would also allow for cost saving through pooling of resources; more impactful advocacy campaigns; larger, more coordinated research and implementation efforts; and ultimately a more compelling and effective mechanism to address chronic diseases in low and middle income countries. Such a unified effort would also help make a more persuasive argument for incorporating chronic disease prevention into, for example, existing infectious disease programs, since both infectious and noncommunicable diseases exert a mutually reinforcing risk of susceptibility on the other, and both sets of conditions share many common upstream risk factors and structural conditions.

In addition, such an integrated approach promises to be appealing to funders and policy makers as it dovetails with current efforts to streamline expensive, disease-specific approaches toward more efficient, integrated approaches that encourage health systems strengthening and promote better primary health care. Because health promotion and risk-factor reduction occur at all levels of the health system—from the individual to the international level—this integrated approach would also strengthen the public health leadership and workforce. These aspects of strategies to address chronic diseases can be coordinated with, rather than compete against, efforts in other areas of global health, such as infectious diseases, maternal and child health, and family planning and reproductive health.

While an integrated approach to shared-risk-factor reduction, health promotion, and health systems strengthening is critical for success, within this approach there remains a need for disease-specific approaches in some areas, such as training the health workforce to effectively implement secondary prevention and treatment. For instance, while shared-risk-factor reduction is vital to combating CVD, investment in scalable CVD-specific diagnostic tools and interventions such as medications for hypertension or dyslipidemia are also critical. Therefore, flexibility is needed to implement these disease-specific strategies simultaneously with the integrated efforts.

Conclusion 8.4: *Many chronic diseases such as diabetes, cancer, and chronic respiratory illnesses share common behavioral risk factors* *with CVD, including smoking, dietary factors, and physical inactivity. Global-level actors for this set of diseases (the World Health Organization, the World Bank, nongovernmental organizations, local and global donors, professional organizations, and advocacy organizations) can maximize their efforts by integrating advocacy, funding, evaluation, and program implementation. This integration can include a shared focus on the relationship between chronic diseases and health systems strengthening and the relationship between existing Millennium Development Goal commitments and chronic disease prevention and control, including the importance of addressing chronic disease prevention within the context of sustainable development.*

Key Players in Tackling CVD

Many players share the responsibility of addressing CVD. They include international, regional, national, and local players. An exhaustive review of all players is beyond the scope of this report, but illustrative examples of the major current and potential roles of key selected players or categories of players are outlined below. The key players and their primary responsibilities are summarized in Table 8.2. While stakeholders will have different relative strengths and different appropriate contributions to a worldwide effort to address the rising disease burden, each player that commits to taking action has the common need to plan strategically as current efforts are expanded or new ones are adopted. Stakeholders of all kinds will have to carefully assess the needs of the population they are targeting, the state of current efforts, the available capacity and infrastructure, and the political will to support the available opportunities for action. This assessment will inform priorities and should lead to specific and realistic goals for intervention strategies that are adapted to local baseline capacity and burden of disease and designed to improve that baseline over time. These goals will determine choices about the implementation of both evidence-based policies and programs and also capacity building efforts. Ongoing evaluation of implemented strategies will allow policy makers and other stakeholders to determine if implemented actions are having the intended effect and meeting the defined goals, and to reassess needs, capacity, and priorities over time.

International Agencies

World Health Organization (WHO)   WHO plays the lead catalytic and advocacy role within the United Nations (UN) system for all health matters. It has the designated role to "conduct" the health orchestra of the UN and, when it does it well, has leveraged the multiple agencies withing

TABLE 8.2 Ideal Responsibilities of Key Stakeholders

	Stakeholder Group	Funding	Advocacy	Leadership	Policy	Implementation	Capacity Building	Research	Monitoring and Evaluation
International	WHO			✓	✓				✓
	World Bank	✓	✓	✓	✓		✓	✓	
	WEF			✓	✓				
	FAO		✓	✓	✓				✓
	UNICEF		✓	✓	✓				✓
	UNGASS			✓					
	International Aid Agencies	✓		✓	✓	✓	✓	✓	
	Global Health Research Initiatives							✓	✓
	U.S. Government	✓		✓	✓	✓	✓	✓	✓
	International NGOs		✓	✓		✓	✓	✓	
	Private Donors	✓		✓					
	Industry	✓		✓				✓	
	PPPs			✓					
Regional	UN/WHO Regional Offices			✓	✓		✓	✓	✓
	Regional Development Banks	✓		✓	✓		✓		
	Regional NGOs		✓	✓		✓	✓		
National/Subnational	National Governments	✓		✓	✓	✓	✓		✓
	Ministries of Health	✓	✓	✓	✓	✓	✓		✓
	National Research Institutes/MRCs	✓		✓			✓	✓	
	Local Governments			✓	✓	✓	✓		✓
	Local NGOs		✓	✓		✓	✓	✓	
	Local Academia			✓			✓	✓	✓
	Local Donors	✓							

NOTE: FAG = Food and Agriculture Organization, MRCs = Medical Research Centers, PPPs = public–private partnerships, UNGASS = United Nations General Assembly Special Sessions, UNICEF = United Nations Children's Fund, WEF = World Economic Forum.

the UN effectively. What happens within the UN very often gets mirrored by governments. An example is the work undertaken early in the development of the FCTC when WHO convened all key agencies of the UN and gained agreement among them about the centrality of all agencies placing tobacco demand reduction as the primary role of the UN within tobacco control. This led to FAO and the World Bank shifting past support for tobacco farmers; and the fact of the debate led United Nations Children's Fund (UNICEF) to recognize its role in addressing those aspects of tobacco control that affect children. The same approach is warranted now for CVD given its multisectoral components.

WHO's leadership in global CVD includes both direct activities related to global CVD and coordinating responsibilities, bringing other stakeholders together in partnership. WHO's global norms and guidelines, its development of monitoring tools, and its support for many Health Days linked to CVD risks (such as World No Tobacco Day) place it in a unique and critical role to enhance advocacy and action for CVD. The recent development of the WHO Action Plan for the Global Strategy for the Prevention and Control of Noncommunicable Diseases provides a framework for action not only for WHO but also for other stakeholders (WHO, 2008a). It should be stressed that the role of WHO should not be restricted to the currently constituted CVD program but needs to enhance many of the related programs, such as those that tackle diets, tobacco, physical activity, and alcohol and those that are involved in improving monitoring, information systems, and research. Increased investment in WHO at the level of Geneva and within regions and countries would be an effective way of stimulating governments and other partners to act faster. Such investment is justified on the basis of the burden of disease and the relatively modest support forthcoming today.

World Bank The World Bank had historically not played an explicit role in CVD, but its work in Eastern and Central Europe led it to become more deeply engaged in the health systems aspects of CVD. The World Bank played a decisive role in providing the economic rationale for action in tobacco control. Now it should consider expanding that role to broader aspects of CVD based upon its recent recognition of the effects of chronic diseases on the poor and in developing countries and its acknowledgement of chronic noncommunicable diseases as a development priority (World Bank, 2007). The World Bank is a major lender and provides technical assistance to developing countries within the health sector. Regional development banks, notably the Inter American Development Bank, have also started to support chronic disease programs. Regional banks for Asia and Africa should similarly expand their efforts to include chronic diseases.

Food and Agriculture Organization (FAO) FAO has historically focused on addressing hunger and has not explicitly considered how it might develop policies aimed at encouraging farmers to grow foods that promote health in general or heart health in particular. There is an unmet need for WHO and FAO to engage on this critical issue. It could well help to revise current reliance on palm oil, slow the dramatic growth underway in the beef and dairy sectors, and provide greater support to farmers to address the need for more vegetables, fruits, and healthy oils. FAO also has a responsibility within its nutrition and economics divisions to help with policy development and program technical assistance.

United Nations Children's Fund (UNICEF) UNICEF has focused on improving under-5 survival through its many programs. It has provided very modest support to tobacco programs for children but has yet to consider the consequences of poor-quality diets, a lack of physical activity, and exposure to tobacco smoke in children under age 5 for their later development and health status as adults. Chapter 6 provided compelling new evidence about the critical role of maternal nutrition and tobacco use and of early childhood factors on adult health. This needs to be incorporated into UNICEF's area of work. UNICEF's work signals what is important to the world of child health. A shift in policy that indicated the importance of an early start for later heart health would have wide implications for the course of the CVD epidemic.

United Nations General Assembly Special Sessions (UNGASS) UNGASS has provided a platform for intersectoral action on major global needs. By bringing together all Member States of the UN in equal representation under the General Assembly, these Special Sessions have the potential to create a platform and agenda for global issues of particular importance. For instance, the 2000 Special Session put forth the Millennium Development Goals. As described earlier in this report, the Millenium Development Goals (MDGs) have helped to spur vast improvements in multiple sectors involving multiple agencies and stakeholders all over the world. These include significant changes in the status of HIV and other infectious diseases.

An UNGASS discussion and resolution calling for action on CVD and broader aspects of chronic diseases could serve to alert governments, NGOs, and corporations of the urgent need to address CVD and, if done right, could inject the same degree of focused action that now characterizes the HIV/AIDS debate. However, success for CVD will require that the specific needs for CVD are well represented in the initiative, that NGOs and the media are fully briefed in the lead-up to UNGASS, that senior foreign policy representative of governments understand the issues since it is they who will represent most of the governments, and that the session is preceded by intensive and sophisticated media messages.

International Nongovernmental Organizations

The international NGOs described below focus on chronic diseases and have evolved in an era of limited resources. They have played a significant role in building the case for action while having minimal resources to take action. The descriptions below outline their potential to move to a new level. This move will require additional and sustained funding. The leading organizations described below also need to take leadership to establish agreements on priority outcomes and common messages and to bring together other NGOs into a broader coalition under a common framework for action to address chronic diseases worldwide.

World Heart Federation (WHF)   The WHF is a membership organization comprised of medical societies and heart foundations from more than 100 countries. Its catalytic and advocacy role for CVD within the NGO community is critical. Its success is a function of how well it can horizontally work with other leaders in the chronic disease NGO world, and how well it can activate its vertical linkages in many countries. The WHF would be well placed to map the strengths and capabilities of these and other related NGOs with the intent of drawing them into a broader coalition to take up the main messages of this report. A recent event held jointly with the International Diabetes Federation and the International Union Against Cancer during the 62nd World Health Assembly in 2009 augurs well for future collaboration (International Diabetes Federation et al., 2009).

The WHF has also played an important global advocacy role for CVD policies. Its national foundations have had an impact in many countries in supporting tobacco control, in placing the heart health needs of women in front of the media and policy makers, and in engaging communities in many events related to World Heart Day. WHF leaders within countries also often serve as physicians to heads of state and the cabinet, and their opinion has deep influence at the highest levels of government. An even stronger WHF with stronger national committees could be a powerful force for progress in tackling the CVD agenda of the future. Despite considerable progress, the WHF has not yet been able to stimulate sufficient urgency about the need for specific actions that influence the entire range of CVD risks. The WHF, in partnership with other organizations mentioned below, can enhance their advocacy capabilities, especially through focused attention on health professionals—without their support and leadership in their own countries, public policy on health rarely moves.

World Hypertension League (WHL) The WHL is another key international organization involved in global efforts to address CVD. The WHL is a federation of leagues, societies, and other national bodies devoted to the goal of promoting the detection, control and prevention of arterial hypertension in populations. The WHL's main activity is to promote the exchange of information among its member organizations and offer internationally applicable methods and programs for hypertension control. This coordinating function has the potential to fit well into the broader goal of greater coordination within a common framework for action to address chronic diseases worldwide.

International Diabetes Federation The International Diabetes Federation has been extremely successful in making the global case for stronger global action on diabetes through the recent UN Resolution. It is a key link to players involved in addressing a growing set of concerns related to overweight and obesity. It also plays an important role in providing deep insights into the long-term changes required within health systems to effectively meet the diagnostic and treatment needs of patients with chronic diseases, including CVD.

International Union Against Cancer The International Union Against Cancer played a key role for many years in stimulating action on tobacco control. It has recently turned its sights toward the role of diet, alcohol, and physical activity in risk for cancer causation. Thus, it shares a common interest in tackling the major chronic disease risks to health. Globally, the worlds of heart and cancer control have not worked together optimally for many reasons. In low and middle income countries, where resources are scarce, the need for closer interaction between these potentially powerful groups needs to be far more fully developed. This could lead to better support to patients and the general public and to enhanced advocacy for effective policies.

Other NGOs There are a myriad of other major NGOs that could have a role in CVD efforts. There is a need to consider which of these would be truly effective partners. This decision should be based on their potential for a shared commitment to act on some aspects of CVD risk. For example, Save the Children is an important example of a global NGO with interests in both under- and overnutrition; the International Pediatric Association is a potential partner with considerable influence on the full range of approaches related to childhood determinants of CVD; the Framework Convention Alliance pulls together 200 national NGOs in support of country action on tobacco; the World Medical Association reaches millions of doctors worldwide; and the International Olympic Committee has influence across the world of sports and physical activity.

There are also many very effective global and national NGOs active in the fields of HIV/AIDS and TB. They have started to address the importance of transforming health systems from their current acute care model to one able to address the long-term needs of chronic disease patients. They increasingly recognize the importance of closer interaction with those active in CVD and diabetes.

Multinational Corporations and Industry

Many intervention approaches designed to change the interrelated determinants that affect chronic diseases are more likely to succeed if public education, government policies, and regulations are complemented by engagement with the private sector. Motivated private-sector leaders at the multinational, national, and local levels in the food industry; the pharmaceutical, biotechnology, and medical device industry; and in the business community have the potential to be powerful partners in the public health challenge to reduce the burden of CVD. The tobacco industry is not a candidate for public health collaborations because its entire portfolio of products is in conflict with public health aims, but—if done with complete transparency—even engagement with tobacco companies may lead to more effective approaches in some narrowly defined policy areas related to tobacco control, such as the shared interest of minimizing illicit trade of tobacco products, which may increase if taxes are implemented.

Until recently, engagement of the pharmaceutical, medical devices, and food manufacturing, retail, and services industries by the CVD prevention communities has been limited. In the past 5 years, a number of pharmaceutical companies and medical device manufacturers have pledged to donate cardiac care equipment and work to improve access to training and care in low and middle income countries, but on the whole, these pledges have been small in scale. Several international and professional organizations, most notably the American Heart Association and the Oxford Health Alliance, have also begun to engage the pharmaceutical industry to explore ways to improve access to care and medications in low and middle income countries. However, as of yet there has been no large-scale pressure placed on the pharmaceutical industry to improve access in low and middle income countries, nor have there been pushes to develop innovative funding mechanisms for CVD drugs as has occurred with many infectious diseases.

As a result of leadership by WHO, pressure from the investment community, and demands by high income country governments, the food manufacturing industry (and to a somewhat lesser degree the food retail and service industries) have begun to implement product reformulation to make their products healthier and to place restrictions on marketing to children (Healthy Weight Commitment Foundation, 2009; International Food and Beverage Alliance, 2009).

Capitalizing on the involvement of the private sector is a critical component of the effort to address CVD, and several stakeholders described below are placed to take on a major role.

World Economic Forum (WEF) The WEF brings together many business sectors. Increasingly it has expanded from a more focused approach on infectious diseases to address chronic diseases. It is able to draw upon members from the food, pharmaceutical, medical device, insurance, and related sectors to build programs and public health partnerships that can be of critical importance to those involved in CVD control. One such effort led to a joint WHO-WEF initiative on workplace wellness that spotlighted the importance of addressing CVD risks and early detection and treatment within workplaces. Meetings have been held on this topic in India, South Africa, Brazil, and China—all in the attempt to draw upon local realities, innovations, and needs. Ongoing interaction between the WEF and WHO will be important to establish solid ground rules to promote public–private interactions that avoid the past era of distrust and concerns about conflicts of interest and move toward leveraging the capabilities of the private sector to "make markets work for CVD." This will require deeper insights within the public sector about the role of incentives and co-regulation in stimulating changes needed.

International Federation of Pharmaceutical Manufacturers and Associations (IFPMA) The IFPMA brings together the research-based pharmaceutical companies, and as such it has a worldwide reach. Its major products are targeted to chronic diseases, including treatment of CVD or its risks. Dialogue between the public sector and the IFPMA and lead global over-the-counter and generic medication groups is needed as the demand for a range of drugs increases. Many CVD drugs are already on the Essential Drug List, off patent, and readily available globally but either not used or underused. The experience of the private sector's efforts in increasing public knowledge regarding the value of statins has yet to be applied more broadly to developing countries. The rise in the use of statins shown in the European Action on Secondary Prevention through Intervention to Reduce Events (EUROASPIRE) data in Chapter 2 demonstrates the potential for corporate efforts in shifting drug use to contribute to reducing population levels of blood pressure and cholesterol.

International Food and Beverage Alliance (IFBA) The newly formed IFBA was explicitly created by several leading food companies to support implementation of the WHO Global Strategy on Diet, Physical Activity, and Health. It has developed plans to restrict the marketing of foods high in salts, sugar, and fats to children under 12 years; to reformulate products to eliminate transfats, lower sodium, and to shift to more healthful oils; to step up support for physical activity programs; and to provide labeling for their products in all countries. This represents an important step forward that, if successful, should lead to the types of alliances described below. The input of food companies is critical to the success of many WHO and government efforts. For example, food company knowledge about sodium and its relationship to population taste preferences can be leveraged to speed up sodium reductions. Industry insights about real constraints to shifting away from palm oil and other sources of saturated fats need to be considered if progress is to happen. In addition, industry capabilities in distribution and marketing, if leveraged in support of CVD goals, could accelerate progress. IFBA is in the process of creating country-specific entities that draw in national and smaller companies and work with national governments and NGOs.

Public–Private Partnerships Public–private partnerships (PPPs) are generally defined as public-sector programs with private-sector participation, and they include a wide variety of arrangements that range from small, single-product collaborations between a government and industry to large entities collaborating with UN agencies or private not-for-profit organizations (WHO, no date). The participation of the private sector in collaborations can serve to achieve health aims if agreements and negotiations are conducted transparently on public health terms under clear ethical guidelines, and if they establish defined goals and timelines that are assessed using independent monitoring mechanisms. Under these circumstances, PPPs have the potential to be an important potential resource base in the global CVD effort (Kraak et al., 2009; Moran, 2005; Widdus, 2001). For example, there are currently new initiatives under way to use commercial marketing mechanisms to promote healthy lifestyles to address the global childhood obesity epidemic (Kraak et al., 2009).

Additional activities of PPPs could include product development, product distribution, strengthening health services, and public education. The CVD community might, for example, increase the number of strategic alliances between the WHF and companies; draw upon companies with expertise and deployed capacity to distribute needed drugs and diagnostics to developing countries; encourage companies to detail staff to work within public health programs both to share their knowledge and to learn better about community needs; co-invest with food companies, foundations, and development agencies in developing healthful oilseeds in developing countries; and create public–private product-focused initiatives to develop more affordable diagnostics and drugs for CVD. The private sector can also be a resource for direct financing to NGOs and academic institutions to enhance capacity in CVD. Many of these approaches have been successfully implemented within efforts to address infectious disease. For example, PPPs have been involved in the area of drug development for neglected diseases, and many of the preliminary results have been promising (Moran, 2005).

Combining different skills and talents of various stakeholders in innovative and productive ways has the potential to improve the production, delivery, and maintenance of improved global health systems. However, some important concerns have been raised about PPPs, such as conflicts of interest regarding industry partners, exclusion of certain countries (with unpopular governments or poor infrastructure) from PPP initiatives, and balance of power between low income country governments and private partners, many of which are based in high income countries (WHO, no date). These concerns need to be addressed and resolved openly as partnerships are formed, roles are defined, and targets and goals are negotiated.

Conclusion 8.5: Private-sector leaders at the multinational, national, and local level in the food industry; pharmaceutical, biotechnology and medical device industry; and the business community have the potential to be powerful partners in the public health challenge to reduce the burden of CVD. The food industry (including manufacturers, retailers, and food service companies) can be engaged to expand and intensify collaboration with international public-sector efforts to reduce dietary intake of salt, sugar, and saturated and transfats in both adults and children, and to fully implement marketing restrictions on these substances. Pharmaceutical, biotechnology, and medical device companies can be enlisted to participate in promoting the rational use of costly interventions and to focus on developing safe, effective, and affordable diagnostics, therapeutics, and other technologies to improve prevention, detection, and treatment efficacy of CVD in low and middle income countries. Global and local businesses can also provide support for implementation of worksite prevention programs and can help establish smoke-free workplace policies and practices.

Recommendation: Collaborate to Improve Diets

WHO, the World Heart Federation, the International Food and Beverage Association, and the World Economic Forum, in conjunction with select leading international NGOs and select governments from developed and developing countries, should coordinate an international effort to develop collaborative strategies to reduce dietary intake of salt, sugar, saturated fats, and transfats in both adults and children. This

process should include stakeholders from the public health community and multinational food corporations as well as the food services industry and retailers. This effort should include strategies that take into account local food production and sales.

Recommendation: Collaborate to Improve Access to CVD Diagnostics, Medicines, and Technologies

National and subnational governments should lead, negotiate, and implement a plan to reduce the costs of and ensure equitable access to affordable diagnostics, essential medicines, and other preventive and treatment technologies for CVD. This process should involve stakeholders from multilateral and bilateral development agencies; CVD-related professional societies; public and private payers; pharmaceutical, biotechnology, medical device, and information technology companies; and experts on health care systems and financing. Deliberate attention should be given to public–private partnerships and to ensuring appropriate, rational use of these technologies.

The Special Role of the U.S. Government

As the world's largest provider of official development aid (OECD, 2009) and the biggest contributor to international health organizations such as The Global Fund to Fight AIDS, Tuberculosis and Malaria (The Global Fund to Fight AIDS, Tuberculosis and Malaria, 2009), the United States has established itself as a leader in global health. This widespread investment and ongoing leadership and dedication to improving the well-being of the world's people places the United States in a unique position of influence over the international community's global health agenda. With this influence comes the opportunity for the U.S. government to take a leadership role to help ensure that the evolving global health agenda includes the threat to health worldwide due to the growth of chronic diseases.

The recent IOM report *The U.S. Commitment to Global Health*, stressed the need for the U.S. government to expand its support for global health to include noncommunicable diseases (IOM, 2009). This represents an important shift from a decade ago. Furthermore, the U.S. government has international obligations related to the MDGs. MDG 6 refers to AIDS, malaria, TB, *and other diseases*. These "other diseases" include the world's biggest killer, CVD. The United States also already has a commitment to WHO in terms of the FCTC. The United States has adopted the treaty but it has not been ratified. It contains requirements that developed countries support tobacco control in developing countries. Finally, the United States' endorsement of the WHO Global Strategy on Diet and Physical Activity and Action Plan for the Global Strategy for the Prevention and Control of Noncommunicable Diseases now also needs to be backed by funding and support for its implementation.

The U.S. government's global health efforts extend across multiple agencies and sectors working independently and in collaboration to achieve a wide array of health policy objectives. The Kaiser Family Foundation recently mapped out these efforts in its 2009 report, *The U.S. Government's Global Health Architecture: Structure, Programs, and Funding* (Kates et al., 2009).

The Centers for Disease Control and Prevention (CDC) includes international health efforts and global health promotion in its overarching goals as an extension of its mandate to protect U.S. health and safety (Kates et al., 2009). A renewed commitment to this area of emphasis was recently demonstrated in a new reorganization that transitioned global health activities from a coordinating office to a new Center for Global Health.

The CDC's global leadership in health surveillance is unequaled, and the CDC has historically supported chronic disease surveillance, especially tobacco surveillance among youth and health professionals, which remains the U.S. government's major commitment to the FCTC. The Global Tobacco Surveillance System is an example of a successful initiative. Established in 1998 as a joint effort by the CDC and the Canadian Public Health Association, the surveillance system helps countries collect data on tobacco use through household and school-based surveys (such as the Global Adult Tobacco Survey and the Global Youth Tobacco Survey). Global Tobacco Surveillance System surveys are a principle source of surveillance data for the Framework Convention and the MPOWER policy package for tobacco control. The CDC is responsible for Global Tobacco Surveillance System survey designs, sample selection, training, developing procedures for implementing the surveys in the field, initial tabulation of survey data, and data management (Warren et al., 2009).

The CDC has also worked closely with WHO, primarily by providing operational support for the negotiation process for the FCTC. In the past the CDC has also detailed staff to strengthen WHO's work on school health worldwide (including prevention of tobacco use and physical activity and healthful eating promotion) and has provided a global leadership role in addressing health within the mega-countries of the world with populations of more than 100 million.

As part of enhanced support for CVD control, the CDC could increase its support for risk-factor surveillance and capacity building beyond tobacco to include other major risks for CVD. The CDC could also reinvest in other aspects of health promotion related to CVD in children through reengaging with WHO's school health program and doing so in close collaboration with UNICEF's school programs. Support to WHO should be primarily focused on building national and regional capacity through technical support.

The NIH is one of the world's leading medical research entities, and global health is included in the activities of its institutes, as well as the Fogarty International Center, which works to train research scientists and to build partnerships among health research institutions in the United States and abroad (Kates et al., 2009). NIH has recently indicated its stepped-up commitment to global health. In a recent address to staff detailing five priority areas in which he would like to increase NIH involvement, Director Francis Collins stressed that NIH should "focus our attention as much as we can on global health" (Collins, 2009). NIH has led the development of innovative approaches to infectious disease control globally and has played a fundamental role in supporting capacity building for research across many content areas in developing countries. It is therefore well placed to continue this leadership role by being at the forefront of an expanded global health focus that includes chronic diseases.

In fact, there has been an increasing effort to shift to a global focus within the areas of CVD and related chronic diseases. The National Heart, Lung, and Blood Institute's (NHLBI's) leadership and commitment within NIH to global chronic diseases has been demonstrated by its recent partnership with UnitedHealth to develop centers of excellence for chronic diseases in developing countries (see Box 8.3) and by its leadership in creating the six-research-institution Global Alliance for Chronic Disease with Canadian, British, Indian, Chinese, and Australian research support agencies. Moving forward in the context of NIH's overall commitment to global health, there is a need to build on this by deepening chronic disease research efforts through collaboration with an even wider number of institutes within NIH that focus on disease with shared risk factors, common outcomes, or common long-term care needs. These include the National Cancer Institute, the National Institute on Aging, the National Institute of Allergy and Infectious Diseases, the National Institute on Alcohol Abuse and Alcoholism, the National Institute of Child Health and Human Development, and the National Institute of Diabetes and Digestive and Kidney Diseases. The Fogarty International Center is also a natural partner as a future leader in global chronic disease efforts and can play a critical role by ensuring that international capacity building efforts include the capacity to meet chronic disease needs.

Development agencies within the U.S. government are a largely underutilized resource for addressing chronic diseases. As the health and economic burden of chronic diseases continues to grow in the developing world, an expanded scope will become critical to truly meet the global health goals of these agencies. The U.S. Agency for International Development (USAID), for example, has to date implemented almost no programs

> **BOX 8.3**
> **UnitedHealth and NHLBI Collaborating Centers of Excellence**
>
> | | |
> |---|---|
> | Institute for Clinical Effectiveness and Health Policy (IECS) | Buenos Aires, Argentina |
> | International Centre for Diarrhoeal Disease Research, Bangladesh (ICDDR, B) | Dhaka, Bangladesh |
> | The George Institute for International Health | Beijing, China |
> | Institute of Nutrition of Central America and Panama (INCAP) | Guatemala City, Guatemala |
> | St. John's Research Institute | Bangalore, India |
> | Public Health Foundation of India | New Delhi, India |
> | Moi University, School of Medicine | Eldoret, Kenya |
> | Universidad Peruana Cayetano Heredia | Lima, Peru |
> | University of Cape Town | Cape Town, South Africa |
> | Department of Epidemiology, University Hospital Farhat Hached | Sousse, Tunisia |
> | Pan American Health Organization (PAHO) U.S.-Mexico Border Office | El Paso, Texas |

to address CVD, and chronic diseases are not included as a technical area of focus for the agency. Program areas such as maternal and child health, food security, infectious diseases, and health systems strengthening are all potential entry points where the scope of activity could be expanded to include chronic diseases. As the burden of chronic diseases continues to rise, this expanded scope will become critical for the agency to truly meet its global health goals.

Similarly, the emerging President's Global Health Initiative makes no specific mention of chronic diseases in its stated goals or its plans for resource allocations. However, the initiative does include a major focus on maternal and child health and nutrition, and on health systems strengthening and sustainable delivery of essential health care and public health programs (U.S. Department of State, 2010). These are all stated priorities for which efforts should incorporate chronic disease needs. Adequate essential primary health care, for example, cannot truly be achieved without attention to risk for chronic diseases. The Global Health Initiative is being developed and refined through ongoing consultations with relevant stakeholders (U.S. Department of State, 2010), which presents an opportunity for the global chronic disease community to make a greater effort to ensure that the needs of chronic disease are included in this process, emphasizing their implicit inclusion in the existing priorities.

There is also an opportunity to build a more synergistic approach with agencies faced with the challenge of developing models of chronic care for HIV/AIDS and TB, especially the U.S. global HIV/AIDS program known as PEPFAR. The CVD community has potentially useful chronic care expertise to offer in support of this effort. In addition, because of the increase in CVD risk factors associated with these diseases, integrated chronic care approaches offer an opportunity to reduce CVD and improve overall health outcomes in this population. The size of the PEPFAR investment could allow for the emergence of novel approaches for all chronic diseases. PEPFAR has also made a commitment to strengthen health systems and to build health workforce capacity, setting targets for the training of new health care workers (Office of Global AIDS Coordinator, 2009). These are two areas in which there are synergistic opportunities to be sure that comprehensive health efforts are not compromised by large disease-specific investments. It will be important, for example, that investments take into account the need to support comprehensive rather than solely disease-specific education of health care workers in order to not inadvertently perpetuate the gaps in curricula that neglect training for chronic diseases.

U.S. embassies also provide technical and financial support in matters of health as part of their international mission in support of foreign governments. The Department of State should consider such support in areas where the United States has made global commitments, such as providing technical support for the implementation of the FCTC and encouraging pharmaceutical companies to find ways to start addressing the lack of access to essential drugs and diagnostics.

The Millennium Challenge Corporation (MCC), with its country compact aid strategy, represents an additional and innovative vehicle for supporting the development of programs that address chronic diseases. As of July 2009, health programs have represented just 2 percent (a total of $179.4 million) of the projects funded under MCC compacts. Chronic diseases do, however, make up a part of the MCC's health portfolio as the agency has invested $17 million (6 percent) of its compact with Mongolia into chronic disease prevention, early diagnosis, and management (Henry J. Kaiser Family Foundation, 2009). With the current administration's stated emphasis on global health (as illustrated by the announcement of the President's Global Health Initiative), increased attention has been paid to the role the MCC plays in supporting global health programs (Henry J. Kaiser Family Foundation, 2009). Although the degree to which the MCC will expand its health portfolio remains unclear, as additional low and middle income countries with high CVD burdens become eligible for MCC compacts, it could become an increasingly significant funder of chronic disease prevention in developing countries and thus should be included at the table when coordinating CVD and chronic disease prevention efforts across U.S. agencies.

The U.S. Department of Agriculture (USDA) also has the potential to contribute to global efforts against chronic diseases, including its strong leverage with FAO. One area in which the USDA can play a role is through funding analytic work aimed at developing agricultural policies and practices that meet nutrition needs while promoting cardiovascular health. This could unify the worlds of agriculture and nutrition and the efforts to address hunger and obesity. Such an effort could inspire widespread and needed changes in priorities that emphasize health-promoting agriculture policies.

National and Subnational Agencies

National Governments Government action is one of the keys to progress on CVD. Among low and middle income countries there is considerable variability in infrastructure, capacity, political will, and power to enact and enforce decisions and to acquire and allocate resources. Nonetheless, national governments have a critical role to play in sustainable solutions that address the multidimensional risk factors that contribute to CVD and related chronic diseases. This potential can be drawn upon in countries with sufficient capacity. In countries with less capacity it may be other stakeholders who need to lead the drive to take action against chronic disease. When feasible, a parallel goal of how these actions are implemented can be to contribute toward raising the level of capacity in national governments as a means to achieve longer-term, sustainable responses.

Governments have the ability to convene many sectors that need to work together through policy approaches such as those outlined in Chapters 5 and 6 of this report. This takes strong leadership and a clear vision about the optimal roles of various government ministries. The health ministry has a critical direct role in supporting public health programs and effective access to diagnosis and treatment as well as a vital leadership role in advocating for action within other ministries whose policies might help or hamper progress on CVD. However, it needs to be supported in these efforts by the finance ministry or treasury. In addition to executive agencies, legislatures are critical for enacting necessary laws and allocating funds and can often be the drivers of change in executive agencies.

For example, tobacco control requires that the finance ministry support annual increases in taxes, that the education ministry support in-school smoking prevention programs, and that the agriculture ministry not subsidize tobacco farmers. Salt reduction requires collaboration among health and agricultural ministries and the ministries of science and technology, as well the leading food manufacturing, retail, and food service companies. Physical activity promotion brings together the sports, urban development, transport, and education ministries if sustainable infrastructural and policy-based interventions are to be implemented.

Governments also have a critical role to play, along with their national research, academic, and NGO partners, in adapting global norms and approaches that are often developed in countries at higher levels of capacity and funding to low-resource settings where there are a broader set of competing health and development challenges. For example, weak regulatory capacity, combined with large informal sectors, pose challenges to the effective implementation of many policies agreed to in WHO meetings.

The presence of a budget line for CVD prevention and control provides visible proof of government commitment to the area. There is a need to develop models for countries to use that would help them allocate funds to CVD in ways that maximize health gains to their populations.

Cities and Local Authorities Cities and other local government authorities around the world provide core services to people and in some countries, have jurisdiction over policies related to many aspects of tobacco, food, and physical activity. Local authorities also can consider opportunities to require more thorough assessments of the potential health impact of future development of cities and urban expansion to promote planning that takes into account the needs of reducing chronic disease risk (Collins and Koplan, 2009). Therefore, in many countries these authorities have great potential to play a crucial role in efforts to combat chronic diseases. Until recently, however, city health departments around the world have focused mainly on environmental health, infectious disease control, and food safety.

The WHO Healthy City initiative has already stimulated many cities to take a broader perspective (WHO, 2009). In addition, some cities in Latin America have led the way in increasing urban walkability, encouraging physical activity, and improving access to healthful foods. As discussed in Chapter 5, São Paulo, Brazil, successfully increased physical activity levels and decreased the percentage of the population considered inactive through the multicomponent Agita São Paulo program (Matsudo et al., 2004). In addition, local authorities have played key roles in implementing smoke-free policies. In 1991, the city of Johannesburg banned smoking in take-out restaurants and mandated no smoking areas in other restaurants, which paved the way for more widespread tobacco control legislation throughout South Africa (de Beyer and Brigden, 2003). In 1996, the state of Delhi banned smoking in public workplaces and the sale or marketing of cigarettes to minors, which prompted several other Indian state governments to pass similar tobacco control laws shortly thereafter (Reddy and Gupta, 2004).

One comprehensive example of an integrated approach to address CVD risks has been developed by the New York City Department of Health and Mental Hygiene over the past decade (Frieden and Bloomberg, 2007; Frieden et al., 2008) (see Box 8.4). Over that time they have systematically targeted key CVD risk factors by collaborating across government sectors to implement and evaluate a range of risk factor-reduction measures. These include efforts to reduce tobacco consumption, increase access to healthful foods, ban transfats, require calories labeling in certain restaurants, and lead a coalition with food companies and NGOs to incrementally and voluntarily reduce sodium levels in foods. Indeed, New York is a clear example of how large-scale interventions can be implemented when the health sector collaborates with the finance, tax, education, and agricultural sectors as well as with industry. The New York City example should inspire local health departments to take action within their own local legal and regulatory frameworks. In doing so they will find that current laws may give them greater leeway to address CVD risks than is at first appreciated.

National and Local NGOs   Unlike their global counterparts, national and local NGOs share an intimate knowledge of the local context, which ensures that they are well placed to support CVD prevention and cardiovascular health promotion programs in local communities. These organizations have played a crucial role in global HIV efforts in terms of service provision, health education, community engagement, political advocacy, and research. As with national government agencies, a multidisciplinary and intersectoral combination of national and local NGOs will be required to effectively respond to the threat of CVD. Ideally, these national and local NGOs would work together in a collaborative manner, bringing to the table their respective strengths, talents, and experiences. In addition, it will be important that these NGOs are supported by their own national governments as well as by international NGOs and multilateral and bilateral aid and public health agencies.

Academia   Within countries, academic leaders and institutions play a leading role in advocating for CVD based upon nationally relevant research and in training future generations of leaders. One strategy to enhance this cultivation of leadership is the creation of academic partnerships between institutions in high income countries and those in low and middle income countries. Examples of such successful academic partnerships exist, built upon the following principles: (1) leveraging the institutional resources and credibility of academic medical centers to provide the foundation to

> **BOX 8.4**
> **New York City: Comprehensive Chronic Disease Risk Reduction at the Local Level**
>
> Since 2002, New York City has systematically implemented a series of interventions aimed at reducing the citywide prevalence of common chronic disease risk factors. This campaign, spearheaded by the New York City Department of Health and Mental Hygiene, has specifically targeted smoking, dietary risk factors, and physical inactivity and has employed regulatory changes, widespread social marketing, and collaboration with the food industry to reduce these factors in the population. These efforts have already resulted in significant declines in smoking prevalence and use of harmful transfats in restaurants.
>
> *Smoking Reduction* New York City increased its cigarette tax from $0.08 to $1.50 per pack, enacted smoke-free legislation prohibiting smoking in almost all indoor workplaces (including bars and restaurants), conducted mass media campaigns warning of the dangers of smoking, and provided quitting assistance by distributing information and nicotine patches and gum to adult smokers. These efforts resulted in significant reductions in smoking prevalence between 2002 and 2007 in both adults (falling from 21.5% to 16.9%) and adolescents (from 17.6% to 8.5%). Notably, from 2002 to 2006, New York City's smoking-related age-adjusted mortality dropped 17%.
>
> *Dietary Risk Factor Reduction* Beginning in 2007, New York City sought to drastically reduce transfat consumption by requiring that all food served in restaurants have less than 0.5g transfat per serving. This resulted in a reduction in the proportion of restaurants using transfat from 51% in June 2006 to 1.6% in December 2008. The city also mandated that chain restaurants clearly post the calorie content of their foods on all menus and menu boards. In January 2010, the city announced the National Salt Reduction Initiative: a partnership with more than 40 city, state, and national health agencies that is working with the food and restaurant industries to reduce Americans' salt intake by at least 20% over 5 years. As an initial step, the initiative has worked with

build systems of care with long-term sustainability; (2) development of a work environment that inspires personnel to connect with others, make a difference, serve those in great need, provide comprehensive care to restore healthy lives, and grow as a person and as a professional; and (3) intensive and sustained professional supervision and training of health care workers at all levels (Einterz et al., 2007; Inui et al., 2007).

Coordinating Action

It would not be practical, efficient, or effective for a single mechanism of coordination to govern all actions to reduce the global burden

> industry to set voluntary salt-reduction targets for pre-packaged and restaurant foods that are significant and achievable. In the next phase, the initiative will finalize these targets and monitor industry achievement and population sodium intake to ensure a gradual reduction in salt content across a range of food categories.
>
> **Physical Activity Promotion** New York City developed guidelines for designs for buildings, streets, and neighborhoods to promote physical activity. The city has also conducted outreach with the Department of Design and Construction and the Department of City Planning to look for ways to improve built environments. In 2008 the city implemented a campaign of posting signs to encourage stair use in public buildings resulting in an increase in stair use from 13% to 22% in buildings where signs were placed.
>
> **Improved Surveillance and Records** In addition to interventions, the Department of Health and Mental Hygiene has strengthened its epidemiological surveillance of chronic disease morbidity, mortality, and risk-factor prevalence through new surveys and reporting requirements. The city has also promoted the adoption of electronic medical records that include registry and clinical decision support for CVD and improved its information dissemination to ensure that physicians are up to date on research and best practices.
>
> New York City's comprehensive approach to chronic disease risk-factor prevention provides an example of how local governments and health departments can take the initiative and make meaningful steps to reduce risk factors. New York's health department had the resources, regulatory authority, and capacity to implement the interventions—factors that many city and regional governments in low and middle income countries lack. Nonetheless, it can still serve as an example of how effective coordination between city departments or local government bureaus can lead to large-scale interventions.
>
> ---
>
> SOURCES: Frieden et al., 2008; NYDHMH, 2010; Silver, 2009.

of chronic diseases. However, sustainable progress on CVD and related chronic diseases can be enhanced if there is greater communication among stakeholders to avoid unnecessary duplication of efforts and if players with complementary functions and goals define shared messages and coordinate their efforts better to take decisive action together. Many emerging mechanisms for coordination at global, regional, and national levels can be strengthened to serve this purpose, while new alliances and partnerships can also be sought.

Global Coordination

Until recently, mechanisms to coordinate global efforts for chronic diseases in general and CVD more specifically have not been up to the tasks at hand. Over the past few years, however, the knowledge that this is the time to act and that well-defined actions exist has started to galvanize a number of groupings of players at the global level. These are illustrative of an emerging system of coordination for chronic diseases, including CVD.

The first is the recently constituted Global Noncommunicable Diseases network (NCDnet), a coalition among WHO, NGOs, and the WEF to address chronic diseases. The aim of NCDnet is to develop a concerted and coordinated approach to chronic diseases in general, with CVD and its major risks explicitly highlighted. The initiative is expected to focus on advocacy for chronic diseases and on funding and support for priority actions contained in the WHO Action Plan (WHO, 2008a). The early involvement of some NGOs and the WEF represents a step toward the type of broad-based coordination that will be required to tackle the complexity of CVD challenges, drawing upon the capabilities and support of civil society organizations including NGOs and the private sector. NCDnet is still in its infancy but deserves continued and future support as it has the potential to reach all governments and to frame the needs of CVD and stimulate funders to invest. If it is able to achieve its mission to unite the currently fragmented efforts in chronic disease prevention and control, this network will fill a critical gap in the leadership of global chronic disease efforts and could be an effective means of building global consensus on the most effective ways of tackling these diseases.

The second global initiative is the recently created Global Alliance for Chronic Disease, which could considerably increase the quality and capacity for research in developing countries (Daar et al., 2009b). The Alliance aims to coordinate research activities to address the prevention and treatment of chronic diseases on a global scale. It includes the lead national research agencies of Australia, Canada, China, India, the United Kingdom, and the United States, specifically NHLBI and Fogarty International Center from NIH. This new initiative is likely to reshape opportunities for high-priority research in many countries and, given its strong CVD base, it will be well positioned to tackle many of the priorities identified in this report. Its close interaction with WHO will allow it to draw upon WHO's Advisory Committee for Health Research's priority-setting process for chronic diseases. The Alliance could represent a turning point in how innovative approaches to CVD are developed if it sets priorities in accord with the messages of this report about the need to research the effectiveness and implementation of a broad range of intervention approaches, including clinical solutions, population-based approaches, intersectoral policy activities, and training programs.

The Initiative for Cardiovascular Health in Developing Countries (IC Health) is another established initiative specifically focused on supporting research on CVD prevention across developing countries. Founded in 1999 as a joint program of the Global Forum for Health Research and WHO, IC Health promotes and prioritizes context-specific research on CVD in low and middle income countries and has quickly established itself as an important convener and collaborator in global CVD prevention efforts. In addition to sponsoring prevention programs in several developing countries in Southeast Asia, IC Health was also a key sponsor of the INTERHEART study discussed in Chapter 2, which established that the same key risk factors are responsible for the vast majority of CVD deaths around the world in both developed and developing countries.

To support these and other emerging mechanisms for global governance, a consistent reporting mechanism at the global level is needed to track progress, to stimulate ongoing dialog about strategies and priorities, and to continue to galvanize stakeholders at all levels. Rather than investing excess additional resources to create duplicative mechanisms, WHO is well suited for a role in global reporting because, with adequate support, it can be accomplished as a component of the existing framework and ongoing activities to report on the Global Strategy for the Prevention and Control of Noncommunicable Diseases, which has an extensive list of proposed measures to track global progress and characterize the different actions underway in Member States (WHO, 2008a). The support from the CDC provided to the FCTC, as well as the general goals and mechanisms for ongoing reporting for the FCTC, offer a useful model. As described in Chapter 4, given the overlapping interest of many of these multilateral organizations, the development of harmonized indicators is an essential next step in leading and coordinating national and regional monitoring and evaluation efforts. An epidemiology reference group has already been working with WHO staff from headquarters and regional offices to develop guidance for chronic disease surveillance systems and to agree on core indicators that will be used to monitor the major chronic diseases and their risk factors (Ala Alwan, World Health Organization, 2009, personal communication). If this effort takes into account the considerations laid out in Chapter 4, it could be a first step in achieving an implementable indicator framework.

Recommendation: Report on Global Progress

WHO should produce and present to the World Health Assembly a biannual World Heart Health Report within the existing framework of reporting mechanisms for its Action Plan for the Global Strategy for the Prevention and Control of Noncommunicable Diseases. The goal of this report should be to provide objective data to track progress in the global effort against CVD and to stimulate policy dialogue. These

efforts should be designed not only for global monitoring but also to build capacity and support planning and evaluation at the national level in low and middle income countries. Financial support should come from the Global Alliance for Chronic Disease, with operational support from the CDC. The reporting process should involve national governments from high, middle, and low income countries; leading international NGOs; industry alliances; and development agencies. An initial goal of this global reporting mechanism should be to develop or select standardized indicators and methods for measurement, leveraging existing instruments where available. These would be recommended to countries, health systems, and prevention programs to maximize the global comparability of the data they collect.

Regional Coordination

Regional efforts provide a much-needed mechanism for countries to share knowledge, innovation, and technical capacity among countries with similar epidemics, resources, and cultural conditions. Regional mechanisms can help disseminate best practices that range from successful health systems and public health program models to successes in developing and implementing legislative strategies and enforcing policies and regulations. Similarities among countries do not necessarily follow geographic boundaries; therefore, "regional" is a term of convenience that is not meant to limit mechanisms for coordination and dissemination to geographical divisions. These mechanisms, especially virtual mechanisms using digital technologies, can also subdivide countries by, for example, risk profile, political system, or economic development status.

WHO and its regional offices have been leading players in supporting regional efforts to promote CVD health. WHO works with regions and individual Member States to develop networks of community-based demonstration programs to promote healthy lifestyles through public policies for healthy living. Major international and regional health and professional organizations such as the WHF, the Oxford Health Alliance, IC Health, the International Union for Health Promotion and Education, and the Pan African Society of Cardiology also convene key meetings to help coordinate regional efforts and help build international support for national-based solutions.

In recent years, the Latin American and Caribbean region has established itself as a model for regional coordination. Since identifying chronic diseases as the top cause of premature death and morbidity in the Latin American and Caribbean region at the 26th Pan American Sanitary Conference in 2002, the Pan American Health Organization (PAHO) has worked quickly to redouble chronic disease prevention and control efforts. In 2006, PAHO published its *Regional Strategy and Plan of Action on an Integrated*

Approach to the Prevention and Control of Chronic Diseases Including Diet, Physical Activity, and Health, which called for a reorientation of regional policies and programs to prioritize chronic disease risk-factor reduction throughout the life course, with a specific focus on targeting the poor and other vulnerable populations. To achieve these goals, the plan highlighted four lines of action: public policy and advocacy, surveillance strengthening, health promotion and disease prevention, and integrated management of chronic diseases and risk factors. The Plan of Action also encouraged national governments to engage stakeholders outside of the health sector, specifically highlighting the education, communications, agriculture, transportation, economic, and trade sectors as important partners for developing effective interventions (PAHO, 2007).

Since the drafting of the PAHO Action Plan, the region has taken a number of concrete steps toward reducing the burden of chronic diseases and their risk factors. In 2007, the Heads of Government of the Caribbean Community (CARICOM) issued the Declaration of Port-of-Spain, at the conclusion of their Regional Summit, which encouraged the establishment of national noncommnicable disease commissions, called for each country to develop comprehensive screening and management plans for chronic diseases, reaffirmed the region's commitment to the provisions of the FCTC, and promised to mandate the reintroduction of physical activity education into the schools (CARICOM, 2007). In 2008, based on the recommendation of the PAHO Task Force on Trans Fat Free Americas (PAHO/WHO Task Force, 2007), leaders of national health ministries, industry, and PAHO issued the Declaration of Rio de Janeiro, which encouraged labeling requirements on processed foods and issued goals for limiting transfats in oils, margarines, and processed foods (PAHO, 2008). PAHO has also begun to address salt reduction, convening an Expert Group on Salt Reduction in September 2009, which will issue recommendations with the intent of establishing a regional initiative. The burden of chronic diseases was highlighted further at the 2009 Summit of the Americas, where regional leaders reaffirmed their commitment to the PAHO Action Plan (*Declaration of Commitment of Port of Spain*, 2009).

The Western Pacific Region has also taken some noteworthy steps in its chronic disease prevention and control efforts. The region was the first to have all Member States ratify the FCTC. Furthermore, in September 2009, Western Pacific Member States voted unanimously in support of a new regional action plan for tobacco control that requires countries to institute indoor smoke-free laws to reduce secondhand smoke, develop action plans for tobacco control, and establish clear indicators to measure regional progress on tobacco control. This was a significant step forward, especially considering that the region includes China, which has the highest number of smokers of any country as well as the largest state-owned tobacco industry (Cheng, 2009).

Recommendation: Disseminate Knowledge and Innovation Among Similar Countries

Regional organizations, such as professional organizations, WHO observatories and chronic disease networks, regional and subregional development banks, and regional political and economic organizations should continue and expand regional mechanisms for reporting on trends in CVD and disseminating successful intervention approaches. These efforts should be supported by leading international NGOs, development and public health agencies, and research funders (including the Global Alliance for Chronic Disease). The goal should be to maximize communication and coordination among countries with similar epidemics, resources, and cultural conditions in order to encourage and standardize evaluation, help determine locally appropriate best practices, encourage innovation, and promote dissemination of knowledge. These mechanisms may include, for example, regional meetings for researchers, program managers, and policy makers; regionally focused publications; and registries of practice-based evidence.

National and Subnational Coordination

As described above, the overlap of efforts to address CVD and other global health issues and the breadth of the determinants that affect CVD mean that in countries it is necessary to coordinate not only within the broader public health and health systems but also with authorities throughout the whole of government. For example, strategies to reduce tobacco use or salt consumption will require actions by a range of governmental agencies (health, agriculture, finance, broadcasting, education) as well as private-sector producers and retailers. The political will to support and the expertise to implement such a broad effort cannot depend on the ministry of health alone. To coordinate these efforts, ensure the allocation of necessary resources, and have the best chance for real impact requires a mechanism at a level that is insulated from the relative influence of different ministries within the government. Coordination and communication within a whole-of-government approach also needs to include legislatures in order to pass laws necessary to implement policies and, in some cases, to initiate changes in the activities of executive agencies. In addition, these efforts must be coordinated with stakeholders in the private sector and civil society as well as donors and agencies providing external development assistance. A useful model for this approach comes from successful efforts to achieve national coordination of efforts in the fight against HIV/AIDS through the formation of national AIDS coordinating authorities. In Uganda, for example, this was a major driver of success in controlling the course of its HIV epidemic (Slutkin et al., 2006). As described above, the Heads of Government of the

Caribbean Community have already called for the establishment of national chronic disease commissions.

Recommendation: Improve National Coordination for Chronic Diseases

National governments should establish a commission that reports to a high-level cabinet authority with the specific aim of coordinating the implementation of efforts to address the needs of chronic care and chronic disease in all policies. This authority should serve as a mechanism for communicating and coordinating among relevant executive agencies (e.g., health, agriculture, education, and transportation) as well as legislative bodies, civil society, the private sector, and foreign development assistance agencies. These commissions should be modeled on current national HIV/AIDS commissions and could be integrated with these commissions where they already exist.

Alliances and Partnerships

A theme that emerges throughout the preceding discussion is that progress in many aspects of what is needed for CVD and related chronic diseases can be accelerated when key stakeholders work together. Partnerships have proven to be a powerful and successful model for solving large-scale public health challenges that require coordination among diverse groups of stakeholders. From ensuring that every child receives life-saving vaccinations to eradicating diseases, successful partnerships have broken through bureaucratic and logistical barriers by bringing together representatives from different sectors to work toward a common goal.

Recent examples include the development of The Global Fund to Fight AIDS, Tuberculosis and Malaria, which provides funds to countries for focused disease control and prevention programs; the International AIDS Vaccine Initiative and Medicines for Malaria Venture, which draws upon public- and private-sector research to develop new technologies for infectious diseases; and the Global Alliance for Improved Nutrition and Global Alliance for Vaccines and Immunisation, which fund and steer implementation of community- and country-based micronutrient and vaccine programs. Relatively few examples of such partnering exist to tackle either the risks for CVD or the treatment needs of those with heart disease and stroke. CVD control could benefit from building analogous alliances and partnerships.

However, if not executed well, partnerships can also be cumbersome, unwieldy, and ineffective. Experience has shown that successful partnerships are marked by several key characteristics, including a well-defined goal, clearly articulated roles for each partner, and effective communication between partners and with the global community (Jean and St-Pierre, 2009; Levine and Kuczynski, 2009). The characteristics of successful partnerships are summarized in Box 8.5.

A clearly defined goal is the starting point of every successful partnership. A well-defined purpose does not mean that the partnership cannot be ambitious; indeed, many of the most acclaimed global health partnerships, such as the global effort to eradicate smallpox in the 1960s and 1970s, have had extraordinarily lofty goals. However, the goal must be focused enough that it is achievable. It is also imperative that the overall goal be clear to all members of the effort to ensure that each partner is working toward a common purpose.

In order to prevent redundancies and improve accountability, partners should be included that provide complementary sets of strengths and areas of expertise that contribute toward the overall goal. Although it is important that key stakeholders be represented in order to assure that the partnership will have clout and credibility, including a partner who does not provide any value-added simply for the sake of inclusiveness can be detrimental to action. It is also critical that each partner's role is well articulated. Clearly defining the appropriate actor for any needed activities ensures that the partnership works efficiently without unnecessary redundancies and also improves accountability within the partnership. While there will

---

BOX 8.5
Characteristics of Successful Alliances and Partnerships

- **A clearly defined goal** The purpose of the collaboration or partnership must be well defined, focused enough to be achievable, and understood by all partners and relevant stakeholders.
- **Carefully selected partners with well-articulated roles** Each partner should have clearly defined roles based on the particular strengths, expertise, and resources they provide. This prevents redundancy and confusion and improves accountability.
- **Accountability** A system of accountability should be established to ensure progress and efficiency. This requires clearly defining the specific actions and actors necessary to achieve intermediate milestones so that progress toward the overall goal can be measured.
- **Effective communication** It is important that partners and key stakeholders communicate and coordinate with one another within the partnership. It is also important for the partnership or collaboration to establish open lines of communication with governments, local communities, the media, advocates, and outside stakeholders in order to raise awareness and build support for the cause.

always be points of disagreement when addressing complex health topics, these disagreements can escalate and impede progress when partners are not clear about their roles.

Once the overall goal, key partners, and roles have been identified, it is important that there be a system for follow-up and accountability to determine if the goals of the partnership are being met. Ensuring accountability can be challenging—especially in partnerships when involved parties are participating in good faith and not for access to funding and other resources. Nonetheless, it is imperative that some system of accountability be agreed upon. Identifying intermediate milestones necessary to achieve the overall goal and delineating which actors are responsible for achieving them will improve internal accountability. This will also help demonstrate progress toward the desired result, both internally and to the public and other stakeholders.

Effective communication, both within and outside of a partnership, is also vital to success. Within the partnership, this communication ensures that each stakeholder is achieving its objectives and that there are no gaps or redundancies. It also promotes flexible and adaptable decision making and effective conflict resolution Outside of the partnership, communication with local communities, the media, advocates, and related sectors can build support for the cause, raise awareness of the partnership's efforts, and correct misinformation or misperceptions.

Finally, it is of critical importance to emphasize that new global alliances and partnerships for CVD should be created in such a way that they do not worsen the current very fragmented architecture of global health aid or increase the fragmentation at the country level and its deleterious effects on country capacity. In particular, it is vital that new global initiatives allocate in a way that is responsive to a country-directed health strategy and that new funding be integrated with existing funding flows.

FINAL CONCLUSION

The early chapters of this report emphasized that CVD is the leading cause of death worldwide, affecting not only developed nations but also the developing world. Indeed, nearly 30 percent of deaths in low and middle income countries are now attributable to CVD, and rates are rising. This health burden is accompanied by significant economic effects that further contribute to the growing burden of CVD. In addition, those chapters laid out the many factors that contribute to the worsening of cardiovascular health worldwide, including behavioral, social, and environmental factors. CVD now threatens once-low-risk regions because of interactions among industrialization, urbanization, and globalization as well as behavioral and lifestyle changes such as westernization of dietary habits, decreased physical activity, and increased tobacco use. There are also significant gaps in the health care infrastructure and in access to health care in many low and middle income countries, which contribute to CVD incidence and mortality.

Despite substantive efforts in the past decade to more accurately document and draw attention to this growing health and economic burden, which have led to a growing recognition that CVD needs to be on the health agenda for all nations, there remains a profound mismatch, or "action gap," between the compelling evidence documenting the burden of CVD and the lack of concrete steps to increase investment and implement global CVD prevention efforts. This chapter has summarized the committee's evaluation of the factors contributing to this "action gap," its assessment of the available evidence on the implementation of intervention approaches in low and middle income countries, and its conclusions about the necessary next steps to move forward. The major messages of this report are summarized in Box 8.6, which were drawn from the report's major conclusions, shown in Box 8.7.

These findings and conclusions have led the committee to define and recommend a limited set of concrete actions for specific stakeholders. These are not intended to be a comprehensive list of all needed actions; indeed, the conclusions of this report and in particular this chapter may lead many stakeholders to develop their own priorities for action. The recommendation of this report, shown in Box 8.8, are intended to be a subset of reasonable steps that should be undertaken in the near term in order to move toward the goal of reducing morbidity and mortality from CVD globally, and specifically in developing countries. To clearly illustrate the roles of key stakeholders and the type of actions required by each recommendation, Table 8.3 maps the recommendations by the essential functions they are each intended to support. Table 8.4 maps the recommendations by the targeted stakeholder group at the international, regional, and local levels.

The committee found that although there is a wealth of knowledge from the successful reductions in CVD that have occurred in the developed world, this knowledge cannot simply be applied directly to implement solutions for the developing world. Local realities matter: low and middle and income countries have resource constraints, cultural contexts, social structures, and social and behavioral norms that are distinct from high income countries and differ across developing countries. To responsibly implement many promising intervention approaches for CVD, there is a need to move beyond what should work and instead move toward determining what does work—what is effective, feasible, and affordable in the settings where intervention is needed. This can be achieved by increasing implementation and health services research in partnership with local governments, researchers, and communities. As knowledge grows, it needs to be disseminated efficiently among countries with similar epidemics, resources, and cultural conditions to achieve widespread implementation.

> **BOX 8.6**
> **Major Messages**
>
> - Alignment of goals and priorities with local epidemic, capacity, resources, and priorities
> - Recognition of the overriding reality of resource constraints
> - Integration across chronic diseases and common risk factors
> - Actions across multiple sectors of government and society
> - Government coordination and leadership
> - Need for more knowledge of effective, economically feasible interventions and programs that can be successfully implemented
> - Integration with health systems strengthening and other existing global health priorities
> - Evaluation and monitoring as a critical component of success

In the near term, donors and governments will want to focus limited resources on efforts with sufficient evidence to suggest economic feasibility, a high likelihood of intervention success, and a large impact on morbidity and mortality. This report describes some policy and population-based intervention approaches that are reasonable for adaptation and implementation in countries with adequate governmental infrastructure, especially in the areas of tobacco control and reducing consumption of salt. In addition, improving clinical prevention in high-risk patients has the potential for high impact where health systems infrastructure is sufficient. Therefore, the CVD community needs to proactively join efforts to improve health systems in developing countries. These efforts should include CVD-specific improvements in education and training as well as generalized efforts to improve primary health care, ensure access, and improve financing. Efforts to improve national and subnational data collection also need to take into account CVD and its related risk factors, as this information will be critical to make decisions based on local priorities.

Ultimately, the committee concludes that better control of CVD worldwide, and particularly in developing countries, is eminently possible. However, achievement of that goal will require sustained efforts, strong leadership, collaboration among stakeholders based on clearly defined goals and outcomes, and an investment of financial, technical, and human resources. Rather than competing against other global health and development priorities, the CVD community needs to engage policy makers and global health colleagues to integrate attention to CVD within existing global health missions because, given the high and growing burden, it will be impossible to achieve global health without better efforts to promote cardiovascular health.

BOX 8.7
Major Conclusions

Conclusion 2.1: Chronic diseases are now the dominant contributors to the global burden of disease, and CVD is the largest contributor to the chronic disease cluster. Although CVD death rates are declining in most high income countries, trends are increasing in most low and middle income countries.

Conclusion 2.2: The broad causes for the rise and, in some countries, the decline in CVD over time are well described. The key contributors to the rise across all countries include tobacco use and abnormal blood lipid levels, along with unhealthful dietary changes (especially related to fats and oils, salt, and increased calories) and reduced physical activity. Key contributors to the decline in some countries include declines in tobacco use and exposure, healthful dietary shifts, population-wide prevention efforts, and treatment interventions.

Conclusion 2.3: The major contributing individual risk factors for CVD are generally consistent across the globe and include abnormal blood lipids, tobacco use and exposure, abdominal obesity, psychosocial factors, hypertension, and diabetes. However, the detailed underlying risk profile differs across populations and varies over time. Interventions and prevention strategies need to focus on current local risk profiles to ensure they are adapted to the specific settings where they will be applied.

Conclusion 2.4: Rheumatic heart disease, Chagas, and infectious pericarditis and cardiomyopathies continue to cause a substantial burden of disease and death in some low and middle income countries despite having been nearly eliminated in high income countries. Their ongoing prevalence in developing countries further widens the gap between the rich and poor, yet they are easily prevented through basic primary health care screenings or proven interventions. Additional surveillance is necessary to obtain a better epidemiological picture of these infectious forms of CVD in developing countries, and efforts to improve health care delivery are needed to facilitate the widespread delivery of existing interventions to prevent and treat these diseases.

Conclusion 3.1: In general, CVD risks are rising among low income countries, are highest for middle income developing countries, and then fall off for countries at a more advanced stage of development. This pattern reflects a complex interaction among average per capita income in a country, trends in lifestyle and other risk factors, and health systems capacity to control CVD. Thus, the challenge facing low income developing countries is to continue to bring down prevalence of infectious diseases while avoiding an overwhelming rise in CVD, especially under conditions of resource limitations. This will require balancing competing population-level health demands while maintaining relatively low overall health expenditures. Investments in health will also need to be balanced with pressing needs to invest in other social needs and industrial development to produce a positive health–wealth trajectory. The challenge facing middle income developing countries is to reverse or slow the rise in CVD in an affordable and cost-effective manner.

Conclusion 3.2: The drivers of CVD extend beyond the realm of the health sector, and a coordinated approach is required so that policies in non-health sectors of government, especially those involved in agriculture, urban development, transportation, education, and in the private sector can be developed synergistically to promote, or at least not adversely affect, cardiovascular health.

Conclusion 3.3: The economic impacts of CVD are detrimental at national levels. Foregone economic output stemming from lower productivity and savings can reach several percent of GDP each year, with a significant cumulative effect. The toll is most severely felt in low and low-middle income countries, which can ill afford the lost economic output in light of already insufficient health resources.

Conclusion 3.4: There is growing evidence that CVD and its risk factors affect the poor within and across countries, both as a cause and as a consequence of poverty. In most countries, CVD hits hardest among the poor, who have greater risk-factor exposure, tend to be uninsured, and have less financial resilience to cope with the costs of disease management.

Conclusion 4.1: Gaining knowledge about the specific nature of the CVD epidemic in individual countries and about what will work in developing-country settings is a high priority. Improved country-level population data would serve to inform policies and programs.

Conclusion 5.1: Context matters for the planning and implementation of approaches to prevent and manage CVD, and it also influences the effectiveness of these approaches. While there are common needs and priorities across various settings, each site has its own specific needs that require evaluation. Additional knowledge needs to be generated not only about effective interventions but also about how to implement these interventions in settings where resources of all types are scarce; where priorities remain fixed on other health and development agendas; and where there might be cultural and other variations that affect the effectiveness of intervention approaches. Translational and implementation research will be particularly critical to develop and evaluate interventions in the settings in which they are intended to be implemented.

Conclusion 5.2: Risk for CVD and related chronic diseases is increased by modifiable behavioral factors such as tobacco use; high intake of salt, sugar, saturated and transfats, and unhealthful oils; excessive total caloric intake; lack of consumption of fruits and vegetables; physical inactivity; and excessive alcohol consumption. For some of these risk factors, behavior modification and risk reduction have been successfully achieved through health promotion and prevention policies and communications programs in some countries and communities. However, most policies and programs with evidence of effectiveness have been developed and implemented in high income countries, and even in these settings little population-level progress has been made in some areas, such as reducing total calorie consumption and sedentary behavior. Adaptations to the culture, resources, and capacities of specific settings will be required for population-based interventions to have an impact in low and middle income countries.

continued

BOX 8.7 Continued

Conclusion 5.3: Reduction of biological risk factors such as elevated blood pressure, blood lipids, and blood glucose can reduce individual risk for CVD. However, implementation of these approaches requires an adequate health systems infrastructure, including a trained workforce and sufficient supplies with equitable access to affordable essential medicines and diagnostic, preventive, and treatment technologies. Many countries do not currently have sufficient infrastructural capacity. Current efforts to strengthen health systems in many low and middle income countries provide an opportunity to improve delivery of high-quality care to prevent and manage CVD, including chronic care approaches that are applicable to other chronic diseases and infectious diseases requiring chronic management, such as HIV/AIDS.

Conclusion 5.4: Developing countries will want to focus efforts on goals that promise to be economically feasible, have the highest likelihood of intervention success, and have the largest morbidity impact. While priorities will vary across countries, the evidence suggests that substantial progress in reducing CVD can be made in the near term through a subset of the goals and intervention approaches, including tobacco control, reduction of salt in the food supply and in consumption, and improved delivery of clinical prevention using pharmaceutical interventions in high-risk patients. Many countries will want to focus their efforts on achieving these goals on the grounds that they have limited financial and human resources and political energy to allocate to CVD programming, that the evidence for lowered CVD morbidity associated with achieving these goals is credible, and that there are examples of successful implementation of programs in each of these focus areas with the potential to be adapted for low and middle income countries.

Conclusion 6.1: Accumulation of cardiovascular risks begins early in life, and strong evidence supports the value of starting cardiovascular health promotion during pregnancy and early childhood and continuing prevention efforts throughout the life course. Maternal and child health programs and other settings that already serve children in low and middle income countries offer an opportunity to provide care that takes into account not only shorter-term childhood outcomes but also long-term healthful behavior and reduction of chronic disease risk.

Conclusion 7.1: Governments need better health-sector and intersectoral economic analysis to guide decision making about resource allocations among health conditions and interventions.

Conclusion 8.1: National and subnational governments as well as international stakeholders will be critical to the success of global CVD control efforts, and it will be important to use the relative and specific strengths of different levels and institutions of government and international agencies.

Conclusion 8.2: Most agencies that provide development assistance do not include chronic diseases as an area of emphasis. Given the compelling health and economic burden, these agencies will not truly meet their goals of improving health and well-being worldwide without committing to address chronic diseases in alignment with their evolving global health priorities. Eliminating this gap at these agencies is a critical first step to encourage a greater emphasis on chronic diseases among all stakeholders and policy makers from the global to national and local levels.

Conclusion 8.3: Organizations investing resources in global health currently focus efforts toward acute health needs, chronic infectious diseases, and maternal and child health. Global donor funding and other forms of assistance are heavily weighted toward such disease entities, but there is a much higher burden of disease that is attributable to CVD and related chronic diseases. To truly improve health globally, funders need to take chronic disease into account, both as an expansion of their primary global health mission and as part of existing programs where objectives overlap, such as early prevention in maternal and child health, chronic care models in infectious disease, health systems strengthening, and health and economic development.

Conclusion 8.4: Many chronic diseases such as diabetes, cancer, and chronic respiratory illnesses share common behavioral risk factors with CVD, including smoking, dietary factors, and physical inactivity. Global-level actors for this set of diseases (the World Health Organization, the World Bank, nongovernmental organizations, local and global donors, professional organizations, and advocacy organizations) can maximize their efforts by integrating advocacy, funding, evaluation, and program implementation This integration can include a shared focus on the relationship between chronic diseases and health systems strengthening and the relationship between existing Millennium Development Goal commitments and chronic disease prevention and control, including the importance of addressing chronic disease prevention within the context of sustainable development.

Conclusion 8.5: Private-sector leaders at the multinational, national, and local level in the food industry; pharmaceutical, biotechnology and medical device industry; and the business community have the potential to be powerful partners in the public health challenge to reduce the burden of CVD. The food industry (including manufacturers, retailers, and food service companies) can be engaged to expand and intensify collaboration with international public-sector efforts to reduce dietary intake of salt, sugar, and saturated and transfats in both adults and children, and to fully implement marketing restrictions on these substances. Pharmaceutical, biotechnology, and medical device companies can be enlisted to participate in promoting the rational use of costly interventions and focus on developing safe, effective, and affordable diagnostics, therapeutics, and other technologies to improve prevention, detection, and treatment efficacy of CVD in low and middle income countries. Global and local businesses can also provide support for implementation of worksite prevention programs and can help establish smoke-free workplace policies and practices.

BOX 8.8
Recommendations

Recommendation 1: Recognize Chronic Diseases as a Development Assistance Priority
Multilateral and bilateral development agencies that do not already do so should explicitly include CVD and related chronic diseases as an area of focus for technical assistance, capacity building, program implementation, impact assessment of development projects, funding, and other areas of activity.

Recommendation 2: Improve Local Data
National and subnational governments should create and maintain health surveillance systems to monitor and more effectively control chronic diseases. Ideally, these systems should report on cause-specific mortality and the primary determinants of CVD. To strengthen existing initiatives, multilateral development agencies and WHO (through, for example, the Health Metrics Network and regional chronic disease network, NCDnet) as well as bilateral public health agencies (such as the CDC in the United States) and bilateral development agencies (such as USAID) should support chronic disease surveillance as part of financial and technical assistance for developing and implementing health information systems. Governments should allocate funds and build capacity for long-term sustainability of disease surveillance that includes chronic diseases.

Recommendation 3: Implement Policies to Promote Cardiovascular Health
To expand current or introduce new population-wide efforts to promote cardiovascular health and to reduce risk for CVD and related chronic diseases, national and subnational governments should adapt and implement evidence-based, effective policies based on local priorities. These policies may include laws, regulations, changes to fiscal policy, and incentives to encourage private-sector alignment. To maximize impact, efforts to introduce policies should be accompanied by sustained health communication campaigns focused on the same targets of intervention as the selected policies.

Recommendation 4: Include Chronic Diseases in Health Systems Strengthening
Current and future efforts to strengthen health systems and health care delivery funded and implemented by multilateral agencies, bilateral public health and development agencies, leading international nongovernmental organizations (NGOs), and national and subnational health authorities should include attention to evidence-based prevention, diagnosis, and management of CVD. This should include developing and evaluating approaches to build local workforce capacity and to implement services for CVD that are integrated with primary health care services, management of chronic infectious diseases, and maternal and child health.

Recommendation 5: Improve National Coordination for Chronic Diseases
National governments should establish a commission that reports to a high-level cabinet authority with the specific aim of coordinating the implementation of efforts to address the needs of chronic care and chronic disease in all policies. This authority should serve as a mechanism for communicating and coordinating among relevant

executive agencies (e.g., health, agriculture, education, and transportation) as well as legislative bodies, civil society, the private sector, and foreign development assistance agencies. These commissions should be modeled on current national HIV/AIDS commissions and could be integrated with these commissions where they already exist.

Recommendation 6: Research to Assess What Works in Different Settings

The National Heart, Lung, and Blood Institute (NHLBI) and its partners in the newly created Global Alliance for Chronic Disease, along with other research funders and bilateral public health agencies, should prioritize research to determine what intervention approaches will be most effective and feasible to implement in low and middle income countries, including adaptations based on demonstrated success in high income countries. Using appropriate rigorous evaluation methodologies, this research should be conducted in partnership with local governments, academic and public health researchers, nongovernmental organizations, and communities. This will serve to promote appropriate intervention approaches for local cultural contexts and resource constraints and to strengthen local research capacity.

A. Implementation research should be a priority in research funding for global chronic disease.
B. Research support for intervention and implementation research should include explicit funding for economic evaluation.
C. Research should include assessments of and approaches to improve clinical, public health, and research training programs in both developed and developing countries to ultimately improve the status of global chronic disease training.
D. Research should involve multiple disciplines, such as agriculture, environment, urban planning, and behavioral and social sciences, through integrated funding sources with research funders in these disciplines. A goal of this multidisciplinary research should be to advance intersectoral evaluation methodologies.
E. In the interests of developing better models for prevention and care in the United States, U.S. agencies that support research and program implementation should coordinate to evaluate the potential for interventions funded through their global health activities to be adapted and applied in the United States.

Recommendation 7: Disseminate Knowledge and Innovation Among Similar Countries

Regional organizations, such as professional organizations, WHO observatories and chronic disease networks, regional and subregional development banks, and regional political and economic organizations should continue and expand regional mechanisms for reporting on trends in CVD and disseminating successful intervention approaches. These efforts should be supported by leading international NGOs, development and public health agencies, and research funders (including the Global Alliance for Chronic Disease). The goal should be to maximize communication and coordination among countries with similar epidemics, resources, and cultural conditions in order to encourage and standardize evaluation, help determine locally appropriate best practices, encourage innovation, and promote dissemination of knowledge. These mechanisms may include, for example, regional meetings for researchers, program managers, and policy makers; regionally focused publications; and registries of practice-based evidence.

continued

BOX 8.8 Continued

Recommendation 8: Collaborate to Improve Diets
WHO, the World Heart Federation, the International Food and Beverage Association, and the World Economic Forum, in conjunction with select leading international NGOs and select governments from developed and developing countries should coordinate an international effort to develop collaborative strategies to reduce dietary intake of salt, sugar, saturated fats, and transfats in both adults and children. This process should include stakeholders from the public health community and multinational food corporations as well as the food services industry and retailers. This effort should include strategies that take into account local food production and sales.

Recommendation 9: Collaborate to Improve Access to CVD Diagnostics, Medicines, and Technologies
National and subnational governments should lead, negotiate, and implement a plan to reduce the costs of and ensure equitable access to affordable diagnostics, essential medicines, and other preventive and treatment technologies for CVD. This process should involve stakeholders from multilateral and bilateral development agencies; CVD-related professional societies; public and private payers; pharmaceutical, biotechnology, medical device, and information technology companies; and experts on health care systems and financing. Deliberate attention should be given to public–private partnerships and to ensuring appropriate, rational use of these technologies.

Recommendation 10: Advocate for Chronic Diseases as a Funding Priority
Leading international and national NGOs and professional societies related to CVD and other chronic diseases should work together to advocate to private foundations, charities, governmental agencies, and private donors to prioritize funding and other resources for specific initiatives to control the global epidemic of CVD and related chronic diseases. To advocate successfully, these organizations should consider (1) raising awareness about the population health and economic impact and the potential for improved outcomes with health promotion and chronic disease prevention and treatment initiatives, (2) advocating for health promotion and chronic disease prevention policies at national and subnational levels of government, (3) engaging the media about policy priorities related to chronic disease control, and (4) highlighting the importance of translating research into effective individual- and population-level interventions.

Recommendation 11: Define Resource Needs
The Global Alliance for Chronic Disease should commission and coordinate case studies of the CVD financing needs for five to seven countries representing different geographical regions, stages of the CVD epidemic, and stages of development. These studies should require a comprehensive assessment of the future financial and other resource needs within the health, public health, and agricultural systems to prevent and reduce the burden of CVD and related chronic diseases. Several scenarios for different prevention and treatment efforts, training and capacity building efforts, technology choices, and demographic trends should be evaluated. These assessments should explicitly establish the gap between current investments and future investment needs, focusing on how to maximize population health gains. These initial case studies should establish an analytical framework with the goal of expanding beyond the initial pilot countries.

Recommendation 12: Report on Global Progress
WHO should produce and present to the World Health Assembly a biannual World Heart Health Report within the existing framework of reporting mechanisms for its Action Plan for the Global Strategy for the Prevention and Control of Noncommunicable Diseases. The goal of this report should be to provide objective data to track progress in the global effort against CVD and to stimulate policy dialog. These efforts should be designed not only for global monitoring but also to build capacity and support planning and evaluation at the national level in low and middle income countries. Financial support should come from the Global Alliance for Chronic Disease, with operational support from the CDC. The reporting process should involve national governments from high, middle, and low income countries; leading international NGOs; industry alliances; and development agencies. An initial goal of this global reporting mechanism should be to develop or select standardized indicators and methods for measurement, leveraging existing instruments where available. These would be recommended to countries, health systems, and prevention programs to maximize the global comparability of the data they collect.

TABLE 8.3 Recommendations by the Essential Functions They Support

Recommendation	Funding	Advocacy	Leadership	Policy	Implementation	Capacity Building	Research	Monitoring and Evaluation
1 Recognize Chronic Diseases as a Development Assistance Priority	✓		✓	✓	✓	✓	✓	✓
2 Improve Local Data						✓	✓	✓
3 Implement Policies to Promote Cardiovascular Health			✓	✓	✓			✓
4 Include Chronic Diseases in Health Systems Strengthening			✓	✓	✓	✓		
5 Improve National Coordination for Chronic Diseases			✓	✓				✓
6 Research to Assess What Works in Different Settings					✓	✓	✓	✓
7 Disseminate Knowledge and Innovation Among Similar Countries			✓		✓		✓	
8 Collaborate to Improve Diets			✓		✓			
9 Collaborate to Improve Access to CVD Diagnostics, Medicines, and Technologies					✓	✓		
10 Advocate for Chronic Diseases as a Funding Priority	✓	✓	✓					
11 Define Resource Needs	✓						✓	✓
12 Report on Global Progress			✓	✓				✓

TABLE 8.4 Recommendations by Targeted Actor

Recommendation	International												Regional			National/Subnational					
	WHO	World Bank	WEF	FAO	UNICEF	International Aid Agencies	Global Health Research Initiatives	U.S. Government	International NGOs	Private Donors	Industry	PPPs	UN / WHO Regional Offices	Regional Development Banks	Regional NGOs	National Governments	Ministries of Health	National Research Institutes / MRCs	Local Governments	Local NGOs	Local Academia
1. Recognize Chronic Diseases as a Development Assistance Priority	✓	✓	✓		✓	✓	✓	✓		✓			✓	✓							
2. Improve Local Data	✓			✓		✓		✓	✓							✓	✓	✓	✓		
3. Implement Policies to Promote Cardiovascular Health		✓	✓		✓		✓	✓	✓	✓			✓	✓	✓	✓	✓	✓	✓	✓	✓
4. Include Chronic Diseases in Health Systems Strengthening	✓		✓					✓	✓							✓	✓	✓	✓		
5. Improve National Coordination for Chronic Diseases																✓	✓				
6. Research to Assess What Works in Different Settings	✓	✓				✓	✓	✓	✓	✓	✓		✓	✓	✓	✓	✓	✓	✓	✓	✓
7. Disseminate Knowledge and Innovation Among Similar Countries	✓	✓					✓		✓	✓	✓		✓	✓	✓	✓	✓	✓	✓	✓	✓
8. Collaborate to Improve Diets	✓		✓	✓	✓	✓		✓	✓			✓	✓				✓		✓		
9. Collaborate to Improve Access to CVD Diagnostics, Medicines, and Technologies	✓	✓	✓				✓		✓	✓	✓	✓	✓	✓	✓	✓	✓	✓	✓	✓	✓
10. Advocate for Chronic Diseases as a Funding Priority									✓						✓					✓	
11. Define Resource Needs							✓	✓													
12. Report on Global Progress	✓					✓	✓	✓	✓		✓					✓	✓		✓		

REFERENCES

Bill & Melinda Gates Foundation. 2008. *Agricultural development fact sheet: Working to break the cycle of hunger and poverty.* http://www.gatesfoundation.org/topics/Documents/agricultural-development-fact-sheet.pdf (accessed March 12, 2010).

Bill & Melinda Gates Foundation. no date. *Bill & Melinda Gates Foundation Global Health Program.* http://www.gatesfoundation.org/global-health/Pages/overview.aspx (accessed June 30, 2009).

Black, R. E., M. K. Bhan, M. Chopra, I. Rudan, and C. G. Victora. 2009. Accelerating the health impact of the Gates Foundation. *Lancet* 373(9675):1584-1585.

CARICOM (Caribbean Community) Heads of Government. 2007. *Declaration of Port-of-Spain: Uniting to stop NCDS.* http://www.caricom.org/jsp/communications/meetings_statements/declaration_port_of_spain_chronic_ncds.jsp (accessed February 9, 2010).

Cheng, M. H. 2009. WHO's Western Pacific Region agrees tobacco-control plan. *Lancet* 374(9697):1227-1228.

Collins, F. 2009. *Constituents meeting with NIH director Dr. Francis Collins.* http://videocast.nih.gov/launch.asp?15263 (accessed November 10, 2009).

Collins, J., and J. P. Koplan. 2009. Health impact assessment: A step toward health in all policies. *Journal of the American Medical Association* 302(3):315-317.

Crisp, N., B. Gawanas, and I. Sharp. 2008. Training the health workforce: Scaling up, saving lives. *Lancet* 371(9613):689-691.

Daar, A. S., P. A. Singer, D. L. Persad, S. K. Pramming, D. R. Matthews, R. Beaglehole, A. Bernstein, L. K. Borysiewicz, S. Colagiuri, N. Ganguly, R. I. Glass, D. T. Finegood, J. Koplan, E. G. Nabel, G. Sarna, N. Sarrafzadegan, R. Smith, D. Yach, and J. Bell. 2007. Grand challenges in chronic non-communicable diseases. *Nature* 450(7169):494-496.

Daar, A. S., E. G. Nabel, S. K. Pramming, W. Anderson, A. Beaudet, D. Liu, V. M. Katoch, L. K. Borysiewicz, R. I. Glass, J. Bell, A. S. Daar, E. G. Nabel, S. K. Pramming, W. Anderson, A. Beaudet, D. Liu, L. K. Borysiewicz, R. I. Glass, and J. Bell. 2009. The Global Alliance for Chronic Diseases. *Science* 324(5935):1642.

de Beyer, J., and L. W. Brigden, eds. 2003. *Tobacco control policy: Strategies, successes, and setbacks.* Washington, DC: World Bank and International Development Research Centre.

Declaration of Commitment of Port of Spain: Securing our citizens' future by promoting human prosperity, energy security, and environmental sustainability. 2009. Port of Spain, Trinidad and Tobago: Fifth Summit of the Americas.

Einterz, R. M., S. Kimaiyo, H. N. Mengech, B. O. Khwa-Otsyula, F. Esamai, F. Quigley, and J. J. Mamlin. 2007. Responding to the HIV pandemic: The power of an academic medical partnership. *Academic Medicine* 82(8):812-818.

Epping-Jordan, J. E., G. Galea, C. Tukuitonga, and R. Beaglehole. 2005. Preventing chronic diseases: Taking stepwise action. *Lancet* 366(9497):1667-1671.

Foundation Center. 2006. *International grantmaking update: A snapshot of U.S. Foundation trends.* http://foundationcenter.org/gainknowledge/research/pdf/intl_update_2006.pdf (accessed June 30, 2009).

Frieden, T. R., and M. R. Bloomberg. 2007. How to prevent 100 million deaths from tobacco. *Lancet* 369(9574):1758-1761.

Frieden, T. R., M. T. Bassett, L. E. Thorpe, and T. A. Farley. 2008. Public health in New York City, 2002-2007: Confronting epidemics of the modern era. *International Journal of Epidemiology* 37(5):966-977.

The Global Fund to Fight AIDS, Tuberculosis and Malaria. 2009. *Pledges and contributions.* http://www.theglobalfund.org/en/pledges/ (accessed December 2, 2009).

Healthy Weight Commitment Foundation. 2009. *About us.* http://www.healthyweightcommit.org/about (accessed March 10, 2010).
Henry J. Kaiser Family Foundation. 2009. *Fact sheet: The Millenium Challenge Corportation & global health.* Washington, DC: Kaiser Family Foundation.
International Diabetes Federation, UICC (International Union Against Cancer), and World Heart Federation. 2009. Time to act: The global emergency of non-communicable diseases. In *Report on Health and Development: Held Back by Non-Communicable Diseases.* Geneva: International Diabetes Federation, UICC, and World Heart Federation.
International Food and Beverage Alliance. 2009. *IFBA update since November, 2008.* Presentation presented to the World Health Organization on August 31, 2009. Geneva, Switzerland.
Inui, T. S., W. M. Nyandiko, S. N. Kimaiyo, R. M. Frankel, T. Muriuki, J. J. Mamlin, R. M. Einterz, and J. E. Sidle. 2007. AMPATH: Living proof that no one has to die from HIV. *Journal General Internal Medicine* 22(12):1745-1750.
IOM (Institute of Medicine). 2009. *The U.S. Commitment to global health: Recommendations for the new administration.* Washington, DC: The National Academies Press.
Jean, M.-C., and L. St-Pierre. 2009. Applicability of the success factors for intersectorality in developing countries. France: IUHPE. Background paper commissioned by the Committee on Preventing the Global Epidemic of Cardiovascular Disease.
Kates, J., J. Fischer, and E. Lief. 2009. *The U.S. Government's global health architecture: Structure, programs, and funding.* Washington, DC: Henry J. Kaiser Family Foundation.
Kraak, V. I., S. K. Kumanyika, and M. Story. 2009. The commercial marketing of healthy lifestyles to address the global child and adolescent obesity pandemic: Prospects, pitfalls and priorities. *Public Health Nutrition*:1-10.
Levine, R., and D. Kuczynski. 2009. *Global nutrition institutions: Is there an appetite for change?* Washington, DC: Center for Global Development.
Madon, T., K. J. Hofman, L. Kupfer, and R. I. Glass. 2007. Public health. Implementation science. *Science* 318(5857):1728-1729.
Matsudo, S. M., V. R. Matsudo, D. R. Andrade, T. L. Araújo, E. Andrade, L. de Oliveira, and G. Braggion. 2004. Physical activity promotion: Experiences and evaluation of the Agita São Paulo program using the ecological mobile model. *Journal of Physical Activity and Health* 1(2):81-94.
McCoy, D., G. Kembhavi, J. Patel, and A. Luintel. 2009. The Bill & Melinda Gates Foundation's grant-making programme for global health. *Lancet* 373(9675):1645-1653.
Moran, M. 2005. A breakthrough in R&D for neglected diseases: New ways to get the drugs we need. *Public Library of Science Medicine* 2(9):e302.
NHLBI (National Heart, Lung, and Blood Institute) Global Health Initiative. 2009. *National Heart, Lung, and Blood Institute Global Health Initiative.* http://www.nhlbi.nih.gov/about/globalhealth/index.htm (accessed June 30, 2009).
Nugent, R., and A. Feigl. 2010. *Scarce donor funding for non-communicable diseases: Will it contribute to a health crisis?* Washington, DC: Center for Global Development (forthcoming).
NYDHMH (New York Department of Health and Mental Hygiene). 2010. *Cut the salt get the facts: The national salt reduction initiative.* http://www.nyc.gov/html/doh/downloads/pdf/cardio/cardio-salt-nsri-faq.pdf (accessed January 12, 2010).
OECD (Organisation for Economic Co-operation and Development). 2009. *Development aid at its highest level ever in 2008 (press release).* http://www.oecd.org/document/35/0,3343,en_2649_34447_42458595_1_1_1_1,00.html (accessed on December 2, 2009).
Office of Global AIDS Coordinator. 2009. *The U.S. President's Emergency Plan for AIDS Relief: Five year strategy.* Washington, DC: Office of Global AIDS Coordinator.

PAHO (Pan American Health Organization). 2007. *Regional strategy and plan of action on an integrated approach to the prevention and control of chronic diseases.* Washington, DC: Pan American Health Organization.

PAHO. 2008. *Trans fat free americas: Declaration of Rio de Janeiro.* Rio de Janeiro, Brazil: Pan American Health Organization.

PAHO/WHO Task Force. 2007. *Trans fat free Americas: Conclusions and recommendations.* Washington, DC: Pan American Health Organization.

PEPFAR (President's Emergency Plan for AIDS Relief). 2009. *The United States President's Emergency Plan for AIDS Relief.* http://www.pepfar.gov/ (accessed June 30, 2009).

Reddy, K. S., and P. C. Gupta. 2004. *Report on tobacco control in India.* New Delhi, India: Ministry of Health & Family Welfare, Government of India, Centers for Disease Control and Prevention, USA, & World Health Organization.

Silver, L. 2009. Multisectoral approaches to preventing cardiovascular disease: The New York experience. Presentation at Public Information Gathering Session for the Institute of Medicine Committee on Preventing the Global Epidemic of Cardiovascular Disease, Washington, DC.

Slutkin, G., S. Okware, W. Naamara, D. Sutherland, D. Flanagan, M. Carael, E. Blas, P. Delay, and D. Tarantola. 2006. How Uganda reversed its HIV epidemic. *AIDS and Behavior* 10(4):351-360.

Sridhar, D., and R. Batniji. 2008. Misfinancing global health: A case for transparency in disbursements and decision making. *Lancet* 372(9644):1185-1191.

Stuckler, D., L. King, H. Robinson, and M. McKee. 2008. WHO's budgetary allocations and burden of disease: A comparative analysis. *Lancet* 372(9649):1563-1569.

UNAIDS (The Joint United Nations Programme on HIV/AIDS). 2005. *Getting the message across: The mass media and the response to AIDS, UNAIDS best practice collection.* Geneva: UNAIDS.

U.S. Department of State. 2010. *Implementation of the Global Health Initiative: Consultation document.* Washington, DC: U.S. Department of State.

Warren, C. W., S. Asma, J. Lee, and M. J. 2009. *The GTSS atlas.* Atlanta: The CDC Foundation.

WHO (World Health Organization). 2002. *The world health report 2002—reducing risks, promoting healthy life.* Geneva: World Health Organization.

WHO. 2005. *Preventing chronic diseases: A vital investment.* http://www.who.int/chp/chronic_disease_report/full_report.pdf (accessed April 23, 2009).

WHO. 2006. WHO country health information. http://www.who.int/nha/country/en/ (accessed February 17, 2010).

WHO. 2008a. *2008-2013 action plan for the global strategy for the prevention and control of noncommunicable diseases.* Geneva: World Health Organization.

WHO. 2008b. *The global burden of disease: 2004 update.* Geneva: World Health Organization.

WHO. 2009. *Healthy cities and urban governance.* http://www.euro.who.int/en/what-we-do/health-topics/environmental-health/urban-health/healthy-cities/who-healthy-cities-network (accessed December 12, 2009).

WHO. no date. *Public-private partnerships for health.* http://www.who.int/trade/glossary/story077/en/ (accessed June 30, 2009).

WHO Department of Chronic Diseases and Health Promotion. 2006. *Stop the global epidemic of chronic disease: A practical guide to successful advocacy.* Geneva: World Health Organization.

WHO Western Pacific Regional Office. 2004. The Establishment and Use of Dedicated Taxes for Health Manila.

Widdus, R. 2001. Public-private partnerships for health: Their main targets, their diversity, and their future directions. *Bulletin of the World Health Organization* 79(8):713-720.

World Bank. 2007. *World development report 2007*. Washington, DC: World Bank.

Yach, D., and C. Hawkes. 2004 (unpublished). *Towards a WHO long-term strategy for prevention and control of leading chronic diseases*. Geneva: World Health Organization.

Appendix A

Statement of Task

The Institute of Medicine (IOM) will convene an ad hoc committee to study the evolving global epidemic of cardiovascular disease (CVD) and offer conclusions and recommendations pertinent to its control and to a range of public- and private-sector entities involved with global health and development. The proposed study should take advantage of the concept frameworks of the 1998 IOM report, the 2004 Earth Institute/IC Health Report, the 2007 "Grand Challenges" report, and a series of global cardiovascular health declarations (Victoria 1992, Catalonia 1995, Singapore 1998, Victoria 2000, Osaka 2001, and Milan 2004). It should synthesize and expand relevant evidence and knowledge based on findings from research and development, with an emphasis on developing pertinent concepts of global partnership and collaborations, and recommending actions targeted at global governmental organizations, nongovernmental organizations, policy and decision makers, funding agencies, academic and research institutions, and the general public. The study should draw upon the rich experience and best practices learned from global collaborations and infrastructure efforts to combat infectious diseases. An emphasis should be placed on multidirectional learning—best practices in one region of the world which can inform multiple other regions and, importantly, lessons learned from global practices that can inform the delivery and practice of medicine in the United States. It is expected that the report of this definitive, didactic, and scientific study will present, to the extent that evidence permits, sound arguments and reasoning for increasing investment in global cardiovascular health promotion and CVD prevention and control. The report should serve to help initiate global dialogue, align global forces, draw public attention, and lead to concerted global and international actions.

The specific aims of the study are as follows:

1. Define the magnitude of the global CVD epidemic by examining, analyzing, and determining the burden of, and trends in, CVD worldwide.
2. Identify current status, capacities, and best practices in CVD prevention and management in developed and developing countries, and determine how these best practices may be applied to other regions with an emphasis on multidirectional learning.
3. Identify elements of success in global public health collaborations and infrastructure development learned from addressing infectious diseases that can be extended to the chronic, noncommunicable diseases.
4. Examine specific gaps and barriers in implementing effective CVD prevention programs.
5. Review existing frameworks and develop a global platform of actions and priorities (including research and development, prevention programs, and training) that may provide health systems (at the global, regional, country, and local levels) and settings (community, school, workplace, and health care), policy makers, and individuals with a specific set of goals and objectives, and performance measures (metrics).
6. Identify current and potential future opportunities for collaboration and partnerships that will better enable individuals, organizations, or countries to enhance their capacities to address cardiovascular health. Develop strategies to enhance global, regional, and international partnerships.
7. Identify and recommend the knowledge and tools that will be needed by individuals, organizations, and countries to anticipate, prevent, recognize, mitigate, and respond to the CVD epidemic.
8. Develop an evaluation plan for monitoring the progress of global actions.

Appendix B

Committee and Staff Biographies

Dr. Valentín Fuster (*Chair*) serves The Mount Sinai Medical Center as Director of Mount Sinai Heart, the Zena and Michael A. Wiener Cardiovascular Institute, and the Marie-Josée and Henry R. Kravis Center for Cardiovascular Health. He is the Richard Gorlin, MD/Heart Research Foundation Professor at the Mount Sinai School of Medicine. Dr. Fuster is the General Director of the Centro Nacional de Investigaciones Cardiovasculares Carlos III in Madrid, Spain. After receiving his medical degree from Barcelona University and completing an internship at Hospital Clinic in Barcelona, Dr. Fuster spent several years at the Mayo Clinic, first as a resident and later as Professor of Medicine and Consultant in Cardiology. In 1981, he joined Mount Sinai School of Medicine as Head of Cardiology. From 1991 to 1994, he was Mallinckrodt Professor of Medicine at Harvard Medical School and Chief of Cardiology at Massachusetts General Hospital. He returned to Mount Sinai in 1994 as Director of the Zena and Michael A. Wiener Cardiovascular Institute and, most recently, he has been named the Director of Mount Sinai Heart. Dr. Fuster is a past President of the American Heart Association, immediate past President of the World Heart Federation, a member of the Institute of Medicine of the National Academy of Sciences, a former member of the National Heart, Lung, and Blood Institute Advisory Council, and former Chairman of the Fellowship Training Directors Program of the American College of Cardiology. Twenty-seven distinguished universities throughout the world have granted Dr. Fuster Honoris Causa. He has published more than 800 articles on the subjects of coronary artery disease, atherosclerosis, and thrombosis, and he has become the lead editor of two major textbooks on cardiology and of three books related to health for the public in Spain (bestsellers, presently being translated into English). Dr. Fuster has been appointed Editor-in-Chief of the *Nature* journal that focuses on cardiovascular medicine. Dr. Fuster is the only cardiologist to receive all four major research awards from the four major cardiovascular organizations: The Distinguished Researcher Award (Interamerican Society of Cardiology, 2005), the Andreas Gruntzig Scientific Award (European Society of Cardiology, 1992), Distinguished Scientist (American Heart Association, 2003), and the Distinguished Scientist Award (American College of Cardiology, 1993). In addition, he has received the Principe de Asturias Award of Science and Technology (the highest award given to Spanish-speaking scientists), the Distinguished Service Award from the American College of Cardiology, the Gold Heart Award (American Heart Association's highest award), and the Gold Medal of the European Society of Cardiology (the highest award, Vienna, September 2007). Dr. Fuster has four ongoing projects as part of the World Heart Federation: "Promoting health as a priority" in children of Bogotá with Sesame Street, "Promoting health as a priority" in adults in The Island of Grenada, polypill developed in Spain for low and middle income countries, and a project with Jeffrey and Sonia Sachs focused on chronic diseases (as an addition to the Millennium project) in the African villages (Rwanda).

Dr. Arun Chockalingam is the Director of Global Health and a Professor in the Faculty of Health Sciences at Simon Fraser University. He recently completed his term as the Associate Director of the Canadian Institutes of Health Research Institute of Circulatory and Respiratory Health. Dr. Chockalingam received his Masters in Biomedical Engineering from the Indian Institute of Technology, (Madras) Chennai, India, after which he moved to Canada and continued his studies at the Memorial University of Newfoundland. There he completed his Ph.D. and later joined the Faculty of Medicine. During his career, Dr. Chockalingam has addressed the diagnosis, epidemiology, and effect of lifestyle on hypertension, both within and outside of Canada. Dr. Chockalingam was the President of the Canadian Coalition for High Blood Pressure Prevention and Control (now Blood Pressure Canada) for 7 years. He has been an active and influential member of the Canadian Hypertension Education Program. He is currently Secretary General of the World Hypertension League and, since 2005, has initiated and organized World Hypertension Day, an annual public awareness campaign, both in Canada and worldwide. Dr. Chockalingam's areas of research are hypertension prevention and control, control of cardiovascular risk factors, ethnicity, gender and cardiovascular diseases, patient education, clinical trials research, methodology, and global determinants of health. In regards to heart health, hypertension, and preventive cardiology, he has organized a number of national and international conferences, has published more than 100 scientific and medical papers, and has received numerous awards to highlight his achievements in these areas. He is the Editor-in-Chief of the World Heart Federation's "White Book" on *Impending Global Pandemic of CVD: Focus on Developing Countries and Economies in Transition* (1999).

Dr. Ciro A. de Quadros has dedicated his career to freeing the world of infectious diseases, especially those that disproportionately affect the health and social development of the world's poorer countries. A pioneer in developing effective strategies for surveillance and containment, Dr. de Quadros served as the World Health Organization's (WHO's) chief epidemiologist for smallpox eradication in Ethiopia in the 1970s. Following the global eradication of smallpox, he became the Director of the Division of Vaccines and Immunization for the Pan American Health Organization, for which he successfully directed efforts to eradicate poliomyelitis and measles from the Western Hemisphere. In 2003, Dr. de Quadros joined the Albert B. Sabin Vaccine Institute and at present is its Executive Vice-President. He is on faculty at the Johns Hopkins School of Hygiene and Public Health and the School of Medicine at George Washington University. He publishes and presents at conferences throughout the world and has received several international awards, including the 1993 Prince Mahidol Award of Thailand, the 2000 Albert B. Sabin Gold Medal, the Order of Rio Branco from his native Brazil, and, most recently, election into the national Institute of Medicine (IOM).

Dr. John W. Farquhar is Professor of Medicine and Health Research and Policy at the Stanford School of Medicine. In 1971 he began the Stanford Three Community Study, a controlled, comprehensive, community-based study of chronic disease prevention, followed by the Stanford Five City Project (1978-1995). The results and methods used in these studies have been disseminated worldwide. In 1992 he chaired the Victoria Declaration, which contained 64 policy recommendations for worldwide reduction of cardiovascular disease. He chaired the Advisory Board of the Catalonia Declaration (1997), the Singapore Declaration (2000), the Osaka Declaration (2001, member), and the Milan Declaration (2004, member). In 2002, he was a founding member of the International Heart Health Society, which provides policy guidance on international health. His research interests include disease prevention, epidemiology of cardiovascular diseases, community-based education for disease prevention, and international health. He is a member of various distinguished organizations, including the Institute of Medicine, the Society of Behavioral Medicine, and the National Forum for Heart Disease and Stroke Prevention. Dr. Farquhar has authored more than 225 publications. He has received many honors related to his work in disease prevention and community-based interventions, including the James D. Bruce Award for Distinguished Contributions in Preventive Medicine, the Charles A. Dana Award for Pioneering Achievements in Health, the American Heart Association's Research Achievement Award, and the Joseph Stokes Preventive Cardiology Award. Most recently he received the Fries Prize in 2005, awarded "for the person who most improved the public's health."

Dr. Robert C. Hornik is the Wilbur Schramm Professor of Communication and Health Policy at the Annenberg School for Communication, University of Pennsylvania in Philadelphia. He has a wide range of experience in mass media communication evaluations, ranging from breastfeeding promotion, AIDS education, and immunization and child survival projects to antidrug and domestic violence media campaigns at the community, national, and international levels. Dr. Hornik has served as a member of the IOM Committee on International Nutrition Programs, the IOM Committee on Prevention of Obesity in Children and Youth, the National Research Council (NRC) Committee on Communication for Behavior Change in the 21st Century: Improving the Health of Diverse Populations, and the NRC Committee to Develop a Strategy to Prevent and Reduce Underage Drinking. He has received the Mayhew Derryberry Award from the American Public Health Association, the Andreasen Scholar Award in social marketing, and the Fisher Mentorship Award from the International Communication Association. He has also been a consultant to other agencies such as the U.S. Agency for International Development (USAID), the United Nations Children's Fund, the Centers for Disease Control and Prevention, the World Health Organization, and the World Bank. Dr. Hornik serves on the editorial boards of several journals, including *Social Marketing Quarterly* and the *Journal of Health Communication*. Dr. Hornik was the Scientific Director for the evaluation of the Office of National Drug Control Policy's National Youth Anti-Drug Media Campaign, and he is currently the Director of the University of Pennsylvania's National Cancer Institute–funded Center of Excellence in Cancer Communication Research. He most recently edited *Public Health Communication,* and he was the author of *Development Communication* and co-author of *Educational Reform with Television: The El Salvador Experience* and *Toward Reform of Program Evaluation.* Dr. Hornik received a Ph.D. in communication research from Stanford University in 1973.

Dr. Frank B. Hu is Professor of Nutrition and Epidemiology at the Harvard School of Public Health and Professor of Medicine at Harvard Medical School. He serves as co-Director of the Program in Obesity Epidemiology and Prevention at Harvard School of Public Health. Dr. Hu received his medical degree at Tongji Medical College in Wuhan, China, and his M.P.H. and Ph.D. degrees at the University of Illinois, Chicago. He completed a postdoctoral fellowship at Harvard University. His research has focused on epidemiology and prevention of diabetes and cardiovascular disease in both developed and developing countries. Dr. Hu is the recipient of the American Heart Association Established Investigator Award. He is also a Yangtze Scholar at Tongji Medical College, Huazhong University of Science & Technology. Dr. Hu's research has focused on diet and lifestyle determinants of type 2 diabetes and cardiovascular disease. He is the Principal Investigator of the diabetes component of the Nurses' Health Study funded by the National Institutes of Health (NIH). His current research has expanded to investigate complex interactions among nutrition, biomarkers, and genetic factors in the development of diabetes and cardiovascular complications. Dr. Hu is also collaborating with researchers from China to study obesity, metabolic syndrome, and cardiovascular disease in Chinese populations. Dr. Hu lectured on controlling noncommunicable diseases for the 2006 China Senior Health Executive Education Program at Harvard School of Public Health. He has published more than 300 original papers and reviews in peer-reviewed journals and is the principle author of the textbook *Obesity Epidemiology* (Oxford University Press, 2008).

Dr. Peter R. Lamptey is based in Accra, Ghana, and is the President of Public Health Programs at Family Health International (FHI) with headquarters in North Carolina. Dr. Lamptey is an internationally recognized public health physician and expert in developing countries, with particular emphasis on communicable and noncommunicable diseases. With a career at FHI spanning more than 25 years, Dr. Lamptey has been instrumental in establishing FHI as one of the world's leading international nongovernmental organizations in implementing HIV/AIDS prevention, care, treatment, and support programs. His experience in HIV/AIDS efforts internationally includes collaboration with the World Bank to design and monitor the China Health IX HIV/AIDS Project. From 1997 to 2007, Dr. Lamptey directed the 10-year Implementing AIDS Prevention and Care (IMPACT) project. The IMPACT project encompassed HIV/AIDS programs in Africa, Asia, Latin America, the Caribbean, Eastern Europe, and the Middle East. He is the former chair of the Monitoring the AIDS Pandemic (MAP) Network, a global network of more than 150 HIV/AIDS experts in 50 countries that was formed in 1996 by the AIDS Control and Prevention project (AIDSCAP), the François-Xavier Bagnoud Center for Health and Human Rights of the Harvard School of Public Health, and the Joint United Nations Programme on HIV/AIDS. Dr. Lamptey delivered the HIV prevention plenary speeches at the world AIDS conferences held in Berlin, Germany, in 1993 and in Durban, South Africa, in 2000. From 1991 to 1997, Dr.

Lamptey directed the AIDSCAP project, funded by United States Agency for International Development (USAID) and implemented by FHI. The largest international HIV/AIDS prevention program undertaken to date, AIDSCAP consisted of more than 800 projects in 50 countries in Africa, Asia, Latin America, and the Caribbean. Prior to AIDSCAP, he directed AIDSTECH, also funded by USAID as a global HIV/AIDS project and implemented by FHI from 1987 to 1992. Born in Ghana, Dr. Lamptey began his career as a district medical officer there, first in the Salaga district, where he was responsible for preventive and clinical health services for 200,000 individuals, and then for the USAID-funded Danfa Comprehensive Rural Health Family Planning Project. He received his medical degree from the University of Ghana, a master's degree in public health from the University of California, Los Angeles, and a doctorate in public health from the Harvard School of Public Health.

Prof. Jean Claude Mbanya is Vice Dean and Professor of Endocrinology and Medicine in the Department of Internal Medicine and Specialties, Faculty of Medicine and Biomedical Sciences, University of Yaoundé I, Yaoundé, Cameroon; Consultant Physician and Chief of Endocrinology and Metabolic Diseases Unit, Hôpital Central Yaoundé, Cameroon; and Director, Health of Population in Transition Research Group, Cameroon. He is a member of the WHO African Advisory Committee on Health Research and Development, the WHO Expert Advisory Panel on Chronic Degenerative Diseases Diabetes, and the WHO Committee on Classification and Diagnosis of Diabetes, and he is President-elect and member of the Board of Management of the International Diabetes Federation. His research interest is in the epidemiology of noncommunicable diseases, especially diabetes and its complications, ethnopharmacology and molecular biology of diabetes, obesity, hypertension, and thyroid diseases and their impact on the health care systems of developing countries. He has a wide span of expertise, but his current focus is on clinical application of basic research and equity of access to care and education and the integration of diabetes and endocrine diseases in the primary health care activities of developing countries. Prof. Mbanya trained in Yaoundé, Cameroon, and Newcastle upon Tyne, England. He is the author of 15 book chapters and more than 75 published papers.

Prof. Anne Mills is Professor of Health Economics and Policy at the London School of Hygiene and Tropical Medicine and Head of the Department of Public Health and Policy. She has more than 30 years of experience of collaborative research on the health systems of low and middle income countries, and she has researched and published widely in the fields of health economics and health systems. Her most recent research interests have been in the organization and financing of health systems, including evaluation of contractual relationships between public and private sectors, and in economic analysis of disease control activities and the appropriate roles of public and private sectors, especially for scaling up malaria control efforts. She has had extensive involvement in supporting capacity development in health economics in low and middle income countries, for example through supporting the health economics research funding activities of the WHO Tropical Disease Research Programme and chairing the Board of the Alliance for Health Policy and Systems Research. She founded, and is Director of, the Health Economics and Financing Programme, which together with its many research partners has an extensive programme of research focused on increasing knowledge of how best to improve health systems in low and middle income countries. She has advised multilateral, bilateral, and government agencies on numerous occasions; acted as specialist advisor to the House of Commons Select Committee on Science and Technology's inquiry into the use of science in UK international development policy; was a member of WHO's Commission on Macro-economics and Health and co-chair of its working group "Improving the Health Outcomes of the Poor"; wrote the communicable disease paper for the first Copenhagen Consensus; and was a member of the Institute of Medicine (IOM) Committee on the Economics of Antimalarial Drugs. In 2006 she was awarded a CBE for services to medicine and elected Foreign Associate of the IOM.

Dr. Jagat Narula is the Professor of Medicine and Chief of the Division of Cardiology at the University of California (UC), Irvine. He has also served as the Associate Dean for Research at UC Irvine. Dr. Narula completed his cardiology training at the All India Institute of Medical Sciences, Delhi, India, and relocated to Massachusetts General Hospital and Harvard Medical School in 1989. After completing his cardiology, heart failure transplantation, and nuclear cardiology fellowships, he joined the faculty at Massachusetts General. In 1997, he moved to the Philadelphia Hahnemann University School of Medicine. At Hahnemann, he was the Thomas J. Vischer Professor of Medicine, Chief of Division of Cardiology, Vice-Chairman of Medicine, Director of the Heart Failure and Transplantation Center, and Director of the Center for Molecular Cardiology until 2003, when he moved to UC Irvine. Dr. Narula has contributed immensely to cardiovascular imaging from experimental molecular imaging to perfecting the techniques for bedside application of various noninvasive imaging modalities and demonstration of their eventual usefulness for prevention of cardiovascular diseases at the population level. He is considered to be an authority in the fields of programmed cell death in heart failure and atherosclerotic plaques that are likely to lead to acute coronary events. He has also contributed substantially to the field of rheumatic fever and rheumatic heart diseases. His research is funded, in part, by National Institutes of Health (NIH) grants. Dr. Narula has authored or presented more than 700 research manuscripts and edited 25 books or journal supplements. He has been awarded as "best young investigator" on several occasions. He serves on various committees of the American Heart Association and the American College of Cardiology. Dr. Narula is currently the Editor-in-Chief of the *Journal of the American College of Cardiology—Cardiovascular Imaging* and an associate editor of the *Journal of the American College of Cardiology*. He was the founding editor of *Heart Failure Clinics of North America*.

Dr. Rachel A. Nugent is the Deputy Director of Global Health for the Center for Global Development (CGD). She is chair of the CGD working group on drug resistance, manages CGD programs on population and economic development, and conducts research on the economics of chronic diseases in developing countries. She also provides economic and policy expertise on a range of other global health topics. She has 25 years of experience as a development economist, managing and carrying out research and policy analysis in the fields of health, agriculture, and the environment. Prior to joining CGD, Dr. Nugent worked at the Population Reference Bureau, the Fogarty International Center of the NIH, and the United Nations Food and Agriculture Organization. She also served as Associate Professor and Chair of the Economics Department at Pacific Lutheran University in Tacoma, Washington. Dr. Nugent's recent publications address the cost-effectiveness of noncommunicable disease interventions, the economic impacts of chronic disease, and the health impacts of fiscal policies.

Dr. John W. Peabody is the Deputy Director of Global Health Sciences, where he heads health policy activities. He is also a Senior Vice President and Medical Director at Sg2, a health intelligence company advising hospitals and physicians on how to measure and advance health care delivery, finance, and planning. Dr. Peabody is currently a Professor in the Departments of Epidemiology, Biostatistics, and Medicine and has been a member of the University of California (UC) faculty since 1995. Dr. Peabody holds a joint appointment in the Department of Health Services at UC Los Angeles in the School of Public Health and holds an honorary faculty appointment at Tulane University. He spent 9 years at RAND working as a Senior Scientist and Principal Investigator. Before RAND, Dr. Peabody worked for the World Health Organization (WHO) in Geneva and Manila for 3 years; he also spent 2 years as Director for Project Hope in China. He is a Fellow of the American College of Physicians (1999). Dr. Peabody has presented to a congressional panel on health and the environment and has also served on previous national panels and blue ribbon committees including the IOM

Committee on Quality of Care. Dr. Peabody is currently the Principal Investigator on a large NIH-funded research project on children where he leads a broad-based social policy experiment to evaluate the impact of insurance and clinical practice on a variety of health outcomes in the Philippines. Dr. Peabody has published more than 190 papers, articles, and books on international health policy, quality of care, measuring and changing provider practice, and changing financial incentives in health care. He is the lead author of *Policy and Health: Implications for Development in Asia*, published by Cambridge University Press. Dr. Peabody is a board-certified internist. He received his M.D. from UC San Francisco, his D.T.M.&H. from the London School of Hygiene and Tropical Medicine, and his M.Phil. and Ph.D. in public policy from the RAND Graduate School.

Prof. K. Srinath Reddy is the President of the Public Health Foundation of India and until recently headed the Department of Cardiology at the All India Institute of Medical Sciences (AIIMS). He graduated from Osmania Medical College, Hyderabad, and later trained at AIIMS, Delhi, where he received his M.D. (medicine) and D.M. (cardiology) degrees, with high academic honors. Professor Reddy is a clinical cardiologist and is also trained in epidemiology (at McMaster University, Canada). Professor Reddy has been involved in several major international and national research studies, including the INTERSALT global study of blood pressure and electrolytes, Indian Council of Medical Research–commissioned national collaborative studies on Epidemiology of Coronary Heart Disease and Community Control of Rheumatic Heart Disease, and the INTERHEART global study on risk factors of myocardial infarction. Professor Reddy served as the Coordinator of the Initiative for Cardiovascular Health Research in the Developing Countries (IC Health), a global partnership program, and presently chairs the Board of IC Health. He has served on many WHO expert panels and as Chair of the Scientific Council on Epidemiology of the World Heart Federation, and he has recently been elected to serve as Chair of the Federation's Foundation Advisory Board. Professor Reddy edited the *National Medical Journal of India* for 10 years and is on the editorial boards of several international and national journals. He has represented India in intergovernmental treaty negotiations on the WHO Framework Convention on Tobacco Control (FCTC) and the Conference of Parties of that treaty. Professor Reddy has been active in organizing school-based health education programs under the Health Related Information Dissemination Amongst Youth Student Health Action Network (HRIDAY–SHAN) program, which he initiated in 1992. HRIDAY has won international recognition for its innovative programs of health awareness and advocacy and was awarded the WHO Global Tobacco Free World Award in 2002. He recently organized the first ever Global Youth Meet on Health (GYM

2006) in New Delhi and facilitated the launch of the Youth For Health (Y4H) global network for health advocacy and action. He has more than 250 scientific publications in international and Indian peer-reviewed journals. Professor Reddy was awarded the WHO Director General's Award for Global Leadership in Tobacco Control (2003), was conferred the national award PADMA BHUSHAN (one of the highest civilian awards conferred by the Government of India) by the President of India (2005), and was conferred the Queen Elizabeth Medal for 2005 by The Royal Society for the Promotion of Health, United Kingdom Professor Reddy is a member of the Institute of Medicine. In 2009 he received the American Cancer Society's Luther Terry Award for Outstanding Leadership in Global Tobacco Control and the Honorary Fellowship of the London School of Hygiene and Tropical Medicine.

Dr. Sylvie Stachenko is currently the Dean of the School of Public Health at the University of Alberta. Dr. Stachenko earned a B.S. degree in biophysics (1971) and an M.D. degree (1975), both from McGill University, and completed her residency in family medicine at the Université de Montréal (1977). She earned a master's degree in epidemiology and health services administration from the Harvard School of Public Health in 1985. Dr. Stachenko was an Associate Professor in the Department of Family Medicine at the Université de Montréal, where she served as Research Director from 1984 to 1988. In 1988, she joined the federal government with the Department of Health and Welfare and, in 1989, was appointed Director, Preventive Health Services. From 1997 to 2002, Dr. Stachenko worked with the WHO Regional Office for Europe, located in Copenhagen, Denmark, as its Director of Health Policy and Services. She was then appointed Director General in the Centre for Chronic Disease Prevention and Control at the Public Health Agency of Canada, a position she held until 2004.

Dr. Derek Yach is Senior Vice President of Global Health Policy at PepsiCo, where he leads the Human Sustainability Leadership Team and engagement with major international policy, research, and scientific groups. Previously he headed global health at the Rockefeller Foundation and was Professor of Public Health and Head of the Division of Global Health at Yale University. Dr. Yach is a former Executive Director of WHO. Dr. Yach has spearheaded several major efforts to improve global health. At WHO he served as Cabinet Director under Director-General Gro Harlem Brundtland. Dr. Yach helped place tobacco control, nutrition, and chronic diseases such as diabetes and heart disease prominently on the agenda of governments, nongovernmental organizations, and the private sector. He led development of WHO's first treaty, the Framework Convention on Tobacco Control, and the development of the Global Strategy on Diet and Physical Activity.

Dr. Yach established the Centre for Epidemiological Research at the South African Medical Research Council, which focused on quantifying inequalities and the impact of urbanization on health. He has authored or coauthored more than 200 articles covering the breadth of global health issues. Dr. Yach serves on several advisory boards, including those of the Clinton Global Initiative, the World Economic Forum, the Pan American Health and Education Foundation, the Oxford Health Alliance, and Vitality USA. Dr. Yach received his M.B.Ch.B. from the University of Cape Town Medical School in 1979 and completed his clinical internship in medicine and surgery at Groote Schuur Hospital in Cape Town in 1980. Dr. Yach also received an M.P.H. from the Johns Hopkins School of Hygiene in 1985. In 2007 Georgetown University presented Dr. Yach with Honoris Causa (D.Sc.). Dr. Yach is a South African national.

IOM STAFF

Dr. Bridget B. Kelly is a Program Officer with the Board on Global Health. She first joined the National Academies as a Christine Mirzayan Science and Technology Policy Graduate Fellow. Prior to joining the Board on Global Health, she worked in the Board on Children, Youth, and Families as staff for the Committee on the Prevention of Mental Disorders and Substance Abuse Among Children, Youth, and Young Adults, the Committee on Depression, Parenting Practices, and the Healthy Development of Children, and the Committee on Strengthening Benefit-Cost Methodology for the Evaluation of Early Childhood Interventions. She received her B.A. from Williams College and completed an M.D. and a Ph.D. in neurobiology as part of the Medical Scientist Training Program at Duke University. In addition to her work in science and health, she has more than 10 years of experience in grassroots nonprofit arts administration.

Collin Weinberger is a research associate at the Board on Global Health. Prior to joining the IOM, he was a Communications Associate at Global Health Strategies, a communications and advocacy consultancy specializing in diseases of the developing world. He also spent a year as a volunteer with Partners in Health/Socios en Salud in Lima, Peru, where he worked with the organization's children's health, multi-drug-resistant tuberculosis, and HIV/AIDS programs. He received his bachelors degree in health and societies from the University of Pennsylvania.

Louise Jordan is a research assistant for the Board on Global Health. She received a B.S. degree from the University of Utah. Prior to joining the Board on Global Health, she worked for the Board on Population Health as staff for the Committee on Review of Priorities in the National Vaccine

Plan and the Roundtable on Environmental Health Sciences, Research, and Medicine.

Kristen Danforth is a Senior Program Assistant with the Board on Global Health. She received her bachelor's degree in international health from Georgetown University in 2008.

Dr. Patrick Kelley joined the IOM in July 2003 as the Director of the Board on Global Health. He has subsequently also been appointed the Director of the Board on African Science Academy Development. Dr. Kelley has overseen a portfolio of IOM expert consensus studies and convening activities on subjects as wideranging as the evaluation of the U.S. emergency plan for international AIDS relief, the role of border quarantine programs for migrants in the 21st century, sustainable surveillance for zoonotic infections, and the programmatic approach to cancer in low and middle income countries. He also directs a unique capacity building effort, the African Science Academy Development Initiative, which over 10 years aims to strengthen the capacity of African academies to advise their governments on scientific matters. Prior to joining the National Academies, Dr. Kelley served in the U.S. Army for more than 23 years as a physician, residency director, epidemiologist, and program manager. In his last Department of Defense (DoD) position, Dr. Kelley founded and directed the DoD Global Emerging Infections Surveillance and Response System (DoD-GEIS). This responsibility entailed managing surveillance and capacity building partnerships with numerous elements of the federal government and with health ministries in more than 45 developing countries. Dr. Kelley is an experienced communicator, having lectured in English or Spanish in more than 20 countries and having published more than 64 scholarly papers, book chapters, and monographs. Dr. Kelley obtained his M.D. from the University of Virginia and his Dr.P.H. in epidemiology from the Johns Hopkins School of Hygiene and Public Health.

Appendix C

Public Session Agendas

PUBLIC INFORMATION-GATHERING SESSION

April 13-14, 2009

Agenda

Monday, April 13, 2009

8:00AM	Welcoming Remarks
	Valentín Fuster, *Committee Chair*

8:10AM–9:25AM	*Panel 1:* Global Trends in Cardiovascular Disease and Related Risk Factors
	Moderator: Arun Chockalingam, *Committee Member*

	Presentation: Overview of global trends in cardiovascular disease
	Derek Yach, *Committee Member*, PepsiCo

	Presentation: Overview of classic and emerging risks for CVD
	Salim Yusuf, McMaster University

	Q&A AND DISCUSSION

9:25AM–9:45AM	BREAK
9:45AM–10:35AM	*Panel 2, Part I:* **Economic Impact of Cardiovascular Disease**
	Moderator: Rachel Nugent, *Committee Member*
	Presentation: Macro- and micro-economic impacts of cardiovascular disease Marc Suhrcke, University of East Anglia
	Presentation: Macro- and micro-economic costs of diabetes in developing countries Jonathan Brown, Kaiser Permanente Northwest
	Q&A AND DISCUSSION
10:35AM–11:45AM	*Panel 2, Part II:* **Economically Efficient Approaches to Address Cardiovascular Disease**
	Moderator: Rachel Nugent, *Committee Member*
	Presentation: Economically efficient approaches to address cardiovascular disease in developing countries Tom Gaziano, Brigham and Women's Hospital
	Presentation: Economic analysis of care models to address cardiovascular disease Stephen Jan, University of Sydney
	Presentation: Cost-effective public policy tools: Lessons learned from tobacco control Prabhat Jha, University of Toronto
	Q&A AND DISCUSSION
11:45AM–12:05PM	**Key Issues in Implementation**
	Presentation: Lessons learned from the Disease Control Priorities Project Prabhat Jha, University of Toronto
	Q&A AND DISCUSSION
12:05PM–1:00PM	LUNCH BREAK
1:00PM–2:10PM	*Panel 3, Part I:* **Health Promotion and Primary Prevention**

Moderator: Frank Hu, *Committee Member*

Presentation: Emerging global dietary habits and the burden of cardiovascular diseases
Dariush Mozaffarian, Harvard University

Presentation: Under- and overnutrition and cardiovascular disease risk
Benjamin Caballero, Johns Hopkins University

Presentation: Physical activity and cardiovascular disease risk
Frank Hu, *Committee Member*, Harvard University

Q&A AND DISCUSSION

2:10PM–3:25PM *Panel 3, Part II:* **Prevention and Health Systems Strengthening**
Moderator: John Farquhar, *Committee Member*

Presentation: Secondary prevention and systems approaches: Lessons from EUROASPIRE and EUROACTION
Kornelia Kotseva, Imperial College

Presentation: Chronic disease management in healthcare systems in middle and low income countries
Sania Nishtar, Heartfile

Presentation: Integration of care within health systems in LMIC
Mukadi Ya Diul, Family Health International

Q&A AND DISCUSSION

3:25PM–3:45PM **BREAK**

3:45PM–4:35PM *Panel 4:* **Monitoring and Evaluation of Health Promotion and Prevention**
Moderator: Jean Claude Mbanya, *Committee Member*

Presentation: Measurement in low and middle income countries: Lessons from monitoring, evaluation and surveillance programs for HIV

and potential for integration of cardiovascular disease and HIV surveillance
Inoussa Kabore, Family Health International

Presentation: Worldwide surveillance
Samira Asma, U.S. Centers for Disease Control and Prevention

Q&A AND DISCUSSION

4:35PM–4:45PM	**Closing Remarks and Adjournment of Public Session** Valentín Fuster, *Committee Chair*

Tuesday, April 14, 2009

8:00AM	**Welcoming Remarks** Valentín Fuster, *Committee Chair*
8:10AM–10:00AM	*Panel 5:* **Approaches to Behavior Change for Cardiovascular Disease Risk Reduction** *Moderator:* Robert Hornik, *Committee Member*

Presentation: Preventing HIV transmission: Successes and disappointments
Tom Coates, University of California, Los Angeles

Presentation: Use of mass media for health communication in the developing world
Bill Smith, Academy for Educational Development

Q&A AND DISCUSSION

Presentation: Use of education-entertainment for health communication in the developing world
Charlotte Cole, Sesame Workshop

Presentation: Social marketing programs in health in developing countries
Brian Smith, Population Services International

Q&A AND DISCUSSION

Presentation: Behavioral incentives
Dean Karlan, Yale University

Q&A AND DISCUSSION

APPENDIX C 455

10:00AM–10:20AM BREAK

10:20AM–12:15PM *Panel 6:* **Multisectoral Involvement: Collaborations to Foster Effective CVD Prevention**
Moderator: John Peabody, *Committee Member*

Roundtable:

CVD prevention in urban settings: New York City
Lynn Silver, NYC Department of Health and Mental Hygiene

CVD prevention in rural, low-income settings: Millennium Villages
Sonia Sachs, Columbia University

Integrated approaches to address obesity
Diane Finegood, Simon Fraser University

Integrated approaches to address community and environmental barriers to physical activity
Vicki Lambert, University of Cape Town

Q&A AND DISCUSSION

Roles of agriculture and food sectors in cardiovascular disease
Rachel Nugent, Committee Member, Center for Global Development

Agriculture and food policy
Corinna Hawkes, Independent Consultant

Food marketing policy
Gerard Hastings, University of Sterling (via telephone)

Q&A AND DISCUSSION

12:15PM–1:15PM **LUNCH BREAK**

1:15PM–2:05PM *Panel 7:* **Advocacy**
Moderator: Peter Lamptey, *Committee Member*

Presentation: Mobilizing student and youth engagement for advocacy
Sandeep Kishore, Weill Cornell/The Rockefeller

University/Sloan-Kettering Institute, Tri-Institutional MD-PhD Program

Presentation: Lessons learned from successful advocacy and engagement of policy makers
Bill Novelli, AARP

Q&A AND DISCUSSION

2:05PM–3:05PM **Panel 8:** Regional Updates on CVD Trends and Actions
Moderator: Sylvie Stachenko, *Committee Member*

Roundtable:
Srinath Reddy, *Committee Member*, Public Health Foundation of India
George Mensah, U.S. Centers for Disease Control and Prevention
Youfa Wang, Johns Hopkins University
Beatriz Marcet Champagne, InterAmerican Heart Foundation

Q&A AND DISCUSSION

3:05PM–3:25PM **BREAK**

3:25PM–5:15PM **Panel 9:** Governance and Coordination of Global Efforts
Moderator: Derek Yach, *Committee Member*

Roundtable:
Ala Alwan and Fiona Adshead, World Health Organization
Valentín Fuster, *Committee Chair*, World Heart Federation
Abdallah Daar, Global Alliance for Chronic Disease
Sir John Bell, Oxford Health Alliance (via telephone)
Stephen Kehoe, International Food and Beverage Association
Michael Engelgau, World Bank
Scott Ratzan, World Economic Forum
Rachel Nugent, *Committee Member*, Center for Global Development

Q&A AND DISCUSSION

APPENDIX C   457

5:15PM–5:30PM   Closing Remarks and Adjournment of Public
                   Session
                   Valentín Fuster, *Committee Chair*

PUBLIC INFORMATION-GATHERING SESSION

July 9, 2009

Agenda

8:00AM   Welcoming Remarks
                   Valentín Fuster, *Committee Chair*

8:10AM–9:30AM   *Panel 1:* Metrics and Measurement for Surveillance
                   and Impact Evaluation
                   Moderator: John Peabody, *Committee Member*

                   Presentations:
                   Philip Setel, Gates Foundation
                   Michael Engelgau, World Bank
                   Sally Stansfield, Health Metrics Network (via
                      videoconference)

                   Q&A AND DISCUSSION

9:30AM–9:40AM   BREAK

9:40AM–11:05AM   *Panel 2:* Implementation Roundtable
                   Moderator: K. Srinath Reddy, *Committee Member*

                   *Roundtable: Challenges and lessons learned for
                   the implementation of programs and policies to
                   address cardiovascular diseases at various levels
                   (local to national)*
                   K.R. Thankappan, Sree Chitra Tirunal Institute for
                      Medical Sciences and Technology, Karala, India
                   Trevor Hassell, National Commission for Chronic
                      Non-Communicable Diseases, Barbados
                   Pascal Bovet, Ministry of Health, Seychelles (via
                      teleconference)

Jacob Plange-Rhule, Komfo Anokye Teaching Hospital, Ghana (via teleconference)
Wu Fan, Shanghai Centers for Disease Control and Prevention, China
Martha Hill, Johns Hopkins University, United States

Q&A AND DISCUSSION

11:05AM–11:15AM **BREAK**

11:15AM–12:45PM *Panel 3:* **U.S. Federal Agency Roundtable**
Moderator: Rachel Nugent, *Committee Member*

Roundtable: Interagency dialog to inform strategies for addressing global cardiovascular disease and related chronic diseases
Cristina Rabadán-Diehl, National Heart, Lung, and Blood Institute
Roger Glass, Fogarty International Center
Yuling Hong, Centers for Disease Control and Prevention
Gloria Steele, USAID Bureau for Global Health
Kathleen Merrigan and Robert Post, U.S. Department of Agriculture

Q&A AND DISCUSSION

12:45PM **Adjournment**
Valentín Fuster, *Committee Chair*

Appendix D

Acronyms and Abbreviations

ACC	American College of Cardiology
ACE	angiotensin-converting enzyme
ACTIVITY	Advancing Cessation of Tobacco in Vulnerable Indian Tobacco Consuming Youth
AHA	American Heart Association
AIDS	aquired immune deficiency syndrome
AIDSCAP	AIDS Control and Prevention
AIIMS	All India Institute of Medical Sciences
ALSPAC	Avon Longitudinal Study of Parents and Children
AMI	acute myocardial infarction
BMI	body mass index
BP	blood pressure
BRFSS	Behavioral Risk Factor Surveillance Study
CABG	coronary artery bypass graft
CAD	coronary artery disease
CBV	cerebrovascular
CDC	Centers for Disease Control and Prevention
CER	cost-effectiveness ratio
CGD	Center for Global Development
CHD	coronary heart disease
CHF	congestive heart failure
COPD	chronic obstructive pulmonary disease
CORIS	Coronary Risk Factor Study

COTPA	Cigarette and Other Tobacco Products Act
CTFK	Campaign for Tobacco Free Kids
CVD	cardiovascular disease
DALY	disability-adjusted life year
DoD	Department of Defense
DOTS	Directly Observed Treatment Short
ECG	electrocardiogram
EUROASPIRE	European Action on Secondary Prevention by Intervention to Reduce Events
EVIPNet	Evidence-Informed Policy Network
FAO	Food and Agriculture Organization
FCTC	Framework Convention on Tobacco Control
FDA	Food and Drug Administration
FHI	Family Health International
GDP	gross domestic product
GNI	gross national income
GSM	Global System for Mobile Communications
GYAT	Global Youth Action on Tobacco
GYM	Global Youth Meet on Health
GYTS	Global Youth Tobacco Survey
HAART	highly active antiretroviral therapy
HDL	high-density lipoprotein
HIV	human immunodeficiency virus
HMN	Health Metrics Network
HPA	hypothalamic-pituitary-adrenal
HRIDAY–SHAN	Health Related Information Dissemination Amongst Youth-Student Health Action Network
IC Health	Initiative for Cardiovascular Health Research in the Developing Countries
ICER	incremental cost-effectiveness ratio
IFBA	International Food and Beverage Alliance
IFPMA	International Federation of Pharmaceutical Manufactureres and Associations
IHD	ischemic heart disease
IHME	Institute for Health Metrics and Evaluation
IMF	International Monetary Fund

APPENDIX D 461

IMPACT	Implementing AIDS Prevention and Care
IOM	Institute of Medicine
ISH	International Society of Hypertension
ISPOR	International Society for Pharmacoeconomics and Outcomes Research
KBD	Kick Butts Day
LBW	low birth weight
LDL	low-density lipoprotein
M&E	measurement and evaluation
MAP	Monitoring the AIDS Pandemic
MCC	Millennium Challenge Corporation
MCH	maternal and child health
m-health	mobile health
MI	myocardial infarction
MRC	medical research center
MSF	Médecins Sans Frontières
MYTRI	Mobilizing Youth for Tobacco Related Initiatives in India
NCD	noncommunicable disease
NCDnet	Global Noncommunicable Diseases network
NGO	nongovernmental organization
NHANES	National Health and Nutrition Examination Survey
NHLBI	National Heart, Lung, and Blood Institute
NIH	National Institutes of Health
NRC	National Research Council
NTCP	National Tobacco Control Program
OECD	Organisation for Economic Co-operation and Development
PAF	population attributable fraction
PAHO	Pan American Health Organization
PE	physical education
PEPFAR	President's Emergency Plan for AIDS Relief
PPP	purchasing power parity
PREMISE	Prevention of Occurrences of Myocardial Infarction and Stroke
PTCA	percutaneous transluminal coronary angioplasty
QALY	quality-adjusted life year

QIDS	Quality Improvement Demonstration Study
R&D	research and development
RCT	randomized controlled trial
RHD	rheumatic heart disease
SAVVY	Sample Vital Registration with Verbal Autopsy
SBP	systolic blood pressure
SCMS	supply chain management system
SDBP	sitting diastolic blood pressure
SIM	subscriber identity module
STEPS	STEPwise Approach to Chronic Disease Risk Factor Surveillance
SuRF	Surveillance of Chronic Disease Risk Factors
TB	tuberculosis
UN	United Nations
UNAIDS	Joint United Nations Programme on HIV/AIDS
UNDP	United Nations Development Program
UNGASS	United Nations General Assembly Special Sessions
UNICEF	United Nations Children's Fund
USAID	U.S. Agency for International Development
USDA	U.S. Department of Agriculture
WCTOH	World Conference on Tobacco or Health
WEF	World Economic Forum
WHF	World Heart Federation
WHL	World Hypertension League
WHO	World Health Organization
WHOSIS	WHO Statistical Information System
WTO	World Trade Organization
Y4H	Youth for Health

Appendix E

World Bank Income Classifications July 2009

Low Income Economies (43)

Afghanistan	Guinea-Bissau	Rwanda
Bangladesh	Haiti	Senegal
Benin	Kenya	Sierra Leone
Burkina Faso	Korea, Dem Rep.	Somalia
Burundi	Kyrgyz Republic	Tajikistan
Cambodia	Lao PDR	Tanzania
Central African Republic	Liberia	Togo
Chad	Madagascar	Uganda
Comoros	Malawi	Uzbekistan
Congo, Dem. Rep	Mali	Vietnam
Eritrea	Mauritania	Yemen, Rep.
Ethiopia	Mozambique	Zambia
Gambia, The	Myanmar	Zimbabwe
Ghana	Nepal	
Guinea	Niger	

Lower-Middle Income Economies (55)

Albania	Honduras	Paraguay
Angola	India	Philippines
Armenia	Indonesia	Samoa
Azerbaijan	Iran, Islamic Rep.	São Tomé and Principe
Belize	Iraq	Solomon Islands
Bhutan	Jordan	Sri Lanka
Bolivia	Kiribati	Sudan
Cameroon	Kosovo	Swaziland
Cape Verde	Lesotho	Syrian Arab Republic
China	Maldives	Thailand
Congo, Rep.	Marshall Islands	Timor-Leste
Côte d'Ivoire	Micronesia, Fed. Sts.	Tonga
Djibouti	Moldova	Tunisia
Ecuador	Mongolia	Turkmenistan
Egypt, Arab Rep.	Morocco	Ukraine
El Salvador	Nicaragua	Vanuatu
Georgia	Nigeria	West Bank and Gaza
Guatemala	Pakistan	
Guyana	Papua New Guinea	

Upper-Middle Income Economies (46)

Algeria	Grenada	Peru
American Samoa	Jamaica	Poland
Argentina	Kazakhstan	Romania
Belarus	Latvia	Russian Federation
Bosnia and Herzegovina	Lebanon	Serbia
Botswana	Libya	Seychelles
Brazil	Lithuania	South Africa
Bulgaria	Macedonia, FYR	St. Kitts and Nevis
Chile	Malaysia	St. Lucia
Colombia	Mauritius	St. Vincent and the Grenadines
Costa Rica	Mayotte	Suriname
Cuba	Mexico	Turkey
Dominica	Montenegro	Uruguay
Dominican Republic	Namibia	Venezuela, RB
Fiji	Palau	
Gabon	Panama	

High Income Economies (66)

Andorra	France	Netherlands Antilles
Antigua and Barbuda	French Polynesia	New Caledonia
Aruba	Germany	New Zealand
Australia	Greece	Northern Mariana Islands
Austria	Greenland	Norway
Bahamas, The	Guam	Oman
Bahrain	Hong Kong, China	Portugal
Barbados	Hungary	Puerto Rico
Belgium	Iceland	Qatar
Bermuda	Ireland	San Marino
Brunei Darussalam	Isle of Man	Saudi Arabia
Canada	Israel	Singapore
Cayman Islands	Italy	Slovak Republic
Channel Islands	Japan	Slovenia
Croatia	Korea, Rep.	Spain
Cyprus	Kuwait	Sweden
Czech Republic	Liechtenstein	Switzerland
Denmark	Luxembourg	Trinidad and Tobago
Estonia	Macao, China	United Arab Emirates
Equatorial Guinea	Malta	United Kingdom
Faeroe Islands	Monaco	United States
Finland	Netherlands	Virgin Islands (U.S.)

SOURCE: http://go.worldbank.org/D7SN0B8YU0.